AF148695

Pocket Guide to Radiology

Dirk Pickuth · John T. Murchison

Pocket Guide
to Radiology

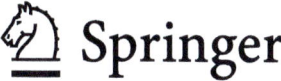 Springer

Dirk Pickuth
Department of Radiology
CaritasKlinikum
Academic Teaching Hospital
of Saarland University
Saarbruecken, Germany

John T. Murchison
Department of Radiology
Edinburgh Royal Infirmary
Edinburgh, UK

ISBN 978-3-031-76519-3   ISBN 978-3-031-76520-9 (eBook)
https://doi.org/10.1007/978-3-031-76520-9

Translation from the German language edition: "Klinische Radiologie Fakten, 9th edition" by Dirk Pickuth, © UNI-MED Verlag AG 2025. Published by UNI-MED Verlag AG, Bremen, Germany. All Rights Reserved.

This Springer imprint is published by the registered company Springer Nature Switzerland AG
The registered company address is: Gewerbestrasse 11, 6330 Cham, Switzerland

If disposing of this product, please recycle the paper.

Preface

Welcome to the 'Pocket Guide to Radiology', a valuable resource for medical students, radiology residents, specialists and radiographers alike. In the fast-paced world of radiology, where precision and efficiency are paramount, we hope this guide will serve as a readily accessible source of concise yet comprehensive knowledge.

Radiology is, at its core, a discipline that combines cutting-edge technology with compassionate patient care. It is a field where every image tells a story, and where changes in size or density can hold the key to accurate diagnosis and treatment. In this book, we have distilled the vast expanse of radiological expertise into a single volume, focusing on details most relevant to everyday practice.

Designed for learning, review and reference, the 'Pocket Guide to Radiology' is structured to meet the needs of busy clinicians. Its format—full of bullet points, tables and diagrams—makes it easy to reference essential information quickly. We have deliberately omitted extraneous detail, ensuring that each word serves a purpose, making this guide both concise and thorough.

While this guide assumes a basic understanding of radiological concepts, it avoids lengthy explanations in favour of associative and abstract presentations. In this way, we aim to provide a seamless transition from theory to application, enabling radiologists to navigate complex cases with confidence.

We would like to express our deep gratitude to all the colleagues, highlighted on the *Acknowledgements* page, who have worked on sections of this book pertaining to their particular fields of expertise. Their specialist insights have greatly enriched this guide and their invaluable contributions have ensured that this edition will be a cornerstone resource for radiology professionals worldwide.

Saarbruecken, Germany   Dirk Pickuth

Edinburgh, UK   John T. Murchison

Acknowledgements

Dr Mark Jones MBChB, FRCR, MRCS
Consultant Thoracic Radiologist
Edinburgh Royal Infirmary
Lungs, Pleura, Mediastinum

Professor Michelle Williams MBChB, BSc, BA, PhD, FRCR, MRCP, FSCCT
Consultant Cardiothoracic Radiologist, Edinburgh Royal Infirmary, and Professor of Cardiothoracic Imaging, University of Edinburgh
Heart

Dr Colum O'Hare MB BCh, BaO, FRCR
Consultant Interventional Radiologist
Edinburgh Royal Infirmary
Vascular, Interventional

Professor Cindy Chew MBChB, PhD, FRCR
Consultant Radiologist, University Hospital Hairmyres, and Honorary Professor, Director of Imaging and Anatomy, University of Glasgow
Oesophagus, Stomach, Small Intestine, Colon

Dr Fiona Minns MBChB, FRCR
Consultant Gastrointestinal Radiologist
Edinburgh Royal Infirmary
Liver, Biliary Tree, Pancreas, Spleen

Dr Allan Green MBChB, FRCR
Consultant Radiologist
Western General Hospital, Edinburgh
Kidneys, Adrenal Glands, Urinary Tract, Prostate, Testes

Dr Tom Fitzgerald MBChB, FRCR
Consultant Radiologist
Edinburgh Royal Infirmary
Uterus, Ovaries

Dr Francesca Camilleri MBChB, FRCR
Consultant Breast Radiologist
Western General Hospital, Edinburgh
Breast

Dr Jennifer Royds MBChB, FRCR
Consultant Breast Radiologist
Western General Hospital, Edinburgh
Breast

Dr Gregor Stenhouse MBChB, FRCR, MRCS
Consultant Musculoskeletal Radiologist
Edinburgh Royal Infirmary
Bones, Joints

Dr Andrew G Murchison BM BCh, MA(Oxon), FRCR, MRCP
Consultant Head and Neck Radiologist
Stoke Mandeville Hospital, Buckinghamshire
Brain, Spinal Cord, Eyes, Ears, Nose, Throat

Dr Emily Stenhouse MBChB, FRCR
Consultant Paediatric Radiologist
Royal Hospital for Children, Glasgow
Paediatrics

About the Authors

Professor Dirk Pickuth, MD, PhD, MDs (honoris causa), FRCR, FFCI, FBCS, FRSPH, IPFPH, SFFMLM (Hon), FRSM, is Chairman of the Department of Diagnostic and Interventional Radiology and former long-standing Medical Director at Caritas Klinikum, Saarbruecken, Germany. He is the founding Director of the Digital Innovation and Strategy Hub (DISH), responsible for driving digital transformation across all radiological, clinical, operational and corporate environments. He also established the International Department of Artificial Intelligence in Medicine and Imaging (id:ai:mi). He is the European Lead for the Faculty of Medical Leadership and Management. He studied in Kiel, London and Edinburgh, undertook a clinical research fellowship at the Royal Marsden Hospital and the Institute of Cancer Research in London, and completed his specialist training in Heidelberg. He is the author of several textbooks on clinical radiology, artificial intelligence and healthcare leadership. He has been awarded numerous visiting and honorary professorships at prestigious European universities. His work has also been independently recognised with honorary doctorates, reflecting the significance and lasting impact of his achievements.

Professor John T. Murchison, MBChB, BSc, PhD, DMRD, FRCR, FRCP, is a Consultant Radiologist at Edinburgh Royal Infirmary and an Honorary Professor at the University of Edinburgh Medical School. He is a former examiner for the FRCR 2A and 2B examinations of the Royal College of Radiologists and a Past President of the Scottish Radiological Society. In 2012, he was appointed the Royal College of Radiologists' Roentgen Visiting Professor. He has published extensively, particularly in the field of thoracic imaging and CT scanning.

Contents

Lungs, Pleura, Mediastinum

Anatomy

Assessing CXR Quality

► Orientation
  • PA projection preferable if possible. Requires patient to be able to stand
  • AP projection performed on immobile or unwell patients
  • Heart and mediastinum are further from the X-ray detector on an AP view
    – Heart and mediastinum may be magnified on an AP view
  • Inner edges of the scapulae clear of the thorax on well-taken PA radiograph
► Rotation
  • Assess by checking spinous processes of upper thoracic vertebrae are equidistant from the medial ends of the clavicles
  • In a normal CXR, both lungs should be of equal lucency
► Penetration
  • First–third thoracic vertebral bodies clearly visible
  • Remaining thoracic vertebral bodies just visible through the mediastinal and cardiac shadow
  • Retrocardiac lung and mediastinal structures visible behind the cardiac shadow

© The Author(s), under exclusive license to Springer Nature Switzerland AG 2026
D. Pickuth, J. T. Murchison, *Pocket Guide to Radiology*,
https://doi.org/10.1007/978-3-031-76520-9_1

▶ Inspiration
  • With poor inspiration heart can appear falsely enlarged and lung bases can appear falsely dense
  • Adequate if dome of the diaphragm projected at or below level of anterior sixth rib on full inspiration

Structures Contributing to Mediastinal Contours on CXR

▶ Right side
  • Superior vena cava
  • Ascending aorta
  • Right pulmonary artery—right hilum
  • Right atrium
▶ Left side
  • Aortic arch
  • Left pulmonary artery—left hilum
  • Left atrial appendage
  • Left ventricle

Heart Valve Location on CXR

▶ Aortic valve
  • PA CXR: Projected over the thoracic spine
  • Lateral CXR: Anterosuperior to a line drawn through the centre of the heart (cardiac axis)
▶ Mitral valve
  • PA CXR: Projected to the left of the thoracic spine at a slightly lower level than the aortic valve
  • Lateral CXR: Posteroinferior to a line drawn through the centre of the heart (cardiac axis)

Trachea

▶ Sections
  • Cervical
  • Thoracic

▶ Anatomical relationships of the thoracic trachea
  • Anterior: Brachiocephalic trunk, left brachiocephalic vein, inferior thyroid vein
  • Posterior: Oesophagus, vagus nerve
  • Left: Aortic arch, left common carotid artery, recurrent laryngeal nerve
  • Right: Right-sided pleura, azygos vein
  • Throughout: Lymph nodes

Bronchi

▶ Basic structure
  • Two main bronchi—origin at carina
    – Right main bronchus runs more vertically than the left main bronchus
    – Right upper lobe bronchus originates laterally from the right main bronchus 2 cm distal to the carina
    – Bronchus intermedius continues for 3–4 cm after the origin of the right upper lobe bronchus and then divides into the middle and right lower lobe bronchi
  • Two left-sided lobar bronchi—upper and lower
  • Three right-sided lobar bronchi—upper, middle and lower
  • Two to five segmental bronchi in each lobe
▶ Segmental bronchi of the right lung
  • Right upper lobe
    – Apical (I)
    – Posterior (II)
    – Anterior (III)
  • Middle lobe
    – Lateral (IV)
    – Medial (V)
  • Right lower lobe
    – Apical (VI)
    – Medial-basal (VII)
    – Anterior-basal (VIII)
    – Lateral-basal (IX)
    – Posterior-basal (X)

▶ Segmental bronchi of the left lung
  • Left upper lobe
    – Apicoposterior (I, II)
    – Anterior (III)
    – Superior lingular (IV)
    – Inferior lingular (V)
  • Left lower lobe
    – Apical (VI)
    – Anterior-medial-basal (VII, VIII)
    – Lateral-basal (IX)
    – Posterior-basal (X)

Lungs

▶ Right lung—three lobes and ten segments
▶ Left lung—two lobes and eight–ten segments
  • Horizontal fissure separates the right upper lobe from the middle lobe
  • Oblique fissure separates the upper lobe from the lower lobe on the left, and the middle and upper lobes from the lower lobe on the right
▶ Accessory fissures
  • Azygos fissure—right upper lobe
  • Inferior accessory fissure—separates medial-basal segment on the right from rest of the lower lobe
  • Superior accessory fissure—separates superior and basal segments of lower lobes
  • Left horizontal fissure—separates lingula from left upper lobe, rare anatomical variant
▶ Hilum
  • Contains bronchi, pulmonary arteries, lymph nodes and nerves
  • Hilar point where outer margins of upper lobe pulmonary vein and descending pulmonary artery cross
  • Right hilar point about 2 cm inferior to left hilar point

► Pulmonary arteries
  • Left pulmonary artery shorter than the right
  • Normal pulmonary trunk 29 mm maximum diameter on CT
  • Right and left main pulmonary artery 24 mm maximum diameter on CT
  • Right interlobar pulmonary artery on CXR maximum diameter at hilum 15 mm in women, 16 mm in men
  • Arteries accompany bronchi and generally run more vertically
  • Veins lie between bronchial segments and generally run more horizontally
► Relations
  • Right lung
    – Ventral: Pericardium, right atrium, ascending aorta, thymus, phrenic nerve
    – Dorsal: Oesophagus, vagus nerve, azygos vein, thoracic duct
    – Cranial: Superior vena cava, azygos vein, right brachiocephalic vein, trachea
  • Left lung
    – Ventral: Pericardium, left ventricle, left atrium, phrenic nerve
    – Dorsal: Descending aorta
    – Cranial: Subclavian artery, subclavian vein, vagus nerve
  • Lung apex
    – Scalene muscle
    – Subclavian artery
    – Subclavian vein
    – Brachial plexus

Diaphragm

► Sections
  • Sternal—attaches to posterior aspect of the xiphoid process
  • Costal—attaches to internal surfaces of 7th–12th ribs

- Lumbar—attaches to medial and lateral arcuate ligaments, L1–3 vertebral bodies and intervening intervertebral discs
▶ Diaphragmatic apertures
  - Aortic hiatus—contains aorta, azygos and hemiazygos veins and thoracic duct—T12 level
  - Oesophageal hiatus—contains oesophagus, vagus nerve, small oesophageal arteries and veins—T10 level
  - Vena caval foramen—contains IVC, branches of right phrenic nerve—T8–9 level
  - Several smaller diaphragmatic apertures also exist allowing passage of the greater and lesser right and left splanchnic nerves, the hemiazygos vein, the sympathetic trunks, the left phrenic nerve and the subcostal nerve and vessels
▶ Congenital diaphragmatic hernia
  - Morgagni—anterior, rare. 90% right-sided
  - Bochdalek—posterior and lateral, more common. Predominantly left-sided, in children associated with pulmonary hypoplasia
▶ Diaphragmatic excursion 3–6 cm
▶ On lateral view, right diaphragmatic dome higher than left, gastric air bubble under left side
▶ Diaphragmatic eventration—due to incomplete muscularisation of diaphragm, smooth hump
  - Congenital usually right-sided
  - Acquired more often left-sided

Lymph Nodes

▶ Paratracheal, retrocaval, aortopulmonary window, preaortic, hilar: Up to 10 mm (short axis)
▶ Subcarinal: Up to 14 mm
▶ Paracardiac: Up to 8 mm
▶ Retrocrural: Up to 6 mm

Mediastinal Lymph Nodes Stations

▶ Supraclavicular nodes—level 1
▶ Superior mediastinal nodes—levels 2–4
  • 2R Upper paratracheal on right
  • 2L Upper paratracheal on left
  • 3 Prevascular and retrotracheal
  • 4R Lower paratracheal on right
  • 4L Lower paratracheal on left
▶ Aortopulmonary nodes—levels 5–6
  • 5 Subaortic
  • 6 Paraaortic
▶ Inferior mediastinal nodes—levels 7–9
  • 7 Subcarinal
  • 8 Paraoesophageal (below carina)
  • 9 Pulmonary ligament
▶ Hilar, lobar and (sub)segmental nodes—levels 10–14
  • 10 Hilar
  • 11 Interlobar
  • 12 Lobar
  • 13 Segmental
  • 14 Subsegmental

Paediatric Radiology: Anatomy

Thorax on CXR

▶ Thorax
  • Thorax width, depth and height approximately the same
  • Ribs almost horizontal
▶ Thymus
  • Thymus overlies heart
  • Normal thymus does not cause tracheal constriction or displacement, even when large in size

▶ Trachea
  • Configuration of the trachea is a good indicator of whether the radiograph has been taken in inspiration or expiration
  • Trachea straight in inspiration, buckled in expiration
  • Carinal angle may be increased
  • Peripheral airways significantly narrower compared to the trachea, thus favouring hyperinflation and reduced ventilation
▶ Variants
  • Ductus bump—ductus arteriosus may appear as a transient left-sided mediastinal convexity on a neonatal CXR
  • Pinpoint calcification in the ligamentum arteriosum

Thymus

▶ Initially convex, later concave shape
▶ Involution with replacement of the parenchyma by fatty tissue
▶ Thymic hyperplasia (rebound phenomenon) can be due to stress, chemotherapy, corticosteroid therapy, hyperthyroidism, acromegaly

Lungs

Hyperlucent Lung on CXR

▶ Unilateral
  • Patient rotation—the side to which the patient is turned is hyperlucent
  • Scoliosis
  • Mastectomy—absent breast shadow and surgical clips
  • Lobectomy—rib defects and surgical clips
  • Ball-valve effect of bronchial obstructing lesion
  • Pneumothorax
  • Swyer-James-MacLeod syndrome—complication of bronchiolitis obliterans

- Poland's syndrome—unilateral congenital absence of pectoral muscles, associated with Sprengel's shoulder
- Pulmonary embolism—Westermark sign
▶ Bilateral
  - Emphysema
  - Asthma

Complete Opacification of One Hemithorax on CXR

▶ With an increase in volume: Pleural effusion
▶ With normal volume: Pneumonia (look for air bronchograms)
▶ With a decrease in volume: Total lung collapse or pneumonectomy (rib resection, surgical clips)

Increased Opacification on CXR with Predominantly Alveolar Pattern

▶ Acute
  - Pulmonary oedema
  - Pneumonia
  - Pulmonary infarct
  - Malignancy
  - Haemorrhage
    – Trauma
    – Vasculitis
    – Goodpasture's syndrome
    – Anticoagulation
  - Aspiration
  - Acute respiratory distress syndrome/diffuse alveolar damage
  - Acute hypersensitivity pneumonitis
▶ Chronic
  - Tuberculosis—usually apical
  - Sarcoidosis—usually perihilar/upper zone
  - Post radiotherapy

Increased Opacification on CXR with Predominantly Reticular Pattern

► Acute
  • Pulmonary oedema
  • Pneumonia
  • Alveolitis
  • Acute respiratory distress syndrome/diffuse alveolar damage
► Chronic
  • Tuberculosis
  • Sarcoidosis
  • Idiopathic pulmonary fibrosis
  • Pneumoconiosis
  • Cystic fibrosis
  • Lymphangitic carcinomatosis
  • Systemic sclerosis
  • Rheumatoid lung

Features Favouring Alveolar Opacification Compared with Interstitial Opacification on CXR

► Coalescing/merging
► Air bronchograms
► Indistinct margins
► Over 5 mm diameter
► Rapid change of appearance

Septal Lines

► Kerley A lines
  • Upper zones
  • Straight
  • 2–6 cm long
  • Rarely more than 1 mm thick
  • Point towards hilum centrally

▶ Kerley B lines
- • Basal—usually just above costophrenic angles
- • Straight
- • <2 cm long
- • Rarely more than 1 mm thick
- • Horizontal
- • Perpendicular to the pleural surface in the lung periphery
- • Most common

▶ Kerley C lines
- • Fine branching linear opacities usually at lung bases
- • Due to Kerley B lines en-face—rarely seen

Atelectasis

▶ Types
- • Obstructive atelectasis
  - – Central: Tumour, foreign body
  - – Peripheral: Exudate—infection, mucus—including asthma and cystic fibrosis
- • Contraction atelectasis
  - – Tuberculosis, sarcoidosis, silicosis, fibrosis
- • Compression atelectasis
  - – Pleural effusion, pneumothorax, tumour, lymphadenopathy

▶ CXR
- • Direct signs
  - – Reduced lucency
  - – Displaced fissures
- • Indirect signs
  - – Ipsilateral diaphragmatic elevation
  - – Compensatory emphysema of non-involved lobe/lung
  - – Mediastinal shift to side of collapse
  - – Hilar displacement towards collapse—downwards for lower lobe, upwards for upper lobe
  - – Narrowed intercostal spaces
  - – Absence of air bronchogram

Solitary Pulmonary Nodules

▶ More common
- Granuloma/tuberculoma
- Bronchogenic carcinoma
- Solitary metastasis
- Intrapulmonary lymph node
- Hamartoma—may have popcorn calcification or fat
- Abscess

▶ Less common
- Round atelectasis associated with pleural disease
- Adenoma
- Carcinoid
- Arteriovenous malformation
- Pulmonary cyst
- Amyloid
- Interlobar effusion
- Round pneumonia—mainly seen in children
- Hydatid cyst
- Pulmonary sequestration—usually medial
- Infarct—usually peripheral
- Rheumatoid nodule

▶ Mimics
- Extrapulmonary causes—nipple, skin nodule, clothing artefact, rib lesion, rib fracture, prominent costal cartilage calcification

Characteristics of Solitary Pulmonary Nodules on CT

▶ Benign
- Calcification
  - Diffuse calcification—granuloma
  - Laminated, central or popcorn calcification—hamartoma
- Fat density—hamartoma
- The smaller the size the more likely to be benign
- Stable size >2 years

- Thin wall when cavitating and smooth—94% benign
- Typical perifissural nodule—smooth, triangular or oval in contact with fissure
- Smooth margin—however one third of smaller malignant nodules can also be smooth

▶ Malignant
  - Larger size
  - Irregular margins
  - Spiculation
  - Diffuse, irregular amorphous calcification
  - Thick irregular wall when cavitating more likely malignant
  - Adjacent pleural retraction
  - Pleural thickening
  - Persisting part solid nodule

Clarification of Solitary Pulmonary Round Foci on CT

▶ Volume CT scan
▶ Differentiation of lesions from vessel cross-sections
  - Detection assisted by
    – Thick slice maximum intensity projections
    – Computer-assisted diagnostic software
▶ Current recommendations and criteria of the Fleischner Society and the American College of Chest Physicians for the management of pulmonary round lesions
▶ Even in groups at high risk for the development of bronchial carcinoma, more than 95% of soft tissue dense foci ≤10 mm are benign
  - Focal infection
  - Granuloma
  - Intrapulmonary lymph nodes
    – Perifissural nodules
▶ Round foci >8 mm
  - Management
    – Early follow-up ideally with CT volumetry
    – PET-CT
    – Endobronchial ultrasound (EBUS) with biopsy

- – CT-guided biopsy
- – Resection
▶ Round foci ≤8 mm
  - • Management
    - – Follow-up with CT volumetry

Multiple Pulmonary Nodules

▶ Small/miliary <2 mm
  - • Miliary tuberculosis
  - • Fungal (histoplasmosis, coccidioidomycosis) and viral
  - • Sarcoidosis—usually perihilar/upper zone—hila may be enlarged
  - • Pneumoconiosis—usually mid/upper zone
  - • Metastases
  - • Langerhans cell histiocytosis—mainly upper zone
  - • Acute hypersensitivity pneumonitis
▶ Medium 2–5 mm
  - • Metastases—breast, thyroid, GI tract, bronchus, melanoma
  - • Pulmonary tuberculosis
  - • Vasculitis
  - • Rheumatoid nodules—usually peripheral
  - • Septic emboli—usually peripheral
  - • Arteriovenous malformations—may be part of hereditary haemorrhagic telangiectasia, HHT
  - • Amyloidosis
  - • Post-transplant lymphoproliferative disease
▶ Large >5 mm
  - • Metastases—renal, thyroid, germ cell tumours, chorio-carcinoma
  - • Wegener's granulomatosis—often with cavitation
  - • Sarcoidosis
  - • Lymphoma
  - • Cryptogenic organising pneumonia—may have reverse halo sign

Cavitating Pulmonary Nodules

▶ Malignant
  • Primary—squamous cell more common
  • Metastasis—squamous cell, colon, transitional cell, sarcoma, lymphoma
▶ Lung infection
  • Tuberculosis—upper lobe and apical segment of lower lobes mainly, thick walled
  • Staphylococcus—usually single and upper lobe
  • Hydatid cyst—mainly right lower zone, water lily sign
▶ Pulmonary infarct—peripheral
▶ Vasculitis—Wegener's granulomatosis
▶ Rheumatoid nodules
▶ Laryngeal papillomatosis—associated with tracheal nodules

Solitary Pulmonary Calcification

▶ Granuloma
▶ Tuberculoma
▶ Hamartoma
▶ Carcinoid—usually central
▶ Solitary metastasis—osteosarcoma, chondrosarcoma
▶ Amyloid

Multiple Pulmonary Calcifications

▶ Tuberculosis
▶ Histoplasmosis—North America
▶ Varicella pneumonia—adult infection, multiple small
▶ Sarcoidosis
▶ Alveolar microlithiasis
▶ Haemosiderosis
▶ Silicosis—bilateral upper zone and perihilar predominant, may also be subpleural
▶ Hypercalcaemia
▶ Mitral stenosis—usually lower zone
▶ Metastasis—osteosarcoma, chondrosarcoma, mucinous carcinoma, thyroid

Lung Nodules with Pneumothorax

▶ Metastatic osteosarcoma
▶ Langerhans cell histiocytosis
▶ Wilms tumour

Lower Zone Fibrosis

▶ Idiopathic pulmonary fibrosis
▶ Connective tissue-related interstitial lung disease
   • May see dilated oesophagus (scleroderma), arthropathy such as erosion of the acromioclavicular joint or shoulder (rheumatoid arthritis) and pleural effusions
▶ Asbestosis—pleural plaques
▶ Drug-related fibrosis
▶ Radiotherapy—may be features of previous cancer, for example, previous breast cancer

Upper Zone Fibrosis

▶ Tuberculosis—may be calcification
▶ Histoplasmosis—North America
▶ Radiotherapy—usually unilateral
▶ Fibrotic hypersensitivity pneumonitis
▶ Stage IV sarcoidosis—may be calcified mediastinal nodes
▶ Progressive massive fibrosis—background upper zone nodularity and calcified mediastinal nodes
▶ Ankylosing spondylitis
▶ Semi-invasive aspergillosis
▶ Drugs—nitrofurantoin
▶ Pleuroparenchymal fibroelastosis (PPFE)

Hilar Enlargement

▶ Pulmonary artery
   • Pulmonary venous hypertension: Bilateral, indistinct, opacified lung periphery
   • Pulmonary hyperperfusion: Bilateral, sharply demarcated, normal lung periphery

- Pulmonary hypoperfusion: Due to massive pulmonary embolism, Westermark sign, unilateral, abrupt cut off
- Pulmonary artery aneurysm
- Post-stenotic dilatation—left-sided
▶ Lymph nodes
  - Unilateral: Bronchial carcinoma, tuberculosis, lymphoma
  - Bilateral: Lymphoma, metastases, tuberculosis, sarcoidosis, pneumoconiosis, Castleman disease, histoplasmosis

Basic Pattern in HR-CT

▶ Increased density
  - Reticular pattern
  - Nodular pattern
  - Ground-glass opacity
  - Consolidation
▶ Decreased density
  - Air trapping
  - Emphysema

Reticular Pattern in HR-CT

▶ Thickened interlobular septa
  - Smooth thickened
    - Interstitial pulmonary oedema
    - Pulmonary haemorrhage
    - Lymphangitic carcinomatosis
    - Alveolar proteinosis—with ground-glass/crazy paving
    - Pneumocystis jirovecii pneumonia
  - Nodular thickened
    - Lymphangitic carcinomatosis
    - Sarcoidosis
    - Pulmonary lymphoma
    - Asbestosis
    - Pneumoconiosis
▶ Honeycomb pattern
  - Clustered, palisaded, walled cysts
    - Peripheral, basal, subpleural: Idiopathic pulmonary fibrosis, asbestosis

- Upper zone: Sarcoidosis
- Mid/upper zone: Fibrotic hypersensitivity pneumonitis
- Anteriorly: Barotrauma after ARDS

Nodular Pattern in HR-CT

▶ Micronodular
  • Random distribution: Sign of haematogenous seeding
    - Haematogenous metastasis
    - Miliary tuberculosis
  • Interlobular and peribronchovascular distribution: Sign of lymphatic pathology
    - Sarcoidosis
    - Lymphangitic carcinomatosis
    - Pneumoconiosis
  • Centrilobular distribution: Sign of endobronchial or vascular disease
    - Bronchiolar infection
    - Endobronchial tumour seeding
    - Angiocentric diseases—haemorrhage, congestion
    - Inhalational—smoking, hypersensitivity pneumonitis, pneumoconiosis

Ground-Glass Opacity in HR-CT

▶ Aetiology: Air content in the affected areas is reduced but not eliminated. It can be due to acute processes with displacement of air from the lung parenchyma by intra-alveolar fluid, interstitial structural proliferation, partial collapse, increased perfusion of the lung parenchyma, or to chronic fibrotic proliferation. If traction bronchiectasis is present—likely fibrotic
▶ Causes
  • Acute
    - Pulmonary oedema
    - Acute pneumonia
    - Aspiration
    - ARDS
    - Pulmonary haemorrhage

- Subacute/chronic
  - Preinvasive lesions
  - Sarcoidosis
▶ Special types
- Interstitial lung disease
- Alveolar proteinosis—ground-glass and septal thickening (crazy paving)
- Diffuse fibrosing alveolitis such as non-specific interstitial pneumonia—ground-glass, with traction bronchiectasis
- Hypersensitivity pneumonitis
▶ CT: Airspace density increases with preserved lung architecture, vessels and bronchi still visible

Focal Opacity on HR-CT with Air Bronchograms

▶ Causes
- Infection, infarction, organising pneumonia
- Adenocarcinoma
- Lymphoma
- Sarcoidosis
▶ CT: Airspace density increases with obscured vessels but bronchi still visible

CT-Guided Lung Biopsy

▶ Indications
- Suspected lung cancer—soft tissue nodule, >10 mm or increasing in size
- Indeterminate pulmonary disease
- Potential to influence clinical management
▶ Procedure
- Core biopsy (16–18 G)
- Contraindications: Poor respiratory reserve, clotting disorder, crossing fissures, adjacent emphysema, proximity to major vessels
▶ Complications: Pneumothorax, haemoptysis, air embolism

Chronic Obstructive Pulmonary Disease

▶ Centrilobular emphysema
- Aetiology: Nicotine, chronic bronchitis, dust
- Blue bloater
- **CXR**
  - Preferential involvement of the upper lobes
  - Irregular increased pulmonary vessels
  - Dirty chest sign
  - Enlarged pulmonary arteries
- **HR-CT**: Usually apical predominance, centrilobular areas destroyed, heterogeneous pattern of destruction

▶ Panlobular emphysema
- Aetiology: α1-antitrypsin deficiency
- Pink puffer
- **CXR**
  - Basal lung predominance
  - Hyperlucent lungs
  - Paucity of pulmonary vessels
  - Reduced diaphragmatic excursion
  - Flattened hemidiaphragms
  - Blunting of costophrenic angles
  - Increased sagittal thoracic (A-P) diameter
  - Barrel chest
  - Widened intercostal spaces
  - Kyphotic sternum with increased retrosternal space
  - Bullae may be visible
  - Narrow elongated heart and mediastinum
- **HR-CT**: Basal predominance, entire lobules destroyed, homogeneous pattern of destruction

▶ Paraseptal emphysema
- **CXR**: May cause spontaneous pneumothorax
- **HR-CT**: Apical predominance, subpleural interlobular septa destroyed, usually single row of subpleural cysts

▶ Bullous emphysema
- **HR-CT**: Peripheral/subpleural bullae >1 cm
  - Variant: Progressive lung dystrophy with giant bullae compressing adjacent normal lung—vanishing lung syndrome

► **Complications**: Pulmonary arterial hypertension, cor pulmonale
► Bronchiectasis
  • Aetiology: Congenital, fibrotic, post-stenotic, post-infectious, toxic
  • Presentation: Productive coughing fits, recurrent broncho-pneumonia, haemoptysis, crackles on auscultation
  • Types
    – Tubular—evenly dilated
    – Varicose—variable diameter
    – Cystic—most severe with cystic change
  • **CXR**
    – Cylindrical or cystic-shaped
    – Air- or mucus-filled
    – Most frequently in the lower lobes
    – Streaky dense bands, absence of peripheral tapering
  • **HR-CT:** Bronchodilatation (diameter greater than adjacent pulmonary artery—signet ring sign), non-tapering bronchial walls (tramline sign), bronchial wall thickening, air trapping in expiratory scan
► Chronic bronchitis
  • **CXR**
    – Thickened non-tapering bronchial walls
    – Non-specific increased lung markings—dirty chest sign
    – Pneumonic infiltrates

Specific Types of Emphysema

► Paracicatricial emphysema
  • Aetiology: Focal emphysema adjacent to an area of scarring
► Swyer-James-MacLeod syndrome
  • Aetiology: Unilateral lobular emphysema due to early bronchiolitis obliterans
  • **CXR**
    – Increased translucency of the affected lung
    – Affected lung area reduced in inspiration and enlarged in expiration—distal airway stenosis with air trapping

▶ Vicariant emphysema
  • Aetiology: Compensatory overinflation after loss of lung volume (e.g. lobectomy, pneumonectomy)

Emphysema: Lung Volume Reduction Procedures

▶ Bronchoscopic lung volume reduction
  • Valves, coils
▶ Surgical lung volume reduction
  • Bullectomy, lobectomy

Asthma

▶ **CXR**
  • Hyperinflation during acute episode
  • Focal atelectasis due to acute bronchiolitis
  • Reversibility of the changes
▶ **Differential Diagnosis**: Pneumothorax, pulmonary embolism, left heart failure, tracheal stenosis
▶ **Complications**: Emphysema, pneumothorax, pneumomediastinum, pneumonia

Pneumonia

▶ Lobar pneumonia
  • Aetiology: Pneumococci, Klebsiella, Legionella
  • Stages: Inoculation (serous), red hepatisation (haemorrhagic), grey hepatisation (fibrinous), yellow hepatisation (purulent), lysis (resorptive), resolution (normal)
  • **CXR/CT**: Extensive infiltrate, lobar, air bronchograms visible
▶ Bronchopneumonia
  • Aetiology: Staphylococci, Streptococci, Pseudomonas
  • **CXR/CT**: Patchy infiltrate, round focal infiltrate, segmental infiltrate
  • Often effusion
  • May develop empyema, abscess, pneumatocele

► Atypical pneumonia
  • Aetiology: Viruses, Mycoplasma, Chlamydia
  • **CXR/CT**: Reticulonodular opacification or consolidation, often bilateral, may be enlarged mediastinal lymph nodes
► Cough, fever, dyspnoea
► Localisation
  • Silhouette sign: Loss of the normally existing contour (silhouette) when two structures of the same X-ray density are adjacent to each other, helps localisation of pathology in lung
    – Middle lobe consolidation: Loss of contour of the right heart border at site of contact
    – Lower lobe consolidation: Loss of contour of the diaphragm at the site of contact
► Reasons for negative X-ray findings despite clinical suspicion of pneumonia
  • Neutropenia
  • Dehydration
  • Pulmonary fibrosis
  • Bullous lung disease
► Investigation in cases of discrepancy between clinical and radiological findings, CT or HR-CT for pneumonia detection and pneumonia differentiation
► **Differential Diagnosis**: Pulmonary oedema can look similar but will often improve following appropriate treatment in a few hours, lepidic adenocarcinoma, cryptogenic organising pneumonia

Typical vs. Atypical Pneumonia

Criteria	Typical pneumonia	Atypical pneumonia
Onset	Sudden	Gradual
Fever	High	Moderate
Leukocytosis	Marked	Mild or absent
Lobar/segmental consolidation	Common	Uncommon
Diffuse/interstitial/bilateral	Uncommon	Common
Pronounced CXR/CT findings with moderate clinical findings	Uncommon	Common
Pleural effusion	Common	Uncommon

Lung Abscess

► Aetiology: Complication of pneumonia
► **CXR/CT**
  • Initially focal consolidation
  • Then necrotic with low attenuation centre due to fluid
  • May develop cavity with air-liquid level visible on CXR and CT
  • May be associated with hilar lymphadenopathy
► **Complications**: Empyema

Legionella Pneumonia

► Aetiology: Legionella pneumophila
► Incubation period from 2 to 10 days
► Nosocomial legionella pneumonia has 50% higher mortality than outpatient legionella pneumonia
► Protracted course with respiratory failure
► **CXR/CT**
  • Alveolar infiltrates—consolidation +/− ground-glass with basal predominance
  • Unilateral or bilateral
  • Pleural effusions common

Acute Respiratory Distress Syndrome

► Aetiology: Multiple causes including sepsis, severe pneumonia, inhalation of toxic substances, major injury
► Fever, severe respiratory symptoms—cough, dyspnoea, sore throat
► **HR-CT**
  • CT changes precede CXR changes
  • Especially lower lobe and periphery
  • Ground-glass-like density progresses to pneumonic consolidations
  • Pleural effusions are unusual

COVID-19

▶ Aetiology: Infection with the coronavirus SARS-CoV-2
▶ Cough, fever, rhinitis, olfactory disturbances, taste disturbances, pneumonia, gastrointestinal symptoms
▶ **CXR**: Patchy progressing to more confluent bilateral opacification mainly peripherally in the mid and lower zones
▶ **CT**
  - Early stage (0–5 days)
    – Normal or mainly ground-glass opacities
  - Progressive stage (6–8 days)
    – Increasing ground-glass opacities/consolidation, bilateral and basal predominance and septal thickening with crazy paving pattern
  - Peak stage (9–13 days)
    – Progressive consolidation
  - Late stage (>14 days)
    – Gradual resolution
    – Signs of fibrosis may develop including parenchymal bands, traction bronchiectasis and architectural distortion
  - Summary of CT findings
    – Initially patchy ground-glass and consolidation which becomes more confluent
    – Dilated pulmonary vessels in the vicinity of consolidation
    – Lymphadenopathy uncommon
    – Usually no pleural or pericardial effusions
    – Typical distribution: Multifocal, bilateral, peripherally and posteriorly in the mid and lower zones
  - Categories of CT findings
    – Category I: Suggestive of COVID-19 pneumonia
    – Category II: COVID-19 pneumonia possible
    – Category III: Suggestive of alternative diagnosis
    – Category IV: No pneumonia
▶ Prognosis correlates with the extent of the findings
▶ **Diagnosis**: PCR
▶ **Complications**: Secondary infection, pulmonary embolism

Fungal Infections

▶ Pneumocystis jirovecii pneumonia
  • Unproductive cough, fever, increasing dyspnoea
  • **CXR:** Bilateral, perihilar reticulonodular and ground-glass densities
  • **HR-CT**
    – Ground-glass pattern, predominantly perihilar and mid-zone
    – Subpleural sparing ~40%
    – Septal thickening—may be crazy paving
    – Pneumatoceles
    – Pleural effusions and lymphadenopathy uncommon
▶ Aspergilloma
  • **CXR:** Rounded density in pre-existing cavity (air-crescent sign)—due to fungal ball
▶ Invasive and semi-invasive pulmonary aspergillosis
  • **CXR**
    – Focal consolidation with ill-defined margins
    – Air bronchogram
  • **HR-CT:** Halo sign—ground-glass rim around dense area of consolidation
▶ Allergic Bronchopulmonary Aspergillosis (ABPA)
  • Occurs in asthmatic, cystic fibrosis and immunocompromised patients
  • **HR-CT:** Central bronchiectasis, fleeting consolidation or ground-glass, often centrilobular, dense 'finger-in-glove' mucoceles
▶ Candida pneumonia
  • **CXR:** Alveolar or interstitial infiltrates
  • **HR-CT**
    – Disseminated, bilateral, irregular, patchy consolidation
    – Focal cavitation may develop
▶ Histoplasmosis, coccidioidomycosis
  • Subclinical course, acute pneumonia or disseminated organ involvement
  • **CXR:** Calcified round foci

Tuberculosis

▶ Aetiology: Mycobacterium tuberculosis
▶ Lungs most common site of infection
▶ Primary tuberculosis
  • Often asymptomatic
  • Focal pneumonia—Ghon focus
  • Focal pneumonia and lymph node involvement—Ghon complex
  • 95% heal spontaneously
  • Can progress to more diffuse and varied disease such as miliary tuberculosis and spread to other organs
  • **CXR**
    – Random location of primary focus
    – Hilar/mediastinal lymphadenopathy—unilateral or bilateral
    – Peripheral nodular infiltrates, atelectasis
    – Tendency to calcification with time—pulmonary, nodal, pleural
    – May develop into progressive tuberculosis which can be varied in appearance, can develop miliary tuberculosis
▶ Post-primary tuberculosis
  • May have minor symptoms such as chronic cough or may have constitutional symptoms such as fever, malaise and weight loss
  • **CXR**
    – Predisposition for apical and posterior segments of the upper lobes and apical segments of the lower lobes
    – Miliary tuberculosis—symmetrical bilateral micronodules
    – Ill-defined nodules of varying size
    – Cavitation of nodules—usually thick walled
  • Tree-in-bud on HR-CT
  • Endobronchial tuberculosis with bronchiectasis and strictures
  • Pleural involvement with pleural thickening and pleural

effusion, pneumothorax, bronchopleural fistula
- Can cross pleural boundaries and involve adjacent tissues or haematogenous spread to other organs, including bone, adrenals, kidneys, liver, brain
    - Tendency to calcification with time—pulmonary, nodal, pleural
▶ Features of active disease
- Cavitation
- Centrilobular ground-glass nodules
- Tree-in-bud attenuation
- Change in disease extent over time
▶ **Differential Diagnosis**: Pneumonia, bronchial carcinoma, lymphangitic carcinomatosis, lymphoma
▶ **Diagnosis:** Combination of imaging, microbiological, molecular biological, immunological and histological examination methods
- Genotypic methods enable early diagnosis
- Phenotypic methods are diagnostic gold standards
▶ **Complications**: Haemoptysis, pneumothorax, sepsis

Nontuberculous Mycobacterial Disease

▶ Aetiology: Mycobacterium avium complex
▶ **CXR**
- Bronchiectasis
- Micronodules, tree-in-bud pattern
- Cavitations
- Propensity for apices of upper lobes and lower lobes

Eosinophilic Lung Disease

▶ Types
- Idiopathic eosinophilic pneumonia—Löffler syndrome
- Eosinophilic pneumonia of known cause
    - Drug allergy
    - Asthma

- Fungal infection
- Parasite infection
- Connective tissue diseases
- Paraneoplastic

▶ Paucity of symptoms, myalgia, blood eosinophilia

▶ CXR: Bilateral, transient, ground-glass opacities, may be peripheral

▶ HR-CT: Reverse bat wing sign

Pulmonary Hydatid (Echinococcosis)

▶ Haemoptysis, dyspnoea

▶ CXR
  - Unilocular or multiple pulmonary round or oval cysts
  - 1–20 cm, mainly lower lobe
  - Echinococcus membrane floating on residual fluid (water lily sign)—may be adjacent consolidation when ruptured

AIDS

▶ CD4 cells/μL > 400
  - Bacteria
    - Streptococcus pneumoniae
▶ CD4 cells/μL < 400
  - Lymphoma
  - Kaposi's sarcoma
  - Tuberculosis
▶ CD4 cells/μL < 200
  - Pneumocystis jirovecii
  - Mycobacterium avium complex
▶ CD4 cells/μL < 50
  - Cytomegalovirus
▶ CD4 cells/μL < 20
  - Aspergillosis

Interstitial Lung Disease

▶ Usual interstitial pneumonia (UIP)
- HR-CT: Typical UIP pattern
  – Basal and subpleural predominance
  – Reticulation
  – Traction bronchiectasis
  – Honeycomb cysts
  – Limited ground-glass
- HR-CT: Probable UIP pattern
  – Basal and subpleural predominance
  – Reticulation
  – Traction bronchiectasis
  – Absence of honeycomb cysts
  – Limited ground-glass
- HR-CT: Indeterminate UIP pattern
  – Basal and subpleural predominance
  – Reticulation
  – Absence of traction bronchiectasis
  – Absence of honeycomb cysts
  – Limited ground-glass
- HR-CT: Alternative diagnosis more likely
  – If upper/mid-zone predominance, peribronchovascular predominance, ground-glass predominance, profuse micronodules, discrete cysts (multiple, bilateral, away from areas of honeycombing), diffuse mosaic attenuation/air trapping (bilateral, in three or more lobes), consolidation in bronchopulmonary segment(s)/lobe(s)
▶ Differential Diagnosis: Chronic hypersensitivity pneumonitis, connective tissue-related ILD, asbestosis, drugs, radiotherapy
▶ Complications: Pneumothorax, malignancy, bronchiectasis, pulmonary arterial hypertension, cor pulmonale
▶ Non-specific interstitial pneumonia (NSIP)
- HR-CT
  – Ground-glass opacification, predominantly peripheral and basal

- Traction bronchiectasis
- May be subpleural sparing
- Cystic honeycombing less common
- Commonly occurs with connective tissue-related ILD

▶ Respiratory bronchiolitis with interstitial lung disease (RB-ILD)
  - Associated with smoking
  - **HR-CT**
    - Centrilobular ground-glass nodules due to acute respiratory bronchiolitis
    - Usually more upper zone—inhalational distribution
    - Scattered peripheral reticulations—the ILD component
    - Evidence of emphysema often present

▶ Desquamative interstitial pneumonia (DIP)
  - Associated with smoking, rare
  - **HR-CT**
    - Diffuse ground-glass attenuation
    - Scattered cysts
    - Usually lower zone predominance

▶ Cryptogenic organising pneumonia (COP)
  - Acute to subacute
  - **HR-CT**
    - Bilateral, peripheral consolidation +/− ground-glass attenuation
    - May be migratory
    - May get reverse halo sign with central ground-glass surrounded by denser consolidation

▶ Acute interstitial pneumonia (AIP)
  - Rapidly progressive fulminant disease of unknown aetiology
  - Also known as diffuse alveolar damage, idiopathic ARDS
  - **HR-CT**
    - Diffuse extensive bilateral airspace consolidation +/− ground-glass attenuation
    - Basal predominance
    - Fulminant progression
    - Diffuse alveolar damage

▶ Lymphoid interstitial pneumonia (LIP)
  • Uncommon—associated with HIV and with connective tis-
    sue disease, especially Sjögren's syndrome
  • **HR-CT**
    – Combination of thin-walled cysts, ground-glass opaci-
      ties and centrilobular nodules
▶ Pleuroparenchymal fibroelastosis (PPFE)
  • **HR-CT**
    – Bilateral apical pleural thickening extending to involve
      the adjacent lung with parenchyma distortion
    – Traction bronchiectasis and thickened interlobular septa

Pneumoconiosis

▶ Aetiology: Inhalation of inorganic dust. These include coal
  dust (coal workers pneumoconiosis), talc (talcosis) and silica
  (silicosis). May be in combination depending on exposure.
  Duration and degree of exposure determines findings
▶ Latency from first exposure usually 20–30 years, but can be
  sooner
▶ Acute silicoproteinosis, rare fulminant complication of intense
  exposure
▶ Caplan's syndrome, pneumoconiosis associated with seroposi-
  tive rheumatoid arthritis
  • Multiple nodules typically 0.5–5 cm, which may cavitate
▶ **CXR/CT**
  • Multiple small bilateral mid and upper zone pulmonary
    nodules. Calcifications in 20% (calcification more common
    with silicosis)
  • May have interlobular septal thickening giving a crazy-
    paving pattern
  • Mediastinal nodal enlargement with peripheral eggshell
    calcification
  • In the chronic stage, conglomerate masses in the lateral
    upper fields (progressive massive fibrosis or complicated
    pneumoconiosis)
▶ Radiological classification according to the International
  Labour Office (ILO)
▶ **Complications**: Silicotuberculosis, bronchial carcinoma

Asbestosis

▶ Aetiology: Asbestos, fibrogenic and carcinogenic effects, first changes after 10–40 years
▶ Cough, exertional dyspnoea, fine crackles on auscultation, nail clubbing
▶ **CXR/CT**
- Diaphragmatic and chest wall pleural plaques, often calcified
- Recurrent pleural effusions
- Diffuse pleural thickening
- Basal pulmonary fibrosis
▶ **HR-CT**
- Pleural plaques, both calcified and non-calcified
- Diffuse pleural thickening
- Subpleural septal thickening, ground-glass attenuation, traction bronchiectasis and cystic honeycombing due to asbestosis
- Coarse subpleural bands and benign folded lung
▶ Radiological classification according to the International Labour Office (ILO)
▶ **Complications**: Asbestosis, bronchial carcinoma, pleural mesothelioma

Hypersensitivity Pneumonitis

▶ Aetiology
- Interstitial lung disease due to repeated inhalation of organic dusts
- Type III and type IV allergic mechanisms
- Examples include farmer's lung, bird fancier's lung, mushroom worker's lung
▶ Acute course with flu-like symptoms
▶ Chronic course with fatigue, dry cough and dyspnoea on exertion
▶ Non-fibrotic hypersensitivity pneumonitis
- **CXR**
  - Diffuse fine nodular or more confluent ground-glass pattern

- **CT**
  - Centrilobular ground-glass nodules
  - Diffuse ground-glass
  - May be geographical areas of reduced attenuation due to air trapping
  - Diffuse reticular and micronodular opacification
▶ Fibrotic hypersensitivity pneumonitis
- **CT**
  - Fibrotic features with peripheral interlobular septal thickening, may be associated with traction bronchiectasis and cystic honeycombing. All zones may be involved but often more marked in the upper zones
  - Multifocal ground-glass opacification which may have established fibrotic and ongoing acute alveolitic components
  - Geographical areas of reduced attenuation due to air trapping
  - Fibrotic features with peripheral interlobular septal thickening, traction bronchiectasis and cystic honeycombing
  - Three density pattern (air trapping, normal lung and ground-glass opacity) in the presence of fibrosis is strongly predictive of fibrotic hypersensitivity pneumonitis

Treatment-Related Lung Pathology

▶ Radiotherapy
- Acute radiation pneumonitis—limited to radiation field, may respond to steroids
- Pulmonary fibrosis—limited to radiation field
- Occasionally, a more diffuse organising pneumonia response involving lung remote from radiation field
▶ Drugs
- Acute bronchiolitis
- Acute interstitial pneumonia
- Eosinophilic pulmonary syndrome
- Diffuse fibrosing alveolitis

▶ Cytotoxic medication
  • Diffuse alveolar damage
  • Organising pneumonia
  • Interstitial pneumonia
▶ Immunotherapeutic medication
  • Immunotherapy-associated pneumonitis

Granulomatosis with Polyangiitis

▶ Formerly known as Wegener's granulomatosis
▶ Aetiology: Vasculitis involving small- and medium-sized vessels with necrotising granulomas in the respiratory tract (nose, sinuses, middle ear, oropharynx, lungs) and renal involvement (glomerulonephritis, microaneurysms)
▶ CXR/CT
  • Pulmonary masses or nodules of varying sizes usually multiple, lower zone predominance. Tendency to cavitate
  • Ill-defined areas of consolidation which may have a rim of ground-glass—halo sign
  • Focal areas of tracheobronchial stenosis may occur
  • Patchy infiltrates due to pneumonia or alveolar haemorrhage
▶ Diagnosis: Detection of cANCA, histology

Connective Tissue Disorders

▶ Systemic sclerosis, dermatomyositis, ankylosing spondylitis, systemic lupus erythematosus, rheumatoid arthritis, Sjögren's syndrome
▶ Stages
  • Early stage
    – CXR: Fine nodular and reticular fibrosis with basal and peripheral predominance
  • Late stage
    – CXR: Basal and peripheral pulmonary fibrosis common, but pattern can vary considerably
▶ Associated findings: Pleural effusion, pericardial effusion, cardiomegaly

Goodpasture's Syndrome

▶ Aetiology: Antibasement membrane antibody disease
▶ Recurrent pulmonary haemorrhage and glomerulonephritis
▶ Stages
  • Acute stage
    – **CXR:** Confluent patchy bilateral coalescent areas of airspace opacification due to pulmonary haemorrhage which usually resolve over a few days
    – **HR-CT:** Diffuse bilateral ground-glass opacification which may be centrilobular. May progress to crazy paving pattern as haem is absorbed into the lymphatics
  • After 2–3 weeks
    – **CXR/HR-CT:** Usually normalisation of CXR and HR-CT findings
  • Recurrent episodes
    – **CXR/HR-CT:** May develop pulmonary fibrosis

Langerhans Cell Histiocytosis

▶ Aetiology: Smoking related
▶ **CXR/HR-CT:** Upper zone predominant, diffuse, bilateral, initially micronodular, develops into irregular thin-walled cysts. Lungs may be hyperinflated
▶ **Complications:** Pneumothorax

Sarcoidosis

▶ Organs which can be involved
  • Most commonly: Hilar lymph nodes, mediastinal lymph nodes, lungs
  • Less commonly: Skin, eyes, liver, lymphatic system, spleen, nervous system, heart, kidneys
▶ Young and middle age
▶ **CXR/CT**
  • Stage I
    – Mediastinal lymphadenopathy only: Usually bilateral hilar, paratracheal, aortopulmonary and subcarinal involvement. Nodes can calcify over time

- Stage II
  - Mediastinal lymphadenopathy plus lung involvement: Most commonly nodular and reticular lung changes in the perihilar regions and upper zones. However, almost any lung changes can be due to sarcoidosis, with nodules being small or large, sparse or numerous and cavitating or solid. On HR-CT, the presence of irregular broncho-vascular bundles in the perihilar regions and irregular thickening of fissures (fissural beading) are supportive of the diagnosis
- Stage III
  - Lung involvement without mediastinal lymphadenopathy
- Stage IV
  - Pulmonary fibrosis: Typically bilateral upper zone/peri-hilar fibrosis with volume loss in the upper lobes and often an element of traction bronchiectasis
▶ **Differential Diagnosis**: Lymphoma, bronchial carcinoma, silicosis, tuberculosis, lymphangitic carcinomatosis
▶ **Complications**: Pulmonary fibrosis, pulmonary arterial hypertension, cor pulmonale

Alveolar Microlithiasis

▶ Aetiology: Tiny microliths in the alveoli
▶ Respiratory insufficiency
▶ **CXR**
  - Very fine, dense, diffuse micronodular pattern
  - Lung basally reduced transparency, apically increased transparency

Benign or Low-Grade Malignant Lung Tumours

▶ Less than 10% of all pulmonary neoplasms
▶ Adenoma
  - Under 50 years
  - Usually central location
  - **CXR**: Bronchial obstruction with post-obstructive pneumonia or atelectasis

▶ Hamartoma
  • **CXR**: Round nodule with popcorn-like calcifications +/− fatty density
  • **CT**: Round with fat content and calcifications
▶ Lipoma
  • **CT**: Round nodule with fat density HU values
▶ Carcinoid
  • **CT**: Round nodule often involving bronchial tree
▶ Papilloma
▶ Leiomyoma
▶ Chondroma

Bronchial Carcinoma

▶ Aetiology: Often smoking related
▶ Types
  • Small cell bronchial carcinoma
  • Non-small cell bronchial carcinoma
    – Squamous cell carcinoma
    – Adenocarcinoma
    – Large cell carcinoma
▶ Persistent cough, haemoptysis, weight loss, dyspnoea
▶ Central bronchial carcinoma
  • Endobronchial growth
  • **CXR**
    – Distal atelectasis or collapse, often lobar in extent
    – Treatment resistant pneumonia or atelectasis due to bronchial stenosis
    – Occasionally distal lung hyperinflation due to ball valve effect
  • Extrabronchial growth
  • **CXR**
    – Unilateral hilar enlargement
    – Convex hilar contour
    – Perihilar infiltration

▶ Peripheral bronchial carcinoma
  • **CXR**
    – Rounded nodule which may have irregular or lobular margin
    – Pleural tagging
    – Spiculation
    – Tumour cavity with irregularly thickened wall when necrotic
    – May have peripheral or eccentric calcification, but if so usually due to involvement of adjacent pre-existing tuberculous granuloma
▶ Pancoast tumour—located at lung apex, invading adjacent soft tissues such as bones and nerves
▶ Tumour invasion of adjacent structures
  • **CT**
    – Loss of intervening fat plane
    – Irregular interface or infiltration
    – Increased extent of tumour contact or encasement
▶ Lymph node metastases
  • **CT**
    – Nodes less likely to be involved if normal size, oval shape, fatty hilum or calcified
    – Skip metastases may occur
  • **Differential Diagnosis**: Azygos vein and superior pericardial recess can mimic nodes
  • Locoregional staging of bronchial carcinoma using endobronchial ultrasound guided transbronchial needle biopsy or mediastinoscopy
▶ **Nuclear Medicine**: 18F-FDG-PET-CT
  • Staging, detection of distant metastasis, detection of recurrence, radiation planning, progress monitoring
▶ **Diagnosis**: Histology by bronchoscopy, endobronchial ultrasound, CT-guided biopsy, video assisted thoracoscopy.

TNM Classification Lung

- ▶ T1a: ≤1 cm
- ▶ T1b: >1 cm to ≤2 cm
- ▶ T1c: >2 cm to ≤3 cm
- ▶ T2: >3 cm to ≤5 cm or ≤2 cm from carina, main bronchus or further distal to the carina or visceral pleura or associated atelectasis or obstructive inflammation up to the hilum
  - • T2a: >3 cm to ≤4 cm
  - • T2b: >4 cm to ≤5 cm
- ▶ T3: >5 cm to ≤7 cm or parietal pleura, chest wall, phrenic nerve, parietal pericardium or separate tumour in the same lobe as the primary tumour
- ▶ T4: Involving diaphragm, mediastinum, heart, great vessels, trachea, carina, recurrent laryngeal nerve, oesophagus, vertebral body or separate tumour in another lobe ipsilaterally
- ▶ N1: Ipsilateral peribronchial/hilar nodal involvement
- ▶ N2: Ipsilateral mediastinal/subcarinal nodal involvement
  - • N2a: Single N2 nodal station involved
  - • N2b: >1 N2 nodal station involved
- ▶ N3: Contralateral mediastinal/hilar, ipsilateral or contralateral supraclavicular nodal involvement
- ▶ M1a: Thoracic metastasis with separate tumour in a contralateral lobe, pleural metastases, pericardial metastases, malignant pleural effusion, malignant pericardial effusion
- ▶ M1b: Single extrathoracic metastasis
- ▶ M1c: More than one extrathoracic metastasis
  - • M1c1: More than one extrathoracic metastasis in a single organ
  - • M1c2: More than one extrathoracic organ involved

Lung Metastases

- ▶ Primary tumours which more commonly produce lung metastases which are:
  - • Small: (miliary) breast carcinoma, thyroid carcinoma, prostate carcinoma
  - • Large (cannonball): Testicular tumour, melanoma, renal cell carcinoma

- Cavitating: Squamous cell carcinoma, sarcoma, colon carcinoma, melanoma, urothelial carcinoma, cervical carcinoma, metastases of all origins during chemotherapy
- Calcified—rare: Sarcomas (osteosarcoma, chondrosarcoma), mucinous carcinomas (breast, ovarian, colon), thyroid carcinoma, testicular tumour
- Endobronchial: Bronchial carcinoma, lymphoma, renal cell carcinoma, breast carcinoma
- Haemorrhagic: Choriocarcinoma, renal cell carcinoma, melanoma, thyroid carcinoma
- Pleural: Bronchial carcinoma, breast carcinoma, thymic carcinoma, lymphoma, ovarian carcinoma

▶ **CXR/CT**
- Solitary round foci or multiple round foci or miliary seeding
- Most often basal and peripheral if haematogenous spread

▶ **Diagnosis**: If necessary, CT-guided biopsy for confirmation

▶ **IR**: Thermal ablation (microwave ablation, radiofrequency ablation)
- **Complications**: Pneumothorax, pulmonary haemorrhage, haemoptysis, infection

Lymphoma

▶ **CXR**: Mediastinal, bihilar lymphadenopathy, especially consider if anterior mediastinal nodes involved or if asymmetrical involvement

▶ **CT**: Infiltrates, masses with or without air bronchograms, may cavitate, pleural masses, pleural effusion, lymphangitic carcinomatosis

Kaposi's Sarcoma

▶ Types
- Central interstitial form
- Peripheral nodular form
- Mixed type

▶ **CT**: Indistinct tumour margins with flame-like extensions (sparkler sign)

Acute Pulmonary Congestion

▶ Aetiology
  - Capillary venous pressure increased, capillary permeability normal: Left heart failure, mitral regurgitation (→ cardiac pulmonary oedema)
  - Capillary venous pressure normal, capillary permeability increased: Inhalation toxins, aspiration toxins (→ non-cardiac, the so-called toxic pulmonary oedema)
  - Capillary venous pressure increased, capillary permeability increased: Narcotic overdose, ARDS (→ non-cardiac pulmonary oedema)
▶ Capillary venous pressure ↑ → basoapical redistribution
  - **CXR**
    – Upper lobe blood diversion
    – Vessel calibre apically equal to or larger than basally
▶ Capillary venous pressure ↑↑ → interstitial pulmonary oedema
  - **CXR**
    – Peribronchial cuffing
    – Perihilar haze
    – Kerley lines
    – Pleural effusions
▶ Capillary venous pressure ↑↑↑ → alveolar pulmonary oedema
  - **CXR**
    – Patchy airspace consolidation
    – May be air bronchograms
    – Later tendency to confluent opacification
    – Whiteout

Pulmonary Oedema

X-ray sign	Cardiac pulmonary oedema	Non-cardiac pulmonary oedema
Cardiac enlargement	Common	Rare
Consolidation	Diffuse, central	Patchy, peripheral
Kerley lines	Common	Rare
Pleural effusion	Common	Rare
Bronchial walls	Thickened	Normal
Air bronchogram	Rare	Common
Indistinct hila	Frequent	Rare

Chronic Pulmonary Congestion

▶ Aetiology: Mitral stenosis
▶ CXR
  • Chronic interstitial pulmonary oedema and alveolar oedema
  • Redistribution of pulmonary blood flow to upper lungs
  • Pulmonary haemosiderosis—small lower zone nodules which can calcify

High Output Cardiac Failure

▶ Aetiology: Left to right shunt, pregnancy, anaemia, fever, hyperthyroidism
▶ CXR
  • Dilated main pulmonary artery trunk
  • Enlarged and dense hila
  • Distended pulmonary arteries and veins

Pulmonary Hypertension

▶ Aetiology: Emphysema, recurrent venous thromboembolism, pulmonary fibrosis, chronic pulmonary congestion, idiopathic pulmonary hypertension, mitral stenosis, systemic sclerosis
▶ **CXR**
  - Enlarged pulmonary arteries
  - Pruning of peripheral pulmonary vessels
  - Right atrium enlarged
  - Elevated cardiac apex—right ventricular hypertrophy

Acute Pulmonary Embolism

▶ Aetiology
  - Venous thromboembolism
  - Septic pulmonary embolism in endocarditis, septic thrombophlebitis
▶ Chest pain, dyspnoea, haemoptysis, circulatory collapse
▶ Most frequently right posterior-basal lung segments
▶ Often not diagnosed clinically
▶ Wells score for estimating the clinical probability of acute pulmonary embolism
  - Pulmonary embolism unlikely with low clinical probability and non-elevated D-dimers
▶ **US**
  - Triangular or spherical pleural lesions
  - Pleural effusion
  - Echocardiography for estimation of right heart strain
▶ **CXR**
  - Chest X-ray may be normal
  - Most positive cases have non-specific abnormalities
  - Focal atelectasis common
    – Occasionally subpleural wedge-shaped consolidation with convex medial border (Hampton's hump)
  - Calibre changes of the pulmonary arteries
    – Localised perihilar oligaemia (Westermark sign)
    – Unilateral hilar enlargement with significant change of calibre (knuckle sign)
  - Pleural effusion—common

▶ **CT**
- Peripheral vascular imaging up to about the seventh vascular order
- Acute embolism
  - Intraluminal filling defects
  - Pleural based atelectasis
  - Mosaic perfusion
  - Pleural effusion

▶ **Nuclear Medicine**
- Perfusion scintigraphy (99mTc-MAA)
- Perfusion defects with normal CXR appearances (mismatch)

▶ **Differential Diagnosis**: Pneumothorax, pneumonia, myocardial infarction, myocarditis, aortic dissection, pancreatitis

▶ Combination of diagnosis of pulmonary embolism by CT pulmonary angiogram and simultaneous CT leg venography is an alternative to using Doppler US of the lower limbs

▶ **IR**: Thrombus fragmentation, thrombus aspiration, thrombolysis

Chronic Pulmonary Embolism

▶ Aetiology: Incomplete lysis, inadequate anticoagulant therapy, recurrent pulmonary embolism

▶ Clinical picture of chronic thromboembolic pulmonary hypertension

▶ **CT/MR**
- Organised thrombi (wall-adherent, crescent-shaped, eccentric, irregular, webs, may calcify)
- Thickened vessel walls
- Reduced peripheral vascularisation
- Mosaic attenuation due to regional hypoperfusion (perfusion heterogeneity) and reduced vessel diameter due to hypoperfusion and vasoconstriction
- Serpiginous peripheral pulmonary arteries
- Pulmonary arterial hypertension
  - Right ventricular wall thickening and may be right heart enlargement
  - Dilated pulmonary trunk (>30 mm) and main pulmonary arteries

▶ **Differential Diagnosis**: Pulmonary arterial angiosarcoma (marked enhancement, dilated vessel), Takayasu's arteritis (aorta also affected)

Superior Vena Cava Thrombosis

▶ **Superior vena cava syndrome**
- Aetiology: Tumours—especially right lung
- Oedema and cyanosis of the neck and head
- May be spontaneous collateralisation via the azygos vein
- **Diagnosis**: CT scan

▶ **Inferior vena cava syndrome**
- Aetiology: Obstruction of the IVC by thrombus or tumour—most commonly renal. Compression of the IVC by neighbouring structures or tumours. Can occur in pregnancy
- Swelling of both legs
- Risk of fatal pulmonary embolism if due to thrombus
- **Diagnosis**: Colour Doppler ultrasound, CT phlebography

Caval Filter

▶ Indications
- Recurrence of pulmonary embolism despite adequate anticoagulant therapy
- Pulmonary embolism when clinical contraindication to anticoagulant therapy
- Prophylactic filter placement after pulmonary embolectomy
- Free floating iliofemoral deep vein thrombosis
- Caval or renal tumours

▶ **Complications**:
- Misplacement
- Filter migration
- Filter perforation
- Filter fracture
- Secondary thrombosis

Acute Respiratory Distress Syndrome

▶ ARDS
▶ Shock lung
▶ Aetiology
  • Direct mechanism of injury: Aspiration, pneumonia, near drowning, intoxication, pulmonary contusion
  • Indirect mechanism of damage: Sepsis, transfusion, shock, burn, consumption coagulopathy
▶ CXR
  • Stage I (initial stage, first hour): Perihilar consolidation
  • Stage II (exudative stage, 1st–24th hour): Interstitial pulmonary oedema
  • Stage III (proliferative stage, day 2–7): Alveolar pulmonary oedema, air bronchograms
  • Stage IV (fibrosing stage, after first week): Coarse parenchymal, later pulmonary fibrosis

Lines and tubes on CXR

▶ **Endotracheal tube**
  • Position with head in neutral position 3–5 cm cranial to the carina
  • **Complications**: Mucosal damage, vocal cord damage, tracheal stenosis, atelectasis, pneumothorax
▶ **Tracheostomy tube**
  • Position with head in neutral position two thirds of the distance between tracheostomy site and carina
  • **Complications**: Mucosal damage, tracheomalacia
▶ **Central venous line**
  • Types
    – Non-tunneled catheters: Single-lumen central venous catheter, multi-lumen central venous catheter, Shaldon catheter, peripherally advanced central venous catheter
    – Port systems: Chemotherapy ports, dialysis port systems, pumps
    – Tunneled catheters: Hickman catheter, Broviac catheter, dialysis catheter

- Position of the central venous catheter in the superior vena cava at the level of the mouth of the azygos vein
- **Complications**: Vascular injury, infection, bacteraemia, sepsis, thrombosis, embolism, pneumothorax, arrhythmias, pericardial tamponade, catheter rupture, catheter dislocation, extravasations

► **Pulmonary artery catheter**
- Location no more than 2 cm distal in the right or left main pulmonary artery trunk
- **Complications**: Vascular injury, infection, thrombosis, pneumothorax, arrhythmias, pericardial tamponade, pulmonary artery rupture, pulmonary artery infarction

► **Nasogastric feeding tube**
- Location 8–10 cm distal to the oesophageal hiatus
- **Complications**: Oesophageal perforation, mediastinitis, reflux, aspiration pneumonia

► **Intercostal drain**
- Location in pneumothorax near the lung apex with antero-superior alignment
- Location in pleural effusion between sixth and eighth rib with posteroinferior alignment
- **Complications**: Surgical emphysema, haematoma, infection, lung laceration, abdominal organ injury

► **Cardiac pacemaker**
- Position of the ventricular wire at the base of the right ventricle left of the midline
- **Complications**: Infection, malfunction, myocardial perforation, embolism

Thoracic Trauma

► **Ribs**
- Fracture—flail segment
- Pneumothorax
- Haemothorax
- Lung contusion
- Thoracic wall surgical emphysema

▶ **Pleura**
- Pneumothorax
- Haemothorax
- Tension pneumothorax

▶ **Mediastinum**
- Mediastinal emphysema
- Mediastinal haematoma
- Traumatic aortic injury
  - Intimal tear (grade I)
  - Intramural haematoma (grade II)
  - Pseudoaneurysm (grade III)
  - Rupture (grade IV)

▶ **Lungs**
- Atelectasis
- Lung contusion
- Traumatic pneumatocele
- Aspiration

▶ **Heart**
- Pericardial haemorrhage/tamponade
- Cardiac contusion
- Cardiac dilatation

▶ **Diaphragm**
- Rupture—may be late complication of bowel herniation and strangulation

---

Paediatric Radiology: Lungs

Chest X-Ray Appearance

▶ **Large opaque thorax**
- Unilateral
  - Pneumonia
  - Massive pleural effusion
  - Large lung tumour
- Bilateral
  - Bilateral pleural effusions
  - Enlarged thymus

► **Small opaque thorax**
- Unilateral
  - Lung agenesis
  - Lung aplasia
  - Total lung collapse

► **Large radiolucent thorax**
- Unilateral
  - Lobar emphysema
  - Pneumothorax
  - Foreign body aspiration
- Bilateral
  - Asthma
  - Cystic fibrosis
  - Bronchiolitis

► **Small radiolucent thorax**
- Unilateral
  - Pulmonary hypoplasia
  - Swyer-James-MacLeod syndrome

Congenital Lung Anomalies

► Congenital lobar overinflation
- Hyperinflation of usually one lobe of the lung, most commonly the left upper lobe, then the right upper lobe
- Dyspnoea, tachypnoea, cyanosis
- **CXR**: Increased radiolucency with mass effect
- **Complications**: Pneumonia, pneumothorax

► Bronchopulmonary sequestration
- Non-aerated lung parenchyma with systemic arterial blood supply mainly from the descending thoracic aorta (70%), abdominal aorta (25%) or intercostal artery (5%)
- Intralobar type
  - Frequent
  - Venous drainage commonly via pulmonary venous system
  - No additional malformations
- Extralobar type
  - Rarer
  - Venous drainage can be systemic via SVC, azygos,

hemiazygos or portal vein into the right atrium
- – Malformations of the heart, diaphragm, kidneys, intestines
- Often recurrent infections
- Mostly left lung
- **CXR**: Soft tissue density mass typically in the posterobasal lower lobe segment
- **Diagnosis**: CT angiography

▶ Bronchogenic cysts
- Disruption of the branching of the tracheobronchial tree
- Mediastinal or intrapulmonary
- **CXR**
  - – Soft tissue density rounded structure in the central middle third of the lung
  - – Can have a connection to the bronchial system following infection resulting in air in the cyst

▶ Congenital cystic adenomatoid malformation (CCAM) or congenital cystic pulmonary airway malformation (CPAM)
- Intralobar mass of disorganised lung tissue
- Classification according to Stocker
  - – I: One or more large cysts
  - – II: Many small cysts
  - – III: Solid mass with tiny cysts
- Asymptomatic up to progressive respiratory distress
- **CXR**: Variable appearance if fluid filled, usually a multi-cystic lesion
- **Complications**: Pneumonia, pneumothorax

▶ Bronchial atresia
- Developmental anomaly typically affecting apico-posterior segmental bronchus of the left upper lobe

▶ Arteriovenous malformation
- Shunt formation between a pulmonary artery and pulmonary vein
- 30% multiple, 10% bilateral
- Predilection for lower lobes
- **CXR**: Rounded non-specific soft tissue density mass which may have prominent feeding and draining vessels
- **Diagnosis**: CT, angiography

- • **Complications**: Cerebral embolism, cerebral abscess, massive haemoptysis
- ▶ Scimitar syndrome
  - • Partial anomalous pulmonary venous return
  - • Hypoplastic right lung drained by an anomalous pulmonary vein into the systemic venous system
  - • Functional left-right shunt

Transient Neonatal Tachypnoea

- ▶ Wet lung disease
- ▶ Aetiology: Delayed resorption of amniotic fluid retained in the neonatal lungs
- ▶ Risk factors
  - • Perinatal asphyxia
  - • Maternal diabetes
  - • Caesarean section
  - • Excessive analgesia
  - • Rapid birth
- ▶ Fluid accumulation in alveoli, interstitium, pleural space
- ▶ Tachypnoea, chest retraction, nasal flaring, cyanosis
- ▶ **CXR**
  - • Perihilar interstitial oedema or streaky opacities
  - • Hazy vessel outline
  - • Small pleural effusions
- ▶ Normalisation of findings in 48–72 h

Meconium Aspiration Syndrome

- ▶ Aetiology: Serious complication of intrapartum or intrauterine asphyxia
- ▶ Severe respiratory depression, cardiovascular insufficiency if severe
- ▶ **CXR**
  - • Patchy pulmonary opacities
  - • Hyperinflation

- Flattened diaphragms
- Extra-alveolar air, i.e. pneumothorax or pneumomediastinum

Respiratory Distress Syndrome

▶ Aetiology: Surfactant deficiency with alveolar collapse in immature lung
▶ Tachypnoea, nasal flaring, expiratory grunting, intercostal retractions, microcirculatory disturbances, temperature instability
▶ CXR
  - Stage I: Diffuse, bilateral granular opacities, low lung volumes
  - Stage II: I plus air bronchograms extending from the heart borders to the lung periphery
  - Stage III: II plus loss of cardiac and diaphragm contours, veil-like reduction in transparency
  - Stage IV: Opaque lung
▶ Therapy monitoring
  - No improvement in findings after surfactant administration
    - Lung immaturity
    - Sepsis
    - PDA
    - Heart defect
  - Unilateral improvement in findings after surfactant administration
    - Uneven surfactant distribution
▶ Differential Diagnosis: Neonatal infection with β-haemolytic streptococcus
▶ Complications: Pulmonary interstitial emphysema, pneumothorax, pneumomediastinum, pneumoperitoneum, pneumopericardium, bronchopulmonary dysplasia

Ventilation Complications

▶ Bronchopulmonary dysplasia
  • Aetiology: Lung immaturity, respiratory trauma, oxygen toxicity
  • Oxygen dependence, dyspnoea, tachypnoea, recurrent bronchopneumonia, psychomotor developmental delay, pulmonary arterial hypertension
  • CXR
    – Reticular opacities
    – Atelectasis
    – Hyperinflation
    – Focal emphysema
    – Cardiomegaly
    – Fibrotic changes
    – Residual changes detectable over months to years
▶ Pulmonary interstitial emphysema
  • Aetiology: Barotrauma due to mechanical ventilation with PEEP, rupture of overstretched alveoli and terminal bronchioles
  • CXR
    – Interstitial radiolucencies radiating from the hilum
▶ Pneumothorax
  • Differential Diagnosis: Patient rotation, superimposition by scapula, skin fold
▶ Pneumomediastinum
  • CXR: Thymus lifted by air (unilateral: Spinnaker sign, bilateral: Angel wing sign)
  • Complications: Pneumopericardium, pneumoperitoneum
▶ Pneumopericardium
  • CXR: Cardiac contour surrounded by air

Lines and Tubes on the Neonatal CXR

▶ Endotracheal tube
  • Tip at middle third of trachea with neck in a neutral position
▶ Umbilical artery catheter

- Course of the catheter is umbilical artery—internal iliac artery—common iliac artery—aorta
- Abdominal position of UAC above aortic bifurcation or thoracic position above hemidiaphragm

▶ Umbilical vein catheter
- Course of catheter is umbilical vein—umbilical recess—ductus venosus—inferior vena cava
- Tip of the UVC should be at the inferior vena cava/right atrium junction

Cystic Fibrosis

▶ Aetiology: Autosomal recessive inheritance, gene defect on the long arm of chromosome 7
▶ System involvement
- Sinopulmonary manifestations
  - Chronic cough, sputum production, dyspnoea, respiratory infections, chronic rhinosinusitis
- Gastrointestinal manifestations
  - Exocrine pancreatic insufficiency, pancreatitis, meconium ileus, rectal prolapse, reflux, constipation, chronic liver disease
- Other manifestations
  - Reduced nutritional status, nephrolithiasis, obstructive azoospermia

▶ Lung disease is the most frequent cause of death
▶ **CXR/CT/MR**
- Predilection for upper lobes
- Pulmonary hyperinflation
- Bullae
- Hilar enlargement
- Small nodular or ring opacities (bronchiectasis with or without mucous plugging)
- Bronchial wall thickening
- Infiltrates
- Atelectasis
  - Classification of the severity of cystic fibrosis with the CF-CT score or CF-MR score

▶ **Diagnosis**: Pilocarpine iontophoresis, genetic analysis
▶ **Complications**: Liver cirrhosis, cor pulmonale, aspergillosis, diabetes mellitus, pneumothorax

Pleura

Pleural Effusion

▶ Aetiology
  • Transudate
    – Raised capillary pressure—left heart failure, fluid overload, constrictive pericarditis
    – Hypoalbuminaemia—liver cirrhosis, nephrotic syndrome
  • Exudate
    – Pneumonia, malignancy (bronchial carcinoma, breast carcinoma, lymphoma), pulmonary embolism
  • Blood
    – Malignancy, trauma, pulmonary embolism
  • Chyle
    – Trauma, malignancy (bronchial carcinoma, breast carcinoma, lymphomas), lymphangiomyomatosis
▶ Pleural effusions are more frequent in the right side of the thorax than in the left because the pleural surface area is larger on the right
▶ Detectability
  • Not seen on PA CXR until ~250 ml fluid present
  • Lateral decubitus view detects smaller volumes ~100 ml
  • Ultrasound/CT/MR when >10 ml
▶ US
  • Confirm presence of effusion and whether loculated
  • Define site for needle aspiration/drain insertion
▶ CXR
  • Blunting of the costophrenic angle
    – Meniscus sign
  • Fluid in horizontal or oblique fissure
  • Compression atelectasis of lung
  • Displacement of mediastinum away from side of effusion

▶ Subpulmonary effusion (infrapulmonary effusion)
- **CXR**
  - – Lateral shift of the dome of diaphragm
  - – Increase distance between gastric fundus and diaphragm on left

▶ Loculated (encysted) effusion
- **CXR**
  - – Caused by partial adhesion of the pleural layers
  - – Non-dependent pleural-based density with obtuse angle
  - – Interlobar encapsulated effusion—oval or rounded related to fissure

▶ Lamellar effusion
- **CXR**
  - – Linear shadow paralleling the lateral chest wall medial to ribs

▶ Pleural effusion
- **Supine CXR**
  - – Insensitive for detecting effusions—with volume underestimated
  - – Detection reduced when bilateral
  - – Veil-like opacification of the hemithorax

Pleural Empyema

▶ Aetiology: Pneumonia, surgery, intervention
▶ **CXR**
- May be indistinguishable from pleural effusion on CXR
- Lenticular shading of the pleura or obtuse angle to pleural surface if loculated
- May contain locules of gas

▶ **CT**
- Stage I: Exudative stage—no thickened pleura, compressed adjacent lung parenchyma
- Stage II: Fibrinopurulent stage—uniformly thickened pleura, septations, pockets of gas, varying degrees of pleural enhancement
- Stage III: Organising phase—increasingly thickened pleura, thickening of epipleural adipose tissue

Pleural Effusion and Pleural Empyema

Criteria	Parapneumonic pleural effusion	Complicated parapneumonic pleural effusion	Parapneumonic pleural empyema
Incidence	Approximately 50% of hospital patients with pneumonia	About 10% of patients with parapneumonic pleural effusion	About 10% of patients with parapneumonic pleural effusion
Pathophysiology	Exudative stage	Fibrinopurulent stage	Organisational stage
Features of pleural fluid	Not infected, echo-free, not septated, not loculated	Infected, echo-rich, septated, loculated	Purulent or leucocyte-rich secretion, loculated, septated, pleural thickening
Pleural aspirate	Clear	Turbid	Purulent
PH value	>7.3	7.1–7.2	<7.1
Neutrophils	+	++	+++
Microbiology	Sterile	Occasional +	Frequent +

Solid Pleural Lesions

▶ Pleural thickening
  • Aetiology: Pleural effusion, pleural empyema (including tuberculosis empyema), pulmonary embolism, haemothorax, previous asbestos exposure
  • **CXR/CT**
    – Thickening of the pleura which can be extensive, most commonly basal, often involving a costophrenic angle
    – Distortion or adjacent lung with parenchymal bands and benign folded lung
▶ Pleural plaques—may be calcified or non-calcified
  • Aetiology: Exposure to asbestos, haemothorax, empyema especially past tuberculosis
  • **CXR/CT**
    – With asbestos exposure, typically smooth, elevated, bilateral involving the hemi-diaphragms, dorsal and anterior pleural surfaces
    – Haemothorax/empyema—usually unilateral—may calcify

▶ Benign pleural tumours
  • Pleural lipoma, pleural fibroma, benign pleural mesothelioma
▶ Malignant pleural tumours
  • Primary: Malignant pleural mesothelioma—most are due to occupational asbestos exposure
  • Secondary: Pleural metastasis due to bronchial carcinoma, breast carcinoma, gynaecological malignancies, gastrointestinal malignancies, thymic carcinoma
  • Metastatic adenocarcinoma is a differential diagnosis for mesothelioma
  • **CXR/CT**
    – Nodular or diffuse pleural thickening
    – May be chest wall invasion
    – Lung tethering
    – Encasement of the hemithorax
    – Calcifications uncommon
    – Pleural effusion is often an early sign
    – Associated mediastinal and hilar lymph node enlargement

Pneumothorax

▶ Aetiology
  • Spontaneous pneumothorax, more common in tall thin adolescent males—rupture of subpleural bleb
  • Secondary to lung disease—for example, asthma, emphysema, cystic fibrosis, neoplasm, Langerhans cell histiocytosis, pulmonary fibrosis
  • Traumatic pneumothorax (rib fracture, knife wound)
  • Iatrogenic pneumothorax (pleural puncture, positive pressure ventilation)
  • Catamenial pneumothorax—thoracic endometriosis—cyclical—females, related to menses
▶ Categories
  • Simple pneumothorax: Lung collapse without mediastinal displacement
  • Tension pneumothorax: Ball-valve mechanism with mediastinal shift away from the side of pneumothorax

▶ **US**
- Pneumothorax ruled out with evidence of lung sliding along the pleural line with sliding z-lines—vertical comet tails running down from the pleural surface
- With pneumothorax, pleural sliding and z-lines are absent—Detection of the lung point sign (transition point between sliding lung and non-sliding lung) is 100% specific for a pneumothorax
- Absence of lung pulse (subtle lung oscillation due to cardiac contraction)

▶ **Erect CXR**
- Visceral pleura visible as a clear thin line parallel to pleural surface which curves at lung apex remaining parallel to chest wall
- When small may only be seen at the lung apex
- Absence of lung markings between lung edge and chest wall
- An expiratory radiograph may help detection by increasing density of normal lung
- CT most sensitive for uncertain cases

▶ **Supine CXR**
- Pneumothorax can be very subtle—gas collects anteriorly and inferiorly
- Deep sulcus sign—air in lateral costophrenic recess
- Sharply defined dome of diaphragm
- A lateral decubitus CXR with suspected side up can help bedbound patients

▶ **Differential Diagnosis**: Skin fold—usually elderly patients with an AP radiograph

▶ Hydropneumothorax
- **CXR:** Air-fluid level—horizontal line separating fluid and gas

▶ Tension pneumothorax
- **CXR**
  – Mediastinal shift away from affected side
  – Diaphragmatic depression on affected side

Mediastinum

Anterior Mediastinal Masses

▶ Thyroid—retrosternal goitre
▶ Thymic tumours
  • Thymoma, thymolipoma, thymic cysts, thymic carcinoma
▶ Lymph nodes
  • Lymphoma, metastasis, for example, small cell lung cancer
▶ Germ cell tumours
  • Dermoid, teratoma, seminoma, choriocarcinoma
▶ Lipomatosis
  • Cushing's disease, steroid therapy, obesity
▶ Pericardial fat pad
▶ Pericardial cyst
▶ Diaphragmatic hump
▶ Morgagni hernia

Middle Mediastinal Masses

▶ Lymph nodes
  • Malignant: Lymphoma, metastases
  • Benign: Infectious disease including tuberculosis, sarcoidosis, benign lymph node hyperplasia (Castleman disease)
▶ Tracheal tumour
▶ Oesophagus
  • Tumour, diverticulum, achalasia, hiatus hernia
▶ Bronchogenic cyst
▶ Foregut duplication cyst
▶ Vascular causes
  • Dilatation or aneurysm of aorta, pulmonary trunk, superior vena cava, azygos vein

Posterior Mediastinal Masses

▶ Neurogenic tumours
  • Children: Neuroblastoma, ganglioneuroma
  • Adults: Neurofibroma, schwannoma

▶ Meningocele—association with neurofibromatosis
▶ Spinal pathology—abscess/expansile metastasis
▶ Extramedullary haemopoiesis—haemolytic anaemias—associated with splenomegaly
▶ Aortic—unfolding/dilatation/aneurysm
▶ Enteric cyst—oesophagus-related duplication cyst
▶ Bochdalek hernia

Diffuse Mediastinal Diseases

▶ Mediastinal lipomatosis
   • Idiopathic or in obesity, Cushing's disease, steroids
▶ Mediastinal fibrosis
   • Tuberculosis, histoplasmosis, sarcoidosis, radiotherapy, methysergide, autoimmune—IgG4 related
   • CT: increased density
   • MRI: low signal on T1 and T2

Acute Mediastinitis

▶ Aetiology: Oesophageal perforation, disseminated inflammation, thoracic trauma
▶ CXR
   • Mediastinal widening
   • Pleural effusion, pneumomediastinum, subcutaneous emphysema
▶ CT: Diffuse fat stranding, oedema and loss of normal fat planes, mediastinal collections which may contain gas

Pneumomediastinum

▶ Associations: Lung contusion, pneumothorax, bronchial rupture, tracheostomy, positive pressure ventilation, acute asthma, pneumonia, oesophageal perforation, mediastinitis, duodenal perforation
▶ Often also surgical emphysema extending into the neck and may track into the retroperitoneum
▶ CXR/CT: Gas evident in the mediastinum

Diaphragm

Diaphragmatic Depression

▶ Hyperinflation
▶ Tension pneumothorax
▶ Large pleural effusion
▶ Expansile mass

Diaphragmatic Elevation

▶ Unilateral
  • Diaphragmatic hump
  • Diaphragmatic eventration
  • Diaphragmatic paresis—phrenic nerve palsy
  • Subphrenic abscess
  • Hepatomegaly
  • Splenomegaly
  • Unilateral lung volume loss/collapse/resection/fibrosis
▶ Bilateral
  • Shallow inspiration—most common
  • Abdominal causes
    – Pregnancy
    – Obesity
    – Ascites
    – Hepatosplenomegaly
    – Bowel distension—ileus
  • Pulmonary causes
    – Interstitial fibrosis
    – Bilateral atelectasis
  • Neuromuscular causes
    – Myasthenia gravis
    – Amyotrophic lateral sclerosis

Diaphragmatic Hump

► Hernias
► Diaphragmatic tumours
► Basal pleural tumour
► Subpulmonary effusion

Hiatus Hernia

► Sliding hernia (95%)
   • Gastro-oesophageal junction above the oesophageal hiatus
   • Often asymptomatic, may be associated with reflux oesoph-
     agitis, retrosternal pain, feeling of pressure
► Paraoesophageal hernia (5%)
   • Intrathoracic fundus
   • Gastro-oesophageal junction at normal location
   • Rarely herniation of colon, spleen, small intestine into the
     thoracic cavity
   • **Complications**: Incarceration, ileus, gastric volvulus

Diaphragmatic Rupture

► Aetiology: Blunt or penetrating chest trauma
► Almost always left hemi-diaphragm
► Herniation of intra-abdominal organs into the thoracic cavity
► Frequently unrecognised
► Lung compression, respiratory failure
► **Diagnosis**: CXR, US, CT

Diaphragmatic Hernias

► Bochdalek hernia
   • Posteriorly located
   • More common on left

▶ Morgagni hernia
  • Anteriorly located
  • More common on right
▶ Traumatic diaphragmatic hernia
  • Left more often than right
  • Can go unnoticed acutely and present late with strangulation

Heart

Anatomy

Heart

- ▶ Atria
  - Right atrium
  - Left atrium
- ▶ Ventricles
  - Right ventricle
  - Left ventricle
- ▶ Direction of flow
  - Flow into the right atrium: Superior vena cava, inferior vena cava, coronary sinus
  - Flow into the left atrium: Right superior pulmonary vein, right inferior pulmonary vein, left superior pulmonary vein, left inferior pulmonary vein
- ▶ Outflow tracts
  - From the right ventricle: Pulmonary trunk
  - From the left ventricle: Aorta
- ▶ Heart valves
  - Aortic valve (tricuspid, three cusps): Between left ventricle and aorta
  - Mitral valve (bicuspid, two leaflets): Between left atrium and left ventricle

© The Author(s), under exclusive license to Springer Nature
Switzerland AG 2026
D. Pickuth, J. T. Murchison, *Pocket Guide to Radiology*,
https://doi.org/10.1007/978-3-031-76520-9_2

- Pulmonary valve (tricuspid, three cusps): Between right ventricle and pulmonary trunk
- Tricuspid valve (tricuspid, three leaflets): Between right atrium and right ventricle

▶ Valve level
  - Aortic valve: Central
  - Mitral valve: Left posterior
  - Pulmonary valve: Left anterior
  - Tricuspid valve: Right posterior

▶ Partitions
  - Interatrial septum
  - Interventricular septum
    - Pars muscularis
    - Pars membranacea
    - Atrioventricular septum

▶ Closure of the foramen ovale by septae
  - Left septum (septum primum): Free edge in the left atrium (valvula foraminis ovalis)
  - Right septum (septum secundum): Free edge in the right atrium (limbus fossae ovalis)

▶ Main layers
  - Endocardium
  - Subendocardial layer
  - Myocardium
  - Subepicardial layer
  - Epicardium

▶ Topography
  - Right atrium: Middle lobe, lower lobe
  - Left atrium: Oesophagus, descending aorta
  - Right ventricle: Sternum, diaphragm, liver
  - Left ventricle: Lingular lobe, lower lobe

Coronary Arteries

▶ Coronary arteries
  - Left coronary artery
    - Left anterior descending
      - Diagonal

- Left circumflex
  - Obtuse marginal
- Right coronary artery
  - Acute marginal
  - Posterior descending artery
▶ Coronary dominance
  - Right dominance (most common)
  - Left dominance
  - Co-dominance

Aorta

▶ Aortic root (sinus of Valsalva, sinotubular junction)
▶ Ascending thoracic aorta
▶ Aortic arch
▶ Descending thoracic aorta

Thoracic Aorta

▶ Coronary arteries
▶ Brachiocephalic trunk
  - Right common carotid artery
    - Internal carotid artery (dorsal, lateral)
    - External carotid artery (ventral, medial)
  - Right subclavian artery
    - Right vertebral artery
    - Internal mammary artery
    - Costocervical trunk
    - Thyrocervical trunk
▶ Left common carotid artery
  - Internal carotid artery (dorsal, lateral)
  - External carotid artery (ventral, medial)
▶ Left subclavian artery
  - Left vertebral artery
  - Internal mammary artery
  - Costocervical trunk
  - Thyrocervical trunk
▶ Intercostal artery
▶ Bronchial artery

ECG

ECG	Excitation process	Duration
P-wave	Activation of the right atrium (initial part) and the left atrium (terminal part)	0.05–0.10 s
PR interval	Atrioventricular conduction (conduction time from the right atrium via the AV node and the bundle of His to the bundle branches and Purkinje fibres)	012–0.20 s
Q-wave	Excitation of the ventricular septum	<0.04 s
QRS complex	Excitation propagation in the ventricles	0.06–0.10 s
ST segment	Complete excitation of the chambers	
T-wave	Repolarisation of the ventricles	
QT interval	Total electrical ventricular action, with increasing heart rate decrease of QT time	
U-wave	Mechanism still unclear, repolarisation of Purkinje fibres or consequence of post-depolarisation	

Echocardiography

▶ Basics
- Phased array transducers
- Frequencies from 2 to 7 MHz

▶ Procedure
- M-mode echocardiography
- 2D echocardiography
- Colour Doppler
- 3D echocardiography
- Hand-held echocardiography

▶ Applications
- Contrast echocardiography
- Stress echocardiography
    - Physical
    - Pharmacological (Dobutamine, adenosine)
- Transoesophageal echocardiography
- Intraoperative echocardiography
- Intracardiac echocardiography

- Intravascular echocardiography
- Doppler echocardiography
▶ Haemodynamics
  - Ejection fraction
  - Regurgitation volume
  - Shunt calculation
  - Pressure gradients
  - Opening area
  - Pressure values
▶ Ventricular function
  - Systolic
  - Diastolic
  - Regional
  - Global

Cardiac Catheter

▶ Cardiac catheter
  - Pressure measurement
  - Measurement of oxygen saturation
  - Measurement of the cardiac output
  - Assessing shunt connections
▶ Angiography
  - Ventriculography
  - Right heart catheterisation
  - Aortography
  - Pulmonary angiography
▶ Coronary angiography
  - Assessment of the location, length, severity and type (atheroma, thrombus, dissection, spasm, muscle bridge) of the obstruction
▶ Additional diagnostics
  - Intravascular ultrasound
    - Assessment of vessel lumen, vessel wall and plaque formation
    - Virtual histology
    - Classification into lipomatous, fibrous and calcified plaque components

- Intracoronary Doppler
  - Assessment of coronary perfusion, haemodynamic relevance of coronary stenosis and coronary physiology
- Intracoronary pressure wire measurement
  - Assessment of the haemodynamic significance of coronary stenosis (fractional flow reserve)

Heart Function

▶ Stroke volume SV = EDV – ESV
▶ Ejection fraction EF = (EDV – ESV)/EDV
▶ Cardiac output CO = SV × heart rate
▶ Myocardial mass MM = Myocardial volume × 1.05 g/ml

Normal Values

Parameter	Men	Women
End-diastolic volume (EDV) [ml]	65–171	55–139
End-systolic volume (ESV) [ml]	15–66	10–48
Ejection fraction (EF) [%]	56–77	61–80
Myocardial mass (MM) [g]	119–190	79–141

Heart

Heart Enlargement

▶ Cardiothoracic ratio
  - Normally 1:2
  - Can vary with degree of inspiration, diaphragm position and shape of chest
  - Pectus excavatum—pseudocardiomegaly
  - No fixed relationship between heart size and heart function
▶ Left atrial enlargement
  - **CXR**
  - PA
    - Enlarged left atrial appendage

- – Double density on right side of heart
- – Splaying of the carina
- Lateral
  - – Dorsal displacement of the oesophagus

▶ Left ventricular enlargement
- **CXR**
- PA
  - – Cardiomegaly
  - – Left heart border displaced laterally, inferiorly and posteriorly
- Lateral
  - – Reduction of the retrocardiac space
  - – Posterior inferior heart contour overhangs vena cava dorsally by more than 2 cm

▶ Right atrial enlargement
- **CXR**
- PA
  - – Can be difficult to detect unless gross
  - – Enlarged globular heart
  - – When gross—increased convexity of lower right heart border
- Lateral
  - – Reduced retrosternal space

▶ Right ventricular enlargement
- **CXR**
- PA
  - – Elevated cardiac apex
  - – Heart enlargement to the right
  - – Left heart border rounded
- Lateral
  - – Reduction of the retrosternal space

Left Heart Failure

▶ Aetiology
- Left ventricular pressure overload
  - Hypertension
  - Aortic stenosis
  - Aortic coarctation
- Left ventricular volume overload
  - Aortic insufficiency
  - Mitral regurgitation
  - Left-right shunt

▶ Main symptom dyspnoea
▶ **CXR**
- Enlargement of the left atrium and ventricle
- Pulmonary venous hypertension

Right Heart Failure

▶ Aetiology
- Right ventricular pressure overload
  - Pulmonary stenosis
  - Pulmonary arterial hypertension
- Right ventricular volume overload
  - Pulmonary insufficiency
  - Tricuspid regurgitation

▶ Main symptom peripheral oedema
▶ **CXR**
- Enlargement of the right atrium and ventricle
- Widening of the SVC and azygos shadows
- Pleural effusions
- Diaphragmatic elevation due to hepatomegaly

Valvular Disease

▶ Aetiology
- Insufficiency → volume load → increased diastolic wall tension → dilatation
- Stenosis → pressure load → increased systolic wall tension → hypertrophy

► Women more likely to have mitral valve disease, men more likely to have aortic valve disease
► Mitral regurgitation
  • Aetiology: Rheumatic, infectious, ischaemic, functional
  • Fatigue, dyspnoea
  • CXR: Mitral configuration with normal lungs
  • MR: Quantification of regurgitation volume
► Mitral stenosis
  • Aetiology: Rheumatic, degenerative
  • Dyspnoea, palpitations, cough, right heart failure
  • CXR: Mitral configuration with pulmonary venous and pulmonary arterial hypertension
  • MR: Determination of mitral valve opening area and pressure gradient
► Aortic valve regurgitation
  • Aetiology: Rheumatic, infectious, traumatic
  • Blood pressure changes, palpitations, reduced performance, dyspnoea
  • CXR: Aortic configuration
  • MR: Quantification of regurgitation volume
► Aortic valve stenosis
  • Aetiology: Degenerative
  • Types
    – Subvalvular
    – Valvular
    – Supravalvular
  • Palpitations, dyspnoea, angina, syncope
  • CXR
    – Aortic configuration
    – Aortic valve calcification
    – Post-stenotic aortic root dilatation
    – When severe, cardiomegaly and features of heart failure
  • MR: Determination of aortic valve opening area and pressure gradient
  • CT: Severity of calcification correlates with stenosis severity

Coronary Heart Disease

▶ Aetiology: Atherosclerosis
  • Stary type I: Incipient intimal thickening
  • Stary type II: Fatty streak
    – Stary type II a: Progression prone
    – Stary type II b: Progression resistant
  • Stary type III: Preatheroma
  • Stary type IV: Atheroma
  • Stary type V
    – Stary type V a: Fibroatheroma
    – Stary type V b: Calcified lesion
    – Stary type V c: Fibrotic lesion
  • Stary type VI
    – Stary type VI a: Surface disruption
    – Stary type VI b: Plaque haematoma
    – Stary type VI c: Plaque thrombosis
▶ Deficient supply (residual perfusion) → Reversible loss of function, blood flow obstruction (ischaemia) → Cell necrosis (myocardial infarction)
▶ Ischaemia cascade
  • Haemodynamically relevant coronary stenosis
  • Perfusion defect
  • Metabolic changes
  • Diastolic functional defect
  • Systolic functional defect
  • ECG changes
  • Clinical anginal symptoms
▶ Ischaemia localisation
  • Subendocardial
  • Transmural
▶ Types
  • Stunned myocardium
    – Aetiology: Temporary reduced perfusion; acute coronary artery occlusion with spontaneous or therapeutic recanalisation
    – Temporary myocardial dysfunction, spontaneous recovery

- Hibernating myocardium
  - Aetiology: Repetitive or chronic reduced perfusion; high-grade stenosis, coronary artery occlusion with collateral supply
  - Chronic myocardial dysfunction, recovery after revascularisation
- Necrotic myocardium
  - Aetiology: Severely reduced perfusion (<20% of resting blood flow) or lack of perfusion; coronary artery occlusion without collateral supply
  - Irreversible myocardial dysfunction, no recovery
▶ In coronary heart disease, the leading symptom is exercise-induced angina; in acute coronary syndrome, such as myocardial infarction, the leading symptom is severe retrosternal pain
  - Acute coronary syndromes at sites with vulnerable plaques
▶ **Diagnosis**
  - Radiology
    - Quantification of coronary calcium (Agatston calcium score, volume calcium score, calcium mass determination; clear relationship between the extent of coronary atherosclerosis and the extent of coronary calcium)
    - Visualisation of coronary artery stenoses by CT coronary angiography (classification according to CAD-RADS)
    - Visually assessed adverse (vulnerable, high risk) plaque characteristics (positive remodelling, low attenuation plaque, punctate calcification, napkin ring sign)
    - Coronary plaque characterisation by CT coronary calcium measurement and CT coronary angiography (low attenuation plaque indicates high-risk plaque)
    - Assessment of the haemodynamic relevance of coronary artery stenosis by CT-FFR (determination of fractional flow reserve by CT, simulated via mathematical models or estimated via artificial intelligence) or MRI, SPECT, PET or CT perfusion

▶ **Nuclear Medicine**
- 99mTc-MIBI, 99mTc-Tetrofosmin (disadvantage: poorer spatial resolution, relatively high radiation exposure)

▶ **Other Imaging**
- Stress echo (disadvantage: operator dependent, peripheral segments, right ventricle, image interpretation)
- Coronary angiography
- Optical coherence tomography
- Intravascular ultrasound with virtual histology

▶ Chest Pain—Triple rule out
- **Contrast CT**: Differentiation of aortic dissection, acute coronary syndrome and pulmonary embolism

Myocardial Ischaemia

Myocardium	Late enhancement	Wall movement (rest)	Wall movement (stress)
Normal myocardium	No	Normal	Normal
Stunned myocardium	No	Normal	High dose: pathological
Hibernating myocardium	No	Pathological	Low dose: pathological
Necrotic myocardium	Yes	Pathological	Pathological

Myocardial Infarction

▶ **MR**
- T2 hyperintense
- Wall movement disorder
- Wall thickness <5.5 mm
- Early enhancement (about 2 min after contrast injection): Visualisation of the microvascular obstruction
- Late enhancement (about 15 min after contrast injection): Visualisation of the myocardial scar
  - Subendocardial late enhancement, transmural late enhancement

- **Differential diagnosis**: Subendocardial myocardial layer always affected in ischaemic myocardial infarction; lack of enhancement in the subendocardial myocardial layer in non-ischaemic myocardial disease

▶ **Stress MR**
- No increase in wall thickness, no improvement in contractility

▶ Accompanying findings
- Thrombus
- Ventricular aneurysm
- Valve insufficiency
- Pericardial effusion

▶ **Differential Diagnosis**: Angina, pericarditis, myocarditis, pleurisy, pulmonary embolism, aortic dissection, hiatus hernia, gastric/duodenal ulcer

▶ **Complications**
- Cardiac arrhythmias, heart failure, pulmonary oedema, shock, recurrent infarction, ventricular septal defect, mitral regurgitation, ventricular aneurysm, ventricular rupture, pericardial tamponade, pericarditis, emboli
- Diffuse hypoxic brain damage after circulatory arrest

Myocarditis

▶ Aetiology: Viral infections (enteroviruses, parvoviruses, hepatitis C viruses, HIV), rheumatic diseases, systemic connective tissue disorders, bacterial infections

▶ Flu like symptoms, heart failure, CK-MB, troponin T

▶ **MR**
- Myocardial oedema
- Focal, patchy, subepicardial late enhancement (acutely inflamed myocardial islets)
  - Contrast agent accumulation due to increased blood flow, extravasation of fluid in areas of inflammation and acute cell damage
- Pericardial thickening
- Pericardial effusion

▶ **Diagnosis**: Clinical presentation, troponin activity, ECG, echocardiography, and endomyocardial biopsy

Cardiomyopathies

▶ Haemodynamic classification
  • DCM: Dilated
    – Systolic pump abnormality
    – Interstitial myocardial fibrosis
  • HOCM or HNCM: Hypertrophic with or without obstruction
    – Diastolic compliance abnormality
    – Interstitial myocardial fibrosis
  • RCM: Restrictive
    – Diastolic compliance abnormality
    – Endomyocardial fibrosis
  • ARVCM: Arrhythmogenic right ventricular
    – Predominantly right ventricular combined pumping defect with ventricular tachycardia
    – Fatty fibrous transformation of the right ventricular myocardium
▶ Aetiological classification
  • Ischaemic, valvular, hypertensive, inflammatory, collagenous, toxic, metabolic, endocrine, neuromuscular, neoplastic, granulomatous, physical, peripartum, alimentary
▶ Heart failure, arrhythmias, cardiac death
▶ MR
  • Uses
    – Anatomical representation of the heart and the adjacent vessels as well as the outflow tract
    – Functional assessment of the wall sections of the two ventricles as well as the outflow tract
  • Findings
    – DCM: Ventricular dilatation, atrial dilatation, wall motion abnormalities, EDV ↑, ESV ↑, EF ↓
    – HOCM/HNCM: Left ventricular myocardial thickening, biventricular myocardial thickening, hypertrophied septum, variable obstruction, EDV ↓, ESV ↓, MM ↑

- RCM: Pericardial thickening, marked enlargement of both atria, paradoxical wall movement of the interventricular septum, pericardial effusion
- ARVCM: Dilated right ventricle, right ventricular trabeculation, regional right ventricular dyskinesia, right ventricular enhancement, fatty fibrous infiltrated myocardium
- Late enhancement of intramural fibrosis, subendocardial and subepicardial myocardium often not affected

Amyloidosis

▶ Protein storage disease
▶ Clinical association with chronic inflammatory diseases and monoclonal gammopathies
▶ Cardiac involvement depending on the corresponding subtype and responsible for the high mortality rate
▶ Often diagnosed at a late stage
▶ Heart failure, arrhythmias, paraesthesia, paresis, constipation, diarrhoea, weight loss, renal failure
▶ MR
  • Myocardial thickening
  • Atrial dilatation
  • Severe diastolic dysfunction
  • Normal systolic function
  • Diffuse late enhancement
  • Increased extracellular volume fraction
▶ Diagnosis: Endomyocardial biopsy

Sarcoidosis

▶ Cardiac involvement common in sarcoidosis, clinical symptoms less common
▶ MR
  • Wall-thickened and wall-thinned segments
  • Regional or global functional impairment
  • Patchy or streaky late enhancement intramural or subepicardial

▶ **Diagnosis**: Endomyocardial biopsy
▶ **Complications**: Sudden cardiac death

Cardiac Tumours

▶ Types
  • Primary cardiac
    – Uncommon
    – Mostly benign (myxoma, lipoma, fibroelastoma), rarely malignant (angiosarcoma, rhabdomyosarcoma, lymphoma)
  • Secondary metastatic
    – More frequent
    – Bronchial carcinoma, breast carcinoma, melanoma, lymphoma
▶ Localisation
  • Intracavitary
    – Myxoma: Pedunculated, no myocardial infiltration, no necrosis, enhancement
    – Sarcoma: Broad-based, myocardial infiltration, necrosis, enhancement
  • Valvular
    – Fibroelastoma: Low signal intensity, moderate enhancement
  • Subendocardial
    – Lipoma: Fat isointense mass, broad myocardial contact
▶ Age
  • Children
    – Rhabdomyoma: Multifocal, T2 hyperintense
    – Fibroma: Solitary, T2 hypointense
  • Adults
    – Metastasis: Invasive, T2 hyperintense, necrosis, enhancement
    – Myxoma: Pedunculated, no myocardial infiltration, no necrosis, enhancement

▶ **Differential Diagnosis**: Thrombus (intracavitary localisation, valvular localisation, age-dependent signal behaviour, no enhancement), crista terminalis as an anatomical variant (fibromuscular band on the posterior wall of the right atrium between the ostia of the superior and inferior vena cava)

▶ **Complications**: Recurrent central and peripheral emboli, especially in myxoma

Paediatric Radiology: Heart

Congenital Heart Defects

▶ 1% of live births
▶ Cyanotic congenital heart disease manifests in infancy, acyanotic at school age or later
▶ Without shunt: 25%, acyanotic
  • Aortic coarctation
  • Pulmonary stenosis
  • Aortic stenosis
▶ With Left-right shunt: 60%, acyanotic
  • Ventricular septal defect
  • Atrial septal defect
    – Septum primum defect
    – Septum secundum defect
    – Sinus venosus defect
  • Patent ductus arteriosus
▶ With right-left shunt: 15%, cyanotic
  • Tetralogy of Fallot
    – Pulmonary stenosis
    – Ventricular septal defect
    – Overriding aorta
    – Right ventricular hypertrophy
  • Transposition of the great arteries
  • Pulmonary atresia
  • Truncus arteriosus

Aortic Coarctation

- ▶ Aetiology: Stenosis at the junction of the aortic arch and the descending aorta, in the immediate vicinity of the ductus arteriosus
- ▶ Mostly men
- ▶ Most common symptom—Upper body hypertension
- ▶ Infantile form (25%)
  - Preductal
  - Blood supply to the lower half of the body via an open ductus arteriosus
- ▶ Adult form (75%)
  - Postductal
  - Blood supply to the lower half of the body via brachiocephalic, internal thoracic and intercostal arteries
- ▶ **CXR/CT/MR**
  - Narrowing of the aorta at the level of the stenosis (reverse 3 sign)
  - Prestenotic dilatation of the ascending aorta
  - Post-stenotic dilatation of the descending aorta
  - Dilatation of the supra-aortic vessels (stag antler sign)
  - Rib notching due to dilated intercostal arteries (usually 4th–8th ribs)

Septal Defects

- ▶ **Atrial septal defect**
  - Aetiology: Congenital defect of the interatrial septum
  - Limited exercise capacity and supraventricular arrhythmias only when shunt haemodynamically significant
  - **MR:** Enlargement of the right atrium and right ventricle
- ▶ **Ventricular septal defect**
  - Aetiology: Defect of the interventricular septum
  - Left heart failure with haemodynamically significant shunt
- ▶ **Diagnosis:** Two-dimensional Doppler echocardiography (transthoracic and transoesophageal)
- ▶ **Complications:** Left-right shunt → volume load lung, pressure load right ventricle → right ventricle. Right-left shunt (Eisenmenger syndrome)

Pericardium

Pericardial Effusion

▶ Aetiology: Pericarditis, autoimmune diseases, tumours, heart failure, anticoagulation, trauma
▶ Localisation between epicardium and pericardium
▶ Different mechanisms for haemodynamic effects
  • Mechanical heart cavity stenosis
  • Inspiratory inflow reduction into the left ventricle due to increased filling of the right ventricle
  • Venous congestion
▶ Detectability from 20 ml by US, from 200 ml on CXR
▶ Echo: Detection of the effusion
▶ CXR
  • Acute findings
    – Cardiomegaly
    – Acute cardiac diaphragm angle
    – Reduced lung perfusion
    – Pulmonary congestion
  • Chronic findings
    – Cardiomegaly
    – Obtuse cardiac diaphragm angle
▶ Echo/CT/MR
  • Minimum effusion: Width <5 mm
  • Moderate effusion: Width 5–10 mm (300–500 ml)
  • Large effusion: Width >10 mm (>500 ml)
▶ Complications: Pericardial tamponade

Constrictive Pericarditis

▶ Aetiology: Viral pericarditis, bacterial pericarditis, tuberculosis, trauma
▶ CXR: Pericardial calcification
▶ CT: Pericardial thickening, pericardial calcification, atrial enlargement, hepatic vein congestion

Vascular, Interventional

Anatomy

Aorta

▶ Aortic root
▶ Ascending aorta
▶ Aortic arch
▶ Descending aorta

Thoracic Aorta

▶ Coronary arteries
▶ Brachiocephalic trunk
  • Right common carotid artery
    – Internal carotid artery (posterior, lateral)
    – External carotid artery (anterior, medial)
  • Right subclavian artery
    – Right vertebral artery
    – Internal thoracic artery
    – Costocervical trunk
    – Thyrocervical trunk
▶ Left common carotid artery
  • Internal carotid artery (posterior, lateral)
  • External carotid artery (anterior, medial)

© The Author(s), under exclusive license to Springer Nature
Switzerland AG 2026
D. Pickuth, J. T. Murchison, *Pocket Guide to Radiology*,
https://doi.org/10.1007/978-3-031-76520-9_3

▶ Left subclavian artery
  • Left vertebral artery
  • Internal thoracic artery
  • Costocervical trunk
  • Thyrocervical trunk
▶ Intercostal arteries
▶ Bronchial artery
▶ Internal mammary artery

Upper Limb Arteries

▶ Axillary artery
  • Thoracoacromial artery
  • Lateral thoracic artery
  • Subscapular artery
  • Anterior humeral circumflex artery
▶ Brachial artery
  • Profunda brachii artery
▶ Radial artery
▶ Deep palmar arch
▶ Ulnar artery
  • Superficial palmar arch

Important Variants

▶ Outflow of the left common carotid artery from the brachioce-
  phalic trunk
▶ Origin of the left vertebral artery directly from the aorta
▶ Aberrant right subclavian artery:
  • Origin of the right subclavian artery directly from the aorta.
    Vessels arise from the aorta in the order right common
    carotid artery, left common carotid artery, left subclavian
    artery, right subclavian artery
  • Right subclavian artery crosses behind the oesophagus to
    the right side (dysphagia lusoria)
▶ High branching of the radial and ulnar arteries

Abdominal Aorta

▶ Paired dorsal branches
- Lumbar artery
- Common iliac artery
▶ Paired lateral branches
- Inferior phrenic artery
- Middle suprarenal artery
- Renal arteries
- Ovarian or testicular artery
▶ Unpaired ventral branches
- Coeliac trunk
    - Common hepatic artery
    - Splenic artery
    - Left gastric artery
- Superior mesenteric artery
- Inferior mesenteric artery

Important Variants

▶ Origin of the hepatic artery from the superior mesenteric artery (hepato-mesenteric trunk)
▶ Origin of the hepatic artery proper from the left gastric artery
▶ Partial blood supply (10%) or full supply (2%) to the liver from the superior mesenteric artery

Pelvic Arteries

▶ Common iliac arteries
▶ Internal iliac artery
- Parietal branches
    - Iliolumbar arteries
    - Lateral sacral artery
    - Superior gluteal artery
    - Inferior gluteal artery
    - Obturator artery
    - Internal pudendal artery

- Visceral branches
  - Umbilical artery with superior vesical arteries and artery of the ductus deferens
  - Inferior vesical artery
  - Uterine artery with vaginal artery
  - Middle rectal artery
▶ External iliac arteries
  - Deep circumflex artery
  - Inferior epigastric artery
▶ Common femoral artery

Lower Limb Arteries

▶ Common femoral artery
▶ Profunda femoris artery
▶ Superficial femoral artery
▶ Popliteal artery—three segments
  - P1: From adductor hiatus to the top of the patella
  - P2: From top of patella to centre of the knee joint
  - P3: Centre of knee joint to anterior tibial artery origin
▶ Anterior tibial artery
  - Dorsalis pedis artery
▶ Tibiofibular trunk
  - Posterior tibial artery
    - Medial plantar artery and lateral plantar artery
  - Peroneal artery

Lower Limb Veins

▶ Superficial venous system
  - Great saphenous vein
  - Small saphenous vein
▶ Perforating veins
  - Cockett group (3) on the lower leg
  - Boyd group (1) at the knee
  - Dodd group (2) on the thigh
  - Connect superficial to deep veins
  - Valves prevent reflux from deep to superficial veins

▶ Deep venous system
- Posterior tibial vein
  – Drains the soleus veins
- Fibular vein
- Anterior tibial vein
- Popliteal vein
  – Drains the gastrocnemius veins and saphenous vein
- Superficial femoral vein
  – In the adductor hiatus (hiatus magnus) often connects to the profunda femoris vein
- Profunda femoris vein
- Common femoral vein
  – Drains the great saphenous vein
  – Duplication of the popliteal vein and femoral vein in 25%
- External iliac vein

Lymphatic System

▶ Lymph
▶ Regional lymph node
▶ Central draining lymph nodes
▶ Lymphatic trunks
- Left lymphatic (thoracic) duct
- Right lymphatic (thoracic) duct
- Lymphatic ducts connect to the subclavian vein, returning lymph to the bloodstream

Arteries

Hypertension (systemic)

▶ Hypertension cascade
- Concentric hypertrophy of the left ventricle
- Dilatation of the left ventricle
- Relative mitral regurgitation
- Pulmonary venous hypertension

▶ **CXR/CT**
  - Left heart enlargement (normal size in early stages)
  - Aortic unfolding
  - Aortic sclerosis
  - Pulmonary congestion

Pulmonary Arterial Hypertension

▶ Pulmonary hypertension
  - Group I: Pulmonary arterial hypertension
    - Idiopathic, hereditary, drug-induced, associated with: Connective tissue diseases, portal hypertension, congenital heart defects, HIV
  - Group II: Pulmonary hypertension due to left heart disease
  - Group III: Pulmonary hypertension due to lung diseases
  - Group IV: Chronic thromboembolic pulmonary hypertension
  - Group V: Pulmonary hypertension due to systemic diseases or with multifactorial causes
▶ Initial assessment by means of echocardiography
▶ **CXR/CT**
  - Dilatation of the main pulmonary artery trunk
  - Dilatation of the central pulmonary arteries
  - Pruning of the peripheral pulmonary arteries and veins
  - Cor pulmonale—right heart enlargement

Acute Arterial Occlusion

▶ Acute ischaemia syndrome
▶ Aetiology
  - Usually arterial embolism
    - Atrial fibrillation
    - Heart attack
    - Endocarditis
    - Aneurysms
    - Plaques

- Rarer causes
  - Local thrombosis
  - Atherosclerosis
- Trauma, external compression (popliteal aneurysm, entrapment syndrome), ergotamine
- Paradoxical embolism from the venous system via a patent foramen ovale
- Septic embolism in endocarditis

▶ (6 P's) according to Pratt: Pain, paleness, paraesthesia, pulselessness, paralysis, prostration

▶ Intense pain at rest in the extremities, most marked about a hand-width proximal to the occlusion

▶ The more acute the occlusion, the less the collateralisation, and the more severe the symptoms

▶ Critical limb ischaemia, non-healing ulcers, pressure-painful muscles, gangrene, and loss of sensory motor function

▶ Arterial embolism
- **CTA/Angiogram**
  - Abrupt occlusion with smooth margin
  - Absent collaterals
  - Paucity of existing plaques

▶ Arterial thrombosis
- **CTA/Angiogram**
  - Tapering towards occlusion with irregular margin
  - Collaterals
  - Plaques

▶ Detection of distal refilling or non-refilling important

▶ **Complications:** Myoglobinuria and renal failure on reopening after more than 4–6 hrs due to rhabdomyolysis and toxins, large fluid losses due to capillary damage after restored distal blood flow (Tourniquet syndrome)

▶ **IR**
- Intra-arterial thrombolysis
  - Multipurpose catheter or multiple side hole infusion catheter
  - Initial dose of 5 mg recombinant tissue plasminogen activator (rtPA) into the occlusion, followed by 1 mg rt-PA via the catheter, additional heparinisation to a target PTT value of 70–80 s
- Mechanical thrombectomy
  - Aspiration catheter
  - Thrombectomy catheter

Thromboangiitis Obliterans

▶ Buerger's disease
▶ Heavy smoking, young men
▶ Often intermittent pain and a feeling of coldness in the feet and hands
▶ Thrombophlebitis saltans, mononeuritis, vascular dementia
▶ **Angiogram**
- Concentric vascular constrictions (filum terminale sign)
- Corkscrew pattern of the collaterals
- Abrupt termination of contrast (cut off sign)
- Otherwise unremarkable vascular system
▶ In the lower leg and foot area, in the case of pathological findings, improved circulation after administration of vasodilators and spasmolytics
▶ **Differential Diagnosis:** Small peripheral emboli, chronic Raynaud syndrome

Peripheral Arterial Occlusive Disease

▶ Chronic ischaemia syndrome
▶ Aetiology
- Atherosclerosis
- Specific types
  - Vasculitides
  - Collagenoses

- – Repetitive trauma
- – External compression
▶ Risk factors of atherosclerosis
  - • Causal: Smoking, diabetes mellitus, hypertension, hyper-cholesterolemia
  - • Predisposing factors: Obesity, inactivity, family history,
▶ Localisation
  - • Upper limb: Shoulder girdle type, upper arm type, peripheral type
    - – Subclavian artery
    - – Forearm and hand arteries
  - • Central type: Coronary arteries, aortic arch, abdominal aorta
  - • Lower limb: Pelvic type (aortoiliac tract), femoral type (femoropopliteal tract), peripheral type (cruropedal tract)
    - – Superficial femoral artery in the adductor canal
    - – Popliteal artery
    - – Trifurcation
    - – Anterior tibial artery, peroneal artery and posterior tibial artery
    - – Lower leg and foot arteries particularly in diabetics
▶ Classification according to Fontaine
  - • I: Symptom free
  - • II: Pain on exertion
    - – II a: Pain-free walking distance >200 m
    - – II b: Pain-free walking distance <200 m
  - • III: Pain at rest
  - • IV
    - – IV a: Trophic disturbances and necrosis
    - – IV b: Secondary infection of necrosis
▶ Vascular diagnostics with the aim of recording the location, length and complexity of the occlusion process
  - • If compression syndrome is suspected, also assess with dynamic studies
▶ **Colour Doppler US**: Readily available, non-invasive, highly examiner-dependent, time-consuming, limitations in assessing the collateral system

▶ **MRA**: Readily available, non-invasive, not examiner-dependent, three-dimensional reconstructions, highest accuracy of the non-invasive methods, tendency to overestimate the degree of stenosis, highest-grade stenoses can look like short-segment occlusions

▶ **CTA**: Readily available, non-invasive, not examiner-dependent, three-dimensional reconstructions, limited informative value in heavily calcified vessels with small diameters

▶ **Angiography**
  • Calibre variations
  • Contour irregularities
    – Atheroma, plaques, ulcerations, mural calcifications
  • Filling defects
  • Local/diffuse, short /long, concentric/eccentric stenoses
  • Occlusion
  • Aneurysms
  • Collaterals
  • Angiographic classification
    – Normal findings: Smooth arterial walls
    – Low-grade stenosis: 30–49% diameter reduction
    – Moderate stenosis: 50–75% diameter reduction
    – High-grade stenosis: 76–99% diameter reduction
    – Occlusion

▶ **Differential Diagnosis:** Lumbar spine syndrome, polyneuropathy, arthritis, arthrosis, root irritation syndrome, Monckeberg medial sclerosis, entrapment syndrome

▶ **IR**
  • Indications
    – No intervention in asymptomatic patients
    – Relative indication: Stage II according to Fontaine
    – Absolute indication: Stages III and IV according to Fontaine
    – Good prognosis in short, circumscribed, concentric, non-calcified stenoses with sufficient distal run-off in stage II a or II b
    – The more distal, the greater the indication; the more distal, the poorer the results

- Requirements
  - Multi-disciplinary team meeting
  - Clinical findings
  - Colour Doppler US examination
  - MRA/CTA of the pelvis to assess supra-inguinal inflow
- Procedure
  - Most commonly 4-6Fr (Sheath)
  - Crossover with crossover catheter and long guidewires
  - Overview angiography of the iliac artery
  - Introduction and manipulation of the wire under fluoroscopy
  - Angiographic control of the wire position for the detection of an intravascular wire position
  - Aortoiliac: Primary stenting
  - SFA: PTA/DEB
  - Popliteal: PTA/DEB
  - Infrapopliteal: Patients being considered for amputation should be assessed for endovascular intervention. Balloon angioplasty may be offered in crural patients
  - Before finishing angiogram while the guide wire is still in place: Check for evidence of adequate recanalisation and exclude peripheral embolism
- Accompanying measures
  - 5000–7500 IU heparin during (or 70 IU/ kg)
  - In case of vasospasm, administer vasodilators during the procedure (e.g. nitroglycerin)
  - 100 mg of acetylsalicylic acid per day as continuous therapy and 75 mg of clopidogrel per day for 6–8 weeks
  - Follow-up of the vascular status
  - Exclusion of complications
  - Monitoring after intervention
- Aftercare
  - Rigorous treatment and control of cardiovascular risk factors

► **Complications**
- Puncture site: Haemorrhage, AV fistula, pseudoaneurysm, arterial occlusion, thrombosis, neurovascular bundle damage
- Access route: Dissection, perforation, vascular occlusion with resultant organ damage
- Interventional site: Dissection, perforation, occlusion, AV fistula, stent malposition
- Distal to the intervention site: Embolism, dissection
- Systemic: Anaphylactic reaction, renal toxicity, thyrotoxic crisis, infection, myocardial infarction, stroke
- Resulting from procedure: Need for surgery, loss of limb, death
- Complication management
  - Aneurysm: Stent graft (pseudoaneurysm—thrombin injection)
  - Dissection: Prolonged balloon inflation, stenting
  - Vessel rupture: Stent graft pseudoaneurysm—thrombin injection covered
  - Wire perforation: Prolonged balloon inflation, coiling
  - Embolisation: Mechanical thrombectomy, drug lysis

Operations for Vascular Occlusions

► Acute arterial occlusion
- Thromboembolectomy
► Peripheral arterial occlusive disease
- Thromboendarterectomy
- Bypass procedure
- Vascular interposition
- Amputation

Angiographic Assessment of Vascular Procedures

▶ Surgical complications
  • Thrombosis
  • Perforation
  • Bypass stenosis
  • Bypass closure
  • Anastomotic stenosis
  • Anastomosis insufficiency
▶ Long-term control
  • Primary patency v secondary patency
  • Aneurysm formation

Carotid Stenosis

▶ Causes:
  • Atherosclerosis
  • Vascular dissection
  • Fibromuscular dysplasia
  • Arteritis
  • Vasospasms
▶ Men, smokers
▶ Transient ischaemic attack, retinal ischaemia cerebral infarction
  • Prevalence of ≥50% carotid stenosis (according to NASCET) in the population of approximately 4%
  • ≥50% asymptomatic carotid stenosis only with low risk of stroke of about 1% per year
  • High risk of stroke only with more than 80% and especially pre-occlusive asymptomatic carotid stenosis
  • Symptomatic carotid stenosis with a risk of stroke of 13% with a stenosis grade of 70–79%, 19% with a stenosis grade of 80–89% and 35% with a stenosis grade of 90–95%
▶ Angiographic classification by means of MRA, CTA or DSA
  • Classification of stenosis according to NASCET (North American symptomatic carotid endarterectomy trial)
    – Ratio of the residual lumen to the vessel diameter above the stenosis (distal degree of stenosis)

- Stenosis grades
  - Low grade stenosis: <50% NASCET
  - Moderate stenosis: 50–69% NASCET
  - High grade stenosis: 70–99% NASCET

▶ **Colour Doppler US**
- Description of vessel sections, anatomical vessel variants, atheromatous wall changes, flow profiles, degree of stenosis, dissections
- Description of plaque interior structure, plaque surface, plaque movement, acoustic shadow, vascularisation, plaque vascularisation
  - Contrast-enhanced US: Evaluation of vascularisation and plaque vascularisation
  - Transcranial US: Examination of the patient in triplex mode (B-scan + colour Doppler + PW Doppler) in retinal ischaemia, transient ischaemic attack
- Multiparametric stenosis criteria for quantification of extracranial internal carotid artery
- Main criteria: B-scan, colour Doppler image, peak systolic velocity at maximum stenosis, peak systolic velocity post-stenotic, collaterals and precursors
  - Additional criteria: Diastolic flow deceleration proximal to the stenosis, disturbed or turbulent flow distal to the stenosis, end-diastolic flow velocity at the point of maximal stenosis, confetti sign, stenosis index

▶ **MR/MRA**
- Assessment of plaque ulcerations and plaque haemorrhages
  - Plaque haemorrhage associated with significantly increased risk of stroke in patients with asymptomatic carotid stenosis
- Detection of the crescent-shaped intramural haematoma, which is highly suggestive of a dissection

▶ **CT/CTA**
- Assessment of plaque ulcerations and plaque haemorrhages

- Plaque morphology
  - lipomatous: -100 to 49 Hounsfield units HU
  - fibrous: 40 to 149 Hounsfield units HU
  - calcified: 150 to 1300 Hounsfield units HU
- Examination protocol including maximum intensity projection and perspective volume rendering

▶ **IR**
- Indications
  - Indication according to the guidelines
  - Consideration of possible risks, (such as symptomatic status, older age or short time interval between symptoms and revascularisation), when determining the indication
  - Evaluation of risks due to vascular anatomy and plaque morphology before intervention
  - In patients with acute stroke and tandem lesions, with extracranial carotid stenosis and concomitant downstream intracranial large vessel occlusion, endovascular treatment with emergency stenting and thrombectomy
- Requirements
  - Multidisciplinary team meeting
  - Supporting clinical findings
  - Angiographic diagnostic confirmation
  - MR of the brain including diffusion weighting before and after intervention
- Procedure
  - Overview angiography of the stenosed carotid and intracranial vessels
  - Catheter flushing exclusively in the descending aorta
  - Primary stenting using self-expanding stents
  - Improve the safety of the intervention with stents by achieving good plaque coverage, filters or endovascular clamping systems
  - Stent diameter at least 1 mm above the largest vessel diameter to be bridged

- Post-dilatation after stent release to achieve the desired vessel diameter against the resistance forces of the plaques
- Final angiography of the dilated carotid artery and intra-cranial vessels with the guide wire in place
- Concomitant medication
  - Prevention of stent thrombosis by self-expanding stents, combined treatment with asprin and clopidogrel before and after the intervention as well as peri-interventional heparinisation
  - 100 mg of asprin and 75 mg of clopidogrel for the three days before intervention until 4 weeks after the intervention. This is then reduced to 100 mg asprin per day as continuous therapy
  - 7500 IU heparin during intervention, then heparinisation for 24 h
  - 1 mg atropine intravenously for prophylaxis of hypotension and bradycardia due to stent pressure on the carotid sinus immediately before the intervention
  - Monitoring by an anaesthetist during the intervention
  - Monitoring in an intermediate care unit for one day after the intervention
- Aftercare
  - Blood pressure control, diabetes management, hyperlipidaemia therapy, nicotine abstinence, weight reduction, exercise

▶ **Complications**: The most significant risk is that of stroke due to embolism

Important Collateral Vascular Systems

▶ Ophthalmic artery
▶ Internal thoracic artery / internal mammary artery
▶ Intercostal arteries
▶ Lumbar artery

► Arc of Riolan connection between middle colic artery from superior mesenteric artery and left colic artery from (inferior mesenteric artery)
► Branches of the internal iliac artery
► Branches of the common femoral artery
► Branches of the profunda femoris artery

Steal Syndrome

► Reverse flow
- In internal iliac artery due to occlusion of the external iliac artery
- Inferior mesenteric artery in occlusion of the proximal abdominal aorta
- In the vertebral artery with occlusion of the proximal sub-clavian artery
  - Brachiocephalic trunk/Aorta → carotid arteries → Circle of Willis → basilar artery → vertebral arteries → subcla-vian arteries
  - Alternatively (without the Circle of Willis) via the verte-bral artery of the opposite side
  - Radicular arteries
  - Thyroid vessels
  - Anastomoses between the internal thoracic (mammary) arteries
► Subclavian steal syndrome
- Cause: Blood flow reduction in the brainstem due to flow reversal in the ipsilateral vertebral artery in cases of high-grade proximal subclavian stenosis or proximal subclavian occlusion
- Dizziness when working with the ipsilateral arm
- Syncope, vertigo, tinnitus, blurred vision
- Load-dependent pain and Raynaud symptoms of the ipsilat-eral arm
- **Colour Doppler US**
  - Flow reversal in the vertebral artery of the affected side
  - Findings augmented by exercise of the ipsilateral arm

– Distal subclavian artery shows parvus-tardus waveform and monophasic waveform
– May be evidence of subclavian stenosis or occlusion but proximal subclavian artery can be difficult to visualise

Leriche Syndrome

▶ Cause: Obstruction at the aortic bifurcation
▶ Buttock pain, bilateral hypotension of the legs, impotence
▶ **Angiogram**: With gradual occlusion, collateralisation from the lumbar arteries (lateral route) or the inferior mesenteric artery (medial route) to the internal iliac artery or profunda femoris artery

Diabetic Angiopathy

▶ Cause: Poor control of diabetes mellitus over a long period of time
▶ **X-ray**: Diffuse arterial calcification due to pronounced medial sclerosis
▶ **Angiography:** Changes of chronic arterial occlusive disease with peripheral arterial tree predominance

Fibromuscular Dysplasia

▶ Young women
▶ Renal artery, internal carotid artery, iliac artery
▶ Types
   • Medial type (frequent)
      – **Angiography**: Pearly with alternating stenoses and dilatations
   • Intimal type (rare)
      – **Angiography**: Short stenoses with post-stenotic dilatations

Raynaud Syndrome

▶ Aetiology
  • Primary
    – Functional disturbance of the vasomotor system
    – Provoked or aggravated by cold and stress
  • Secondary
    – Vasospastic conditions with pre-existing underlying disease
    – Arterial occlusive disease, thromboangiitis obliterans, arterio-arterial embolisms, thoracic outlet syndrome, trauma, collagen-vascular disease, medication
    – Often first manifestation of systemic sclerosis
▶ Seizure-like ischaemia of the fingers or toes with reactive hyperaemia
▶ Pain, skin turns white, numbness
▶ Classification
  • I: Initial cyanosis
  • II: Secondary white colouration
  • III: Post-ischaemic redness
▶ Angiography first with cool, then with warmed extremities
▶ **Angiography MR or digital subtraction**
  • Bilateral findings
  • Involves small vessels
    – Narrowing and tapering of affected digital vessels

Thenar Hammer Syndrome

▶ Aetiology: Microtrauma of the radial artery
▶ Reduced perfusion of fingers 1–3, necrosis of the scaphoid
▶ **Angiography:** Thrombosis or occlusion of the radial artery, microaneurysms

Hypothenar Hammer Syndrome

▶ Aetiology: Microtrauma of the ulnar artery
▶ Reduced perfusion of the fingers 3–5, necrosis of the hamate
▶ **Angiography**: Thrombosis or occlusion of the ulnar artery, microaneurysms

Vascular Compression Syndromes

▶ Thoracic outlet syndrome
  • Aetiology
    – Neurological type: Compression of the brachial plexus (paraesthesia, pain)
    – Arterial type: Compression of the subclavian artery (cold sensation)
    – Venous type: Compression of the subclavian vein (arm vein thrombosis)
    – Mixed type: Neurovascular shoulder girdle compression syndrome
  • Compression by cervical ribs, cervical transverse processes, clavicle, scalenus triangle, pulmonary apex process, pectoralis minor muscle
  • Neuropathy, loss of strength, rapid fatigability, severe syndrome, muscular atrophy
  • Typically pain on the back of the shoulder, discomfort in the axilla with radiation to the inside of the arm, paraesthesia at night with the arm falling asleep, pain when working overhead
  • Abduction-elevation-external rotation (AER) with fist closure exercises as provocation test
  • **X-ray**
    – Cervical rib
  • **MR**
    – Compression of the brachial plexus
    – Occlusion of the subclavian artery on hyperabduction of the arms
    – Stenosis of the subclavian vein

- **Angiography** also functional diagnostics with provocation test (apron bandage position, elevated arm, weight bearing)
- **Complications**: Arterio-arterial embolism
► Entrapment syndrome
  - Aetiology: Compression of the popliteal artery by the gastrocnemius muscle
  - Claudication or acute vascular occlusion
  - Angiography with provocation test (dorsiflexed foot)
  - **Angiography:** Segmental smooth-bordered stenoses with unremarkable upstream and downstream vessel segments
► Bone tumours
► Soft tissue tumours
► Metastases
► Haematomas

Vasculitis Classification

► Primary vasculitides
  - Vasculitides of large vessels
    – Giant cell arteritis
    – Takayasu arteritis
  - Vasculitides of medium-sized vessels
    – Polyarteritis nodosa
    – Kawasaki syndrome
  - Vasculitides of small vessels
    – ANCA-associated vasculitides
    – Immune complex vasculitides
  - Vasculitides of variable vessels
    – Behçet's disease
    – Cogan syndrome
  - Vasculitides of individual organs
    – Cerebral vasculitis
    – Testicular vasculitis
► Secondary vasculitides
  - Vasculitis in lupus erythematosus
  - Vasculitis in rheumatoid arthritis
  - Vasculitis in sarcoidosis

- Vasculitis associated with allergy
- Vasculitis associated with drugs
- Vasculitis associated with tumour

Vasculitides

▶ Giant cell arteritis
  - Large vessels
  - Older women
  - Classic temporal arteritis
    - Temporal artery and central retinal artery
    - Headache, visual disturbances, claudication, cerebral ischaemia
    - Often additionally polymyalgia rheumatica
    - Temporal artery thickened, painful, tortuous
    - Absent or laterally different pulsation of the temporal artery
  - Extracranial giant cell arteritis
    - Aorta, subclavian artery, carotid artery, vertebral artery
    - Aortic aneurysm, aortic dissection
  - **US**
    - Inflammatory, echo-poor wall thickening in arteritis of the small cranial vessels (halo)
    - Disappearance of the halo after steroid therapy
  - **MR**
    - Increased wall thickness in inflamed segments
    - Mural enhancement of the affected vessels
    - Three-layered vessel wall with 'target appearance'
    - Perivascular enhancement
    - Perivascular oedema
  - **MRA**
    - Vascular stenoses
    - Vascular occlusions
  - **Nuclear Medicine**
    - 18F-FDG-PET in fever or inflammation of unclear aetiology

- – Typical periarticular FDG uptake at shoulders and hips in polymyalgia rheumatica
- **Diagnosis**: Biopsy of temporal arteries (necrotising arteritis with mononuclear cell infiltrates, granulomas with giant cells)
- **Complications**: Loss of visual acuity due to anterior ischaemic optic neuropathy or central retinal artery occlusion, cerebral ischaemia, aortic complications
- **IR**: Percutaneous transluminal angioplasty

▶ Takayasu arteritis
- Large vessels
- Younger women, Asian population
- Muscle complaints, arm pain, dizziness, visual disturbances
- Claudication, pulse attenuation at brachial arteries, systolic blood pressure difference between both arms
- **US**: Homogeneously hypoechoic, smoothly limited, regularly circular vessel wall thickening
- **MR**: Clear enhancement of the affected wall sections
- **Angiography**: Stenoses, occlusions and aneurysms of the subclavian, aortic arch and carotid arteries
- **IR**: Percutaneous transluminal angioplasty

▶ Polyarteritis nodosa
- Medium-sized vessels
- Multiple microaneurysms of the medium-sized arteries of various organs
- Especially renal, hepatic, splenic, mesenteric arteries
- Fever, weight loss, myalgias, arthralgias, polyneuropathy, skin manifestations
- **Angiography**: Multiple aneurysms, especially at vessel branch points
- **Complications**: Aneurysm rupture with intra- and extraparenchymal haemorrhage

Aneurysm Classification

▶ True aneurysm
- Aetiology: Atherosclerosis, arteritis, mycotic

- Bulging of all wall layers (intima, media, adventitia)
- Fusiform extension
▶ Pseudoaneurysm
  - Aetiology: Trauma, surgery
  - Interruption of intima/media, but contained by the adventitia
  - Saccular extension

Aneurysms

▶ Dissecting Aortic aneurysm
  - Aetiology: Atherosclerosis, hypertension
  - Tear in intima/media, formation of a false lumen
  - Entry, Dissection flap, Reentry
  - Stanford classification
    – Type A
      - Includes De Bakey Type I and II
      - Involves any part of the ascending aorta proximal to the left subclavian artery
      - Risk of coronary artery involvement and cardiac tamponade
      - Absolute indication for surgery
    – Type B
      - De Bakey Type III
      - Tear in aorta distal to left subclavian artery, further distal dissection propagation possible
      - Blood pressure reduction; surgical indication for cardiac complications, compression of renal and visceral vessels, increasing vessel diameter
  - True lumen
    – Narrow, oval, internal aortic curvature, rarely thrombosis
  - False lumen
    – Large, sickle-shaped, external aortic curvature, frequent thrombosis
  - **CXR**: Mediastinal widening
  - **MR**
    – Increased outer vessel diameter

- – T1 intramural haematoma (acute isointense wall thickening, subacute hyperintense wall thickening)
  - – Lumen narrowing
- **Diagnosis**: CT, transoesophageal echocardiography
- **Complications**: Aortic rupture, pericardial tamponade, aortic insufficiency, myocardial ischaemia
▶ Thoracoabdominal aortic aneurysm
  - Crawford Classification
    - – I: Extension caudal of the left subclavian artery to cranial of the renal artery
    - – II: Extension caudal to the left subclavian artery to the bifurcation of the aorta
    - – III: Extension from the middle descending aorta to the aortic bifurcation
    - – IV: Extension from the diaphragm to the aortic bifurcation
  - Initially no symptoms, then symptoms due to vessel occlusion and compression effects, finally symptoms due to aneurysm perforation (covered rupture, free rupture, rupture into a hollow organ)
  - **Differential Diagnosis**: Aortic dissection, myocardial infarction, pulmonary embolism, pneumonia
  - **IR**: Stenting
▶ Abdominal aortic aneurysm
  - Incidence significantly higher in men than women
  - Dilatation of the diameter of the aorta over >3 cm
    - – Significant risk of rupture if diameter >5 cm or growth rate >0.5 cm per annum
    - – Further increase in the risk of rupture due to saccular morphology, arterial hypertension, smoking, family history and advanced age
  - Localisation
    - – Located below the renal arteries in 95%
    - – Bifurcation and iliac arteries involved in 20%
  - Non-ruptured mostly incidental finding, ruptured present with pain, abdominal distension and shock

- Peripheral embolism relatively common, rare aortocaval fistulas (right heart failure, cyanosis) or aorto-duodenal fistulas (haematemesis, melena)
- **Complications**: Rupture, fistulae
- **IR**: Endovascular aneurysm repair (EVAR)
  - **Complications**: Prosthesis infection, prosthesis kinking, endoleaks, prosthesis migration, prosthesis occlusion
- Classification of endoleaks
  - I: Perigraft leak; at proximal or distal attachment sites; proximal (I a), distal (I b), leak around an iliac occluder plug (I c)
  - II: Collateral leak; retrograde flow from aortic side branches; single feeding vessel (II a), multiple feeding vessels (II b)
  - III: Midgraft leak; leakage between modules; junctions (III a), endograft fracture (III b)
  - IV: Graft porosity leak; seepage bleeding due to porosity
  - V: Endotension; expansion of the aneurysm
▶ Inflammatory aortic aneurysm
  - Thickened aortic wall, perianeurysmal fibrosis
  - **CT**: Ventral, strongly contrast enhancing, horseshoe-shaped tissue layer
▶ Visceral aneurysm
  - Occurrence
    - Splenic artery: Arteriosclerotic, pancreatitic
    - Hepatic artery: Traumatic
    - Superior mesenteric artery: Mycotic, pancreatitic
  - Types
    - Saccular
    - Fusiform
  - Asymptomatic or with aneurysm rupture: Acute abdomen with haemorrhagic shock and gastrointestinal bleeding
  - **IR**: Embolisation (coils), elimination (stent graft)
▶ Peripheral aneurysm
  - Arteriosclerotic, postoperative (graft aneurysm), iatrogenic (puncture), posttraumatic
  - Popliteal fossa, CFA

- **Complications**: Thrombosis, arterio-arterial embolism, rupture
▶ Popliteal aneurysm
  - Aetiology: Atherosclerosis
  - **Complications**: Embolism, acute thrombotic occlusion, rupture, compressed adjacent structures
  - **IR**: Treat with a stent graft

Arteriovenous Fistulas

▶ Aetiology: Congenital, post-traumatic, post-operative
▶ Pathological short-circuit connections between arterial and venous circulation
▶ Local pulsating varices, vibration thrill, audible bruit
▶ Systemic right heart failure, cor pulmonale, congestive dermatitis
▶ Classification
  - I: No detectable reduction of contrast in the artery distal to the fistula
  - II: Slightly reduced contrast in the artery distal to the fistula
  - III: Marked reduction of contrast in the artery distal to the fistula
  - IV: Absence of contrast of the distal artery

Osler-Rendu-Weber Disease

▶ Aetiology: Autosomal dominant inheritance
▶ Perioral telangiectasia, epistaxis, gastrointestinal bleeding
▶ Arteriovenous fistulas and malformations in the respiratory and gastrointestinal tracts

Haemangiomas

▶ Types
  - Capillary
    – Marked enhancement

- Cavernous
  - Network of vessels
  - Pooling of blood
  - Phleboliths

▶ **MR**
- T2 hyperintense
- Capillary haemangiomas: Rapid contrast enhancement
- Cavernous haemangiomas: Slow contrast enhancement

Trauma-Related Vascular Changes

▶ Arterial injury
- Direct
  - Open injury
  - Closed injury
- Indirect
  - Overextension trauma
  - Deceleration trauma

▶ Findings which may be associated
- Bleeding
- Thrombosis
- Embolism
- Ischaemia
- Dissection
- Compartment syndrome
- Aneurysm
- Fistula
- Infection
- Occlusion

Traumatic Aortic Rupture

▶ Aetiology: Road traffic accidents
▶ In the case of deceleration trauma, abrupt displacement of the intrathoracic mediastinum due to sudden deceleration
▶ Most common site is at the aortic isthmus on the inferior side of the proximal descending aorta which is tethered by the ligamentum arteriosum

▶ Classification according to Parmley
  • I: Subintimal haemorrhage
  • II: Tear of the intima with subintimal haemorrhage
  • III: Tear of the media
  • IV: False aneurysm
  • V: Complete vessel rupture
  • VI: Complete vascular rupture with para-aortic haemorrhage
▶ Initially no symptoms, then chest pain, dyspnoea and dysphagia, finally mediastinal haemorrhage, haemothorax and haemorrhagic shock
▶ **Differential Diagnosis:** Rib fractures, lung injury, pneumothorax, aneurysm rupture
▶ **IR:** Stenting

Dissection of Head and Neck Vessels

▶ Aetiology
  • Tearing of the intima with formation of a false lumen and bleeding into the arterial wall
  • Spontaneous, fibromuscular dysplasia, traumatic
▶ Sites where more commonly occur
  • Internal carotid artery at the base of the skull
    – Unilateral neck, head, face and orbital pain
    – Ischaemia of the cerebrum or retina
    – Horner's syndrome
  • Vertebral artery at the atlas loop
    – Headache and neck pain
    – Ischaemia of the lateral medulla oblongata
    – Wallenberg syndrome
▶ **US**
  • Direct morphological criteria
    – Stenosis
    – Low echo wall haematoma
    – Dissection membrane
    – Double lumen

- Indirect haemodynamic criteria
  - Flow acceleration
  - Pendulum flow, sloshing phenomenon
  - Closure

▶ **MR**
  - Lumen constriction
  - String sign (stenosis) or string and pearl sign (stenosis and pseudoaneurysms)
  - Wall haematoma

▶ **Angiography**
  - Irregular narrowing of the artery at a typical location
  - Tapered stenosis with otherwise normal contour
  - Double lumen or intimal flap occasionally visible

▶ **Differential Diagnosis**: Atherosclerosis, fibromuscular dysplasia without dissection, thrombosis

Tumour-Related Vascular Changes

▶ **US/CT/MR**
  - Atypical vascular architecture
  - Microaneurysms
  - Vascular neoplasms
  - Collateral vessels
  - Encasement
  - Vascular displacement
  - Arteriovenous shunts

Veins

Deep Venous Thrombosis

▶ Aetiology: Virchow triad (blood clotting disorder, stasis, vein wall damage)

▶ Risk factors: Surgery, immobilisation, tumour, obesity, pregnancy, contraceptives, coagulopathies

▶ Pain, heaviness, oedema, cyanosis

▶ Lowenberg sign (cuff pressure pain), Bisgaard sign (splint pressure pain), Homans sign (calf pain with dorsiflexion of the ankle), Payr sign (plantar pain), circumference sign (circumferential difference)

▶ Scoring systems, D-dimers
- Venous thrombosis ruled out with extremely high probability if D-dimer is negative

▶ Special types
- Paget-Schroetter syndrome
  - Aetiology: Thoracic inlet syndrome (costoclavicular inflow obstruction in normotensives, muscle hypertrophy, weakness, cachexia), fractures, catheters, port systems, pacemaker systems, dialysis shunts, tumours
  - Arm and shoulder girdle vein thrombosis
  - Swelling, livid skin discolouration, venous rete axillaris, severe pain, feeling of heaviness
  - High spontaneous resolution due to good collateralisation
- Phlegmasia cerulea dolens
  - Aetiology: Extensive thrombotic occlusion of the entire venous drainage of an affected limb with arterial compression
  - Resulting ischaemia can lead to gangrene and sepsis
  - Bluish discolouration of the leg, swelling, blistering, petechial haemorrhages, pain, risk of shock, acute leg ischaemia

▶ **US**
- Distended lumen
- Lack of compressibility
- Lack of respiratory modulation
- Stationary internal echoes
  - Fresh thrombus usually echo-poor
  - Older thrombus more echo-rich
- Lack of wave variation on Valsalva manoeuvre

▶ **Colour Doppler US:** Absence of flow signal

▶ **Venography/CT venography** (rarely now used for DVT)
- Acute thrombosis
  - Cylindrical filling defect

- – Define proximal extent
- Postthrombotic syndrome
  - – Irregular vein course
  - – Incompetent valves
  - – Vein wall changes
  - – Variable vein lumen calibre
  - – Collateral circulation
  - – Secondary varicosis
- ▶ **Complications**: Post-thrombotic syndrome, pulmonary embolism

Interventional Techniques for Deep Venous Thrombosis

- ▶ Most DVTs are treated with anticoagulation therapy but percutaneous treatment of venous thrombosis can be an effective therapy for extensive DVT
  - Rapid revascularisation of iliofemoral and ilio-caval thromboses with preservation of valve function and reduction of post-thrombotic syndrome
- ▶ Procedure
  - Local thrombolysis
  - Pharmacomechanical thrombolysis
  - Mechanical thrombectomy
  - Balloon dilatation
  - Stent implantation
  - Filter implantation

Primary Varicose Veins

- ▶ Aetiology: Age, disposition, orthostasis, obesity, gravidity
- ▶ Women
- ▶ Feeling of heaviness, pain, tension
- ▶ CEAP classification (clinical, etiological, anatomical, pathophysiological) of varices
  - Clinical
    - – C1: Telangiectasia
    - – C2: Varicosis
    - – C3: Oedema

- C4: Trophic skin changes
- C5: Healed ulcerations
- C6: Florid ulcerations
- Aetiological
  - Ec: Congenital
  - Ep: Primary (idiopathic)
  - Es: Secondary (post-thrombotic)
  - En: Non-venous
- Anatomical
  - As: Superficial veins
  - Ap: Perforating veins
  - Ad: Deep veins
- Pathophysiological
  - Pr: Reflux
  - Po: Obstruction
  - Pro: Reflux and obstruction

▶ Truncal varicosities
- Varicose veins 4 mm or larger are defined as truncal
- Usually involves the long or short saphenous veins or tributaries
- Truncal venous insufficiency with varicosities are by far the most common cause of chronic venous insufficiency
- Stages in the long saphenous vein type, depending on the distal point of insufficiency
  - I: Insufficiency of the saphenofemoral junction
  - II: Reflux up to above the knee joint
  - III: Reflux to below the knee joint
  - IV: Reflux to the ankle
- Stages in the short saphenous vein type, depending on the distal point of insufficiency
  - I: Insufficiency of the confluence
  - II: Reflux to the middle of the lower leg
  - III: Reflux to the ankle
- Triplex mode US (B-scan + colour Doppler + PW Doppler)
- US
  - Vein morphology
  - Blood flow
  - Detection of reflux

  - Insufficiency points
  - Truncal veins
  - Perforating veins
  - Side branch veins
► Therapy of truncal varicosis
  • Open surgical
    - Crossectomy
    - Stripping
    - CHIVA
    - Valvuloplasty
  • Endovenous thermal
    - Radiofrequency
    - Laser
  • Endovenous non-thermal
    - Vein glue
    - Mechanochemical ablation
    - Foam sclerotherapy
► Therapy of perforating varicosis
  • Open ligation
► Therapy of side branch varicosis
  • Miniphlebectomy
  • Foam sclerotherapy

Secondary Varicose Veins

► Aetiology: Post-thrombotic syndrome
► **Phlebography**
  • Damaged venous valves
  • Recanalisation
  • Collateralisation
  • Perivascular fibrosis

Lymphatic Vessels

Lymphoedema

▶ Aetiology
- Primary
  - Congenital
  - Non-congenital, occurring for the first time in puberty (praecox) or adulthood (tarda) (agenesis, aplasia, hypoplasia of lymphatic vessels)
- Secondary
  - Tumour
  - Trauma
  - Operation
  - Radiotherapy
  - Venous thrombosis
  - Lymphangitis
  - Erysipelas
  - Parasites

▶ Types
- Mechanical insufficiency
  - Organic damage to the lymphatic system
  - Functional damage to the lymphatic system
- Dynamic insufficiency
  - Lymphatic load higher than transport capacity of the intact lymphatic vascular system
- Combined insufficiency

▶ Classification
- I: Spontaneously reversible lymphoedema, doughy swelling, Stemmer sign negative
- II: Spontaneously irreversible lymphoedema, marked fibrosis, Stemmer's sign positive
- III: Irreversible lymphoedema, lymphostatic elephantiasis

▶ **Differential diagnosis**: Lipoedema, thrombophlebitis

▶ **Complications**: Lymphocele, lymph cyst, lymph fistula, lymphatic varix, lymphangitis

Lymphoceles

▶ Aetiology: Complication after lymphadenectomy or trauma
▶ Cystic masses with smooth and thin walls in the former surgical area (especially axilla and groin)
▶ Spontaneous regression of smaller lymphoceles in a few weeks
▶ **Complications**: Lymphatic blockage, chronic lymphoedema, abscess formation, lymphatic fistula
▶ IR: Percutaneous aspiration or catheter drainage

Lymphatic Drainage Scintigraphy

▶ 99mTc nanocolloid
▶ Functional lymph scintigraphy
  • Investigation of limb lymphoedema
    – Fluorescence lymphography with indocyanine green as an alternative
    – Sentinel node scintigraphy
▶ Diagnosis of the sentinel lymph node
  • Breast carcinoma, melanoma, vulvar carcinoma, penile carcinoma
  • Marking of the sentinel lymph node, removal during surgery, assessment of histology

Oesophagus, Stomach, Small Intestine, Colon

Anatomy

Oesophagus

- ▶ Cervical
- ▶ Thoracic
- ▶ Abdominal

Oesophageal Indentations

- ▶ Lower cricoid cartilage
- ▶ Aortic arch
- ▶ Left main bronchus
- ▶ Diaphragm

Oesophageal Peristalsis

- ▶ Primary peristalsis
  - • Triggered by swallowing a bolus
  - • Transport function
- ▶ Secondary peristalsis
  - • Due to irritation of the mucous membrane
  - • Clearing function

© The Author(s), under exclusive license to Springer Nature
Switzerland AG 2026
D. Pickuth, J. T. Murchison, *Pocket Guide to Radiology*,
https://doi.org/10.1007/978-3-031-76520-9_4

▶ Tertiary peristalsis
- Due to trauma, surgery, infection, neuropathy, myopathy, collagenosis as well as physiologically in old age
- Irregular contractions without transport function

Swallowing Process

▶ Swallowing centres
- Cortical swallowing centre
- Pontine swallowing centre
- Medullary swallowing centre
▶ Swallowing phases
- Oral phase: Can be influenced at will, duration about 0.5 s
- Pharyngeal phase: Reflexive, duration about 0.5 s
- Oesophageal phase: Peristaltic, duration about 3–10 s

Stomach

▶ Sections
- Cardia
- Fundus
- Body
- Antrum
- Pylorus
▶ Curvatures
- Lesser curve
- Greater curve
▶ Gastric mucosal surface
- Areae gastricae: Stomach folds
- Foveolae gastricae: Gastric pits
▶ Arteries
- Common hepatic artery
  - Right gastric artery
- Splenic artery
- Left gastric artery
▶ Lymph nodes
- Perigastric lymph nodes
- Right and left gastroepiploic nodes

- Splenic hilum nodes
- Suprapancreatic nodes
- Hepaticoduodenal ligament nodes
- Root of superior mesenteric artery nodes
- Coeliac nodes
- Para-aortic nodes

▶ Topography
  - Liver
  - Diaphragm
  - Spleen
  - Pancreas
  - Duodenum
  - Transverse colon
  - Aorta
  - Kidneys

Gastric Mucosa

Wall layer	Layer	Sonography findings
1	Mucosa	Hyperechoic
2	Muscularis mucosae	Hypoechoic
3	Submucosa	Hyperechoic
4	Muscularis propria	Hypoechoic
5	Serosa	Hyperechoic

Duodenum

▶ Sections
  - First part—Superior (duodenal cap)
  - Second part—Descending
  - Third part—Horizontal
  - Forth part—Ascending

▶ Arteries
  - Gastroduodenal artery with superior pancreaticoduodenal artery (from common hepatic artery)
  - Inferior pancreaticoduodenal artery (from superior mesenteric artery)

► Topography
  • Pancreas
  • Liver
  • Gallbladder
  • Kidneys
  • Stomach
  • Transverse colon
  • Spine

Small Intestine

► Sections
  • Jejunum
    – Lumen width up to 30 mm
    – 4–8 folds per 2.5 cm segment
  • Ileum
    – Lumen width up to 30 mm
    – 2–4 folds per 2.5 cm segment
► Gross anatomy
  • Duodeno-jejunal (DJ) flexure—left upper abdomen anterior to aorta to left of L2
  • Terminal ileum: Right lower abdomen
► Arteries
  • Inferior pancreaticoduodenal artery (from superior mesenteric artery)
  • Jejunal artery (from superior mesenteric artery)
  • Ileal arteries (from superior mesenteric artery)
  • Ileocolic artery (from superior mesenteric artery)
  • Right colic artery (from superior mesenterica artery)
  • Middle colic artery (from superior mesenteric artery)
► Topography
  • Colon
  • Mesocolon transversum
  • Lesser sac
  • Greater omentum
  • Mesenteric root

Colon

▶ Sections
- Caecum
- Ascending colon
- Transverse colon
- Descending colon
- Sigmoid colon
- Rectum

▶ Components
- Taniae coli—three bands of longitudinal smooth muscle on colon surface
- Haustrae
- Appendices epiploicae

▶ Arteries
- Right hemicolon
  - Superior mesenteric artery with ileocolic artery, right colic artery and middle colic artery
- Left hemicolon
  - Inferior mesenteric artery with left colic artery, rectosigmoid artery and superior rectal artery
- Watershed—splenic flexure region between the supply areas of the mesenteric arteries
- Lower two-thirds of the rectum from the internal iliac artery

▶ Topography of the appendix
- Iliopsoas muscle
- Iliac fascia
- Abdominal wall
- Right ovary

Rectum

▶ Sections
- Rectal ampulla
- Anal Canal
  - Rectum S shaped

▶ Flexures
- Sacral and perineal
- Rectal folds
  - Superior, middle, inferior (Houston's valves)
- Anorectal junction

▶ Anal sphincters
- Muscles
  - Internal anal sphincter
  - External anal sphincter
  - Levator ani

▶ Arteries
- Superior rectal artery (from inferior mesenteric artery)
- Middle rectal artery (from internal iliac artery)
- Inferior rectal artery (from internal pudendal artery)

▶ Lymph nodes
- Superior rectal nodes
- Perirectal nodes
- Internal iliac nodes
- Inguinal nodes

▶ Topography
- Ventral: Urinary bladder, prostate, seminal vesicles, vagina, uterus
- Dorsal: Sacrum, coccyx
- Lateral: Ureter, fallopian tubes, ovaries
- Caudal: Pelvic floor

▶ Upper third intraperitoneal

▶ Middle third retroperitoneal

▶ Lower third extraperitoneal—below the pelvic diaphragm which consists of levator ani and coccygeal muscles

Peritoneal Locations of Structures

▶ Intraperitoneal
- Stomach
- Jejunum
- Ileum
- Caecum

- Appendix
- Transverse colon
- Sigmoid colon
- Liver
- Spleen
- Uterus
- Fallopian tubes
- Ovaries
▶ Retroperitoneal
  - Primary retroperitoneal
    - Kidneys
    - Adrenal glands
    - Ureters
  - Secondary retroperitoneal
    - Duodenum
    - Ascending colon
    - Descending colon
    - Pancreas
▶ Subperitoneal
  - Urinary bladder
  - Rectum
  - Prostate
  - Seminal vesicles
  - Cervix

Inguinal Canal

▶ Walls
  - Anterior wall: External oblique muscle
  - Posterior wall: Parietalis abdominal fascia
  - Above: Transversus abdominis muscle, Internal oblique muscle
  - Below: Inguinal ligament
▶ Content
  - Female: Round ligament
  - Male: Spermatic cord
  - Both: Ilioinguinal nerve, genital branch of the genitofemoral nerve

Retroperitoneum

▶ Anterior pararenal space
  • Duodenum, pancreas, ascending colon, descending colon, great vessels
▶ Perirenal space
  • Kidneys, adrenal glands
▶ Posterior pararenal space
  • Psoas muscle

Oesophagus

Achalasia

▶ Aetiology: Motility disorder of the oesophagus with loss of propulsive peristalsis of the tubular oesophagus, increase in resting pressure of the lower oesophageal sphincter and loss of relaxation of the lower oesophageal sphincter
▶ Aetiology
  • Primary achalasia
    – Idiopathic
    – Familial
  • Secondary achalasia
    – Paraneoplastic
    – In sarcoidosis, amyloidosis, post-vagotomy, chronic intestinal pseudo-obstruction
    – Chagas disease
▶ Types (based on manometric pattern)
  • I: (Classic) hypomotile, minimal contractility
  • II: Intermittent pan-oesophageal pressure increase
  • III: (Spastic) abnormal strong distal oesophageal contractions
▶ Untreated achalasia leads to increased risk of squamous cell carcinoma of the oesophagus
▶ Dysphagia, retrosternal pain, regurgitation, nocturnal cough, weight loss

▶ **X-ray**
- Delayed contrast passage
  - Quantification with Timed Barium Oesophagography
- Smooth mucosal contour
- Acute stenosis
- Often air-fluid level

▶ **Nuclear medicine**: Quantitative assessment by oesophageal function scintigraphy with 99mTc colloid

▶ **Differential Diagnosis**: Oesophageal stricture, oesophageal carcinoma, eosinophilic oesophagitis, gastric carcinoma, aortic aneurysm

▶ **Diagnosis**: Endoscopy, fluoroscopic video swallow, Manometry,
- Motility assessment of the oesophagus with high resolution manometry (HRM)

▶ **Complications**: Nocturnal aspiration, secondary pneumonia, malnutrition, oesophageal carcinoma

Oesophageal Spasm

▶ Aetiology: Uncoordinated, prolonged, spastic contractions of the oesophagus after swallowing (tertiary peristalsis) without disturbance of the lower oesophageal sphincter

▶ Intermittent dysphagia, spasmodic retrosternal pain

▶ **X-ray**: Corkscrew-like configuration of the oesophagus

▶ **Diagnosis**: Manometry, video-fluoroscopy, fluoroscopic barium swallow

Oesophageal Diverticulum

▶ Pulsation diverticulum
- Acquired
- False diverticula, only involves mucosa and submucosa
- Narrow neck, variable shape, not fixed
- Predilection sites: Cervical, epiphrenic

▶ Traction diverticulum
- Aetiology: Retraction due scarring of mediastinal lymph nodes (tuberculosis)
- True diverticula, all wall layers involved

- Wide neck, not variable in shape, fixed
- Predilection site: Thoracic
▶ Pharyngeal pouch (Zenker's diverticulum)
  - Pulsation pseudodiverticulum
  - Herniation of mucosa and submucosa through the posterior wall of the pharyngo-oesophageal junction (weak point, so-called Killian dehiscence between oblique and transverse fibres of the cricopharyngeus muscle)
  - Small diverticula in the midline, larger diverticula postero-laterally on left
  - Grades
    - I: 2–3 mm
    - II: 4–10 mm
    - III: >10 mm without compression of the oesophagus
    - IV: >10 mm with compression of the oesophagus
  - Older men
  - Dysphagia, regurgitation, foetor, aspiration
  - X-ray: Contrast medium pooling in a posterolateral diverticulum in the distal pharynx around C5-6 level

Oesophageal Stenoses

▶ Webs
  - Thin, asymmetrical, oesophageal bands
  - Mostly anterior wall of the cervical oesophagus
▶ Vascular causes
  - Aberrant right subclavian artery from the left aortic arch
  - Double aortic arch
  - Left-sided aortic arch
  - Atypical course of the left pulmonary artery

Systemic Sclerosis

▶ Aetiology: Motility disorder due to fibrosis of the submucosa
▶ X-ray: Dilated patulous oesophagus with delayed emptying and dysmotility
▶ Nuclear medicine: Quantitative assessment of oesophageal function—scintigraphy with 99mTc colloid

Oesophageal Varices

▶ Aetiology: Most frequently portal hypertension
▶ Types
  • Uphill varices: Varicose dilatations of the venous plexus in the lower third of the oesophagus in cirrhosis of the liver, obstruction of the inferior vena cava and splenic vein thrombosis
  • Downhill varices: Varicose dilatations of the venous plexus in the upper third of the oesophagus in the case of obstruction of the superior vena cava
▶ Plexus-like dilatations of the subepithelial or submucosal veins
▶ Anterior part usually connected to the short gastric vein, posterior part to the azygos vein or hemiazygos vein
▶ **Diagnosis:** (and treatment)—usually by endoscopy
▶ **Barium swallow**
  • Serpiginous filling defects in the middle and lower thirds of the oesophagus
  • Better demonstrated with head-down position or Valsalva manoeuvre

Oesophageal Foreign Body

▶ Areas of physiological narrowing in
  • Upper oesophageal sphincter—includes cricopharyngeal muscle
  • Middle oesophagus where crosses the aortic arch
  • Lower oesophageal sphincter
▶ Most common in children
▶ In children usually upper oesophageal sphincter level
▶ In adults usually lower oesophageal sphincter level
▶ Chest pain, ache or vague discomfort, stinging and pressure behind the larynx or sternum, gagging and choking
▶ **CXR +/− lateral cervical X ray**
  • If the foreign body is radiopaque, the radiograph will help determine the object, the location and possible complications

- • If not radiopaque. X-ray after swallowing oral contrast may help clarify the presence and location of the object and diagnose obstruction (Use water-soluble contrast if suspected perforation)
- ▶ **Complication**: Oesophageal perforation

Oesophageal Perforation

- ▶ Aetiology: Chemical burn, radiation, tumour, iatrogenic trauma (endoscopy, probing, use of a bougie)
- ▶ Mediastinitis—retrosternal or interscapular pain
- ▶ Mallory-Weiss syndrome
    - • Intramural mucosal tear in the distal oesophagus or proximal cardia with severe bleeding
    - • Precursor of Boerhaave's disease
    - • A cause of upper gastrointestinal bleeding
- ▶ Boerhaave's disease
    - • Rupture in the distal oesophagus due to intra-abdominal pressure increase (vomiting, coughing)
    - • Severe retrosternal pain
    - • Mediastinal emphysema, mediastinitis, fever, leukocytosis
- ▶ **X-ray/CT**
    - • Widening of the paravertebral soft tissue shadow
    - • Loss of the descending aortic contour
    - • Left pleural effusion
    - • Pneumomediastinum
    - • Soft tissue emphysema
- ▶ **Complication**: Mediastinitis

Reflux Oesophagitis

- ▶ Aetiology: Reflux of gastric contents into the oesophagus due to dysfunction of the oesophageal sphincter
- ▶ Gastro-oesophageal reflux disease (GORD)
    - • Oesophageal syndromes
        - – Reflux oesophagitis, reflux stricture, Barrett's oesophagus, oesophageal carcinoma

- Extraesophageal syndromes
  - Reflux cough, reflux laryngitis, reflux asthma, dental erosions
  - Sinusitis, pharyngitis, pulmonary fibrosis, middle ear infections
▶ Heartburn, retrosternal burning, acid regurgitation, retrosternal pain, epigastric pain, belching
▶ Increased pain when bending over, lying down, after meals
▶ Endoscopic stages
  - I: Reflux disease without reflux oesophagitis
  - II: Minor patchy mucosal defects
  - III: Confluent mucosal lesions
  - IV: Circular confluent mucosal lesions
  - V: Peptic stenosis
▶ **Diagnosis**: Endoscopy, impedance pH-metry, manometry
▶ **Complications**: Ulcer, bleeding, perforation, stricture, carcinoma

Oesophageal Candidiasis

▶ Aetiology: Antibiosis, AIDS, leukaemia, lymphoma, diabetes
▶ Dysphagia, pain on swallowing, retrosternal pain, white plaques in mouth
▶ Often affects the entire oesophagus
▶ **Barium swallow**: Multiple fine punctate, or round mucosal ulcerations, irregular linear or irregular plaque-like lesions with longitudinal orientation
▶ **Diagnosis**: Endoscopy—white plaques on red background

Barrett's Oesophagus

▶ Aetiology: Replacement of the squamous epithelium in the distal oesophagus with a metaplastic cylindrical epithelium
▶ **X-ray**: Deep ulcers with irregular ulcer base
▶ **Complications**: Increased risk of oesophageal adenocarcinoma

Benign Oesophageal Tumours

- ▶ Leiomyoma
- ▶ Lipoma
- ▶ Neurofibroma
- ▶ Fibroma

Malignant Oesophageal Tumours

- ▶ Aetiology: Smoking, alcohol, Barrett's oesophagus, reflux oesophagitis,
- ▶ Types
  - Squamous cell carcinoma
  - Adenocarcinoma
- ▶ Older people, mostly men
- ▶ Dysphagia, weight loss, retrosternal pain, regurgitation, heartburn
- ▶ Locoregional staging (CT, transoesophageal endo-ultrasound with targeted endo-ultrasound guided fine-needle aspiration biopsy)
- ▶ **Barium swallow**
  - Polypoidal mass
  - Irregular stricture
  - Shouldering of edge of stricturing mass
  - Ulcerated mucosa
  - Prestenotic dilatation
- ▶ **CT**
  - Local infiltration of aorta, tracheobronchial system or pericardium
  - Para-oesophageal, mediastinal, supraclavicular, and upper abdominal lymph node metastases
  - Hepatic, pulmonary and bone metastases
- ▶ T-stage
  - Over staging with endo-sonography due to accompanying inflammatory reactions
  - Under staging with CT/MR due to lack of visualisation of microscopic infiltrates

- N-stage
  - Assessment of locoregional lymph nodes with endosonography
  - Imaging of the abdominal lymph nodes with CT/MR
- **Diagnosis**: Endoscopy, CT and PET CT to define local and metastatic spread
- **Complications**: Oesophageal obstruction, tracheoesophageal fistula, tumour haemorrhage

TNM Classification Oesophagus and Gastro-Oesophageal Junction Cancers

- T1a: Lamina propria, muscularis mucosae
- T1b: Submucosa
- T2: Muscularis propria
- T3: Adventitia
- T4a: Pleura, pericardium, azygos vein, diaphragm, peritoneum
- T4b: Aorta, vertebral body, trachea
- N1: 1 to 2 regional
- N2: 3 to 6 regional
- N3: ≥7 regional
- M1: Distant metastases

Stomach

Gastric Ulcer

- Aetiology: Stress, smoking, Helicobacter pylori, NSAIDs, steroids
- Upper abdominal pain
- Most commonly on lesser curve/ gastric body and antrum (90–95%) Greater curve rare (5%)
- Post bulbar ulcers very rare—consider Zollinger-Ellison syndrome especially if multiple
- **Barium meal** (only now used when contraindication to endoscopy)
  - >2–3mm oval mucosal defect (crater)
  - Thin gastric folds radiating towards the crater

- Ulcer outside the gastric contour on profile imaging
- Smooth margins
- Thin smooth raised ring of oedema around the ulcer crater (Hampton line)

▶ **Diagnosis**: Endoscopy—primary investigation of choice, biopsy

▶ **Complications**: Bleeding, invasion, perforation, stenosis

Gastric Tumours

▶ Types of tumour
- Benign: Adenoma, polyp, leiomyoma, lipoma, neurinoma, fibroma
- Malignant: Carcinoma, sarcoma, lymphoma

▶ Non-specific epigastric fullness, nausea, vomiting, weight loss

▶ **Diagnosis**: Endoscopy with biopsy primary investigation of choice

Gastric Polyp

▶ **Barium meal** (only in the event endoscopy is contraindicated)
- Smooth surface
- Broad-based sessile or stalked
- Protruding into the gastric lumen
- Suspicious of malignancy if the surface is irregular, the diameter is more than 1 cm and the base is retracted

▶ **Diagnosis**: Endoscopy +/− biopsy

Gastric Carcinoma

▶ Adenocarcinoma

▶ Classification according to Laurén
- Intestinal (polypoid)
- Diffuse (infiltrative)

▶ Classification according to Borrmann
- I: Non-infiltrating, polypoid
- II: Non-infiltrating, locally fungating

- III: Infiltrating, locally ulcerating
- IV: Diffusely infiltrating

▶ Mostly antrum, lesser curve, fundus

▶ Upper abdominal discomfort, loss of appetite, weight loss, anaemia, melaena

▶ **Endoscopic Ultrasound (EUS)**
  - Symmetrical or asymmetrical gastric wall thickening, reduced or absent gastric wall elasticity, lumen narrowing, polypoidal mass, submucosal masses
  - Detection of submucosal gastric tumours, differentiation of extra-gastric processes, clarification of enlarged gastric folds, assessment of locoregional staging
    - Assessment of the current infiltration depth
    - Assessment of local lymph node involvement

▶ **Barium meal appearances of malignant ulcer**
  - – Rarely now used unless contraindication to endoscopy
    - Ulcer which does not protrude beyond the gastric contour
    - Irregular ulcer border
    - Carman meniscus sign
    - Nodular gastric folds

▶ **CT**
  - Detection of lymph node metastases
    - Level 1: Perigastric
    - Level 2: Coeliac
    - Level 3: Periportal, retroduodenal, retropancreatic, mesenteric

▶ **Diagnosis**: High-resolution video endoscopy and sampling for histological confirmation

TNM Classification Gastric Cancer

▶ T1a: Lamina propria, muscularis mucosae
▶ T1b: Submucosa
▶ T2: Muscularis propria
▶ T3: Subserosa
▶ T4a: Serosa

▶ T4b: Neighbouring structures
▶ N1: 1 to 2 regional
▶ N2: 3 to 6 regional
▶ N3a: 7 to 15 regional
▶ N3b: ≥16 regional
▶ M1: Distant metastases

Gastric Surgery

▶ Surgical procedure
  • Billroth I resection
    – End-to-end anastomosis or end-to-side anastomosis of the gastric remnant with the duodenum
  • Billroth II resection
    – Anastomosis of the gastric remnant with a retrocolic or antecolic raised jejunal loop
    – In the antecolic procedure, the inflow and outflow loops can be short-circuited by a Braun foot point anastomosis
  • Roux-en-Y gastroenterostomy or jejunostomy
    – Connection of the gastric remnant with a jejunal loop
    – Distal to the Treitz ligament, an upper jejunal loop is severed, i.e. eliminated from the food passage, with end-to-end anastomosis of the distal portion and the gastric remnant
    – The proximal part of the jejunal loop is anastomosed end-to-end with the distal part in a Y-shape
    – The duodenal stump is closed by sutures
▶ Progress monitoring
  • Postoperative complications
    – Anastomotic stenosis
    – Anastomotic leak
  • Delayed complications
    – Functional, dumping syndrome, anaemia, nutritional deficiencies
    – Pathological changes: Stenosis, ulcer, intussusception, internal hernia, fistula, tumour recurrence

▶ Syndromes after gastric surgery
  • Early dumping syndrome
    – Reduced plasma volume with postprandial collapse due to rapid, undiluted and hyperosmolar food passage into the jejunum
  • Late dumping syndrome
    – Hypoglycaemic attacks due to excessive insulin release
  • Blind loop syndrome
    – Due to stasis and drainage obstruction, bacterial colonisation and retention in the blind loop with debris, sudden bilious vomiting and diarrhoea

Gastrointestinal Stromal Tumour

▶ Aetiology: Mesenchymal tumour of the gastrointestinal tract from interstitial cells
▶ Most often stomach and small intestine, rarely colon and rectum
▶ Bleeding, anaemia, pain, abdominal bloating
▶ **CT/MR**
  • Small GISTS are often submucosal
  • Large GISTS are often exophytic
  • Smooth boundary
  • Usually strongly enhancing
  • Central necroses
  • Hepatic, mesenteric and omental metastases
▶ Positive response to treatment on CT scan (Choi criteria)
  • 10% decrease in unidimensional length (size criterion)
  • 15% decrease in lesion CT attenuation (density criterion)

TNM Classification Gastrointestinal Stromal Tumour

▶ T1: ≤2 cm
▶ T2: >2 cm to ≤5 cm
▶ T3: >5 cm to ≤10 cm
▶ T4: >10 cm
▶ N1: Regional
▶ M1: Distant metastases

Small Intestine

Coarsening of the Duodenal Folds

▶ Inflammatory
  • Ulcer
  • Duodenitis
  • Hyperplasia of Brunner's glands
  • Ectopic gastric mucosa
  • Ectopic pancreatic tissue
▶ Neoplastic
  • Carcinoma
  • Sarcoma
  • Lymphoma
  • Carcinoid
  • Metastases
▶ Intramural haemorrhage
▶ Whipple's disease
▶ Amyloidosis
▶ Varices

Duodenal Lumen Narrowing

▶ Duodenal atresia
▶ Pyloric stenosis
▶ Annular Pancreas
▶ Duodenal diverticulum
▶ Duodenal tumour

Loss of Small Intestinal Folds

▶ Celiac disease in the jejunum
▶ Crohn's disease, atrophic stage
▶ Tuberculosis, end stage
▶ Focal bowel ischaemia
▶ Chronic radiation enteritis

Lumen Narrowing of the Small Intestine

▶ Extrinsic
- Adhesion
- Hernia
- Metastasis
- Carcinoid
- Abscess
▶ Intrinsic
- Tumours
- Inflammation
- Crohn's disease
- Ischaemia
- Radiation stricture
- Intussusception

Duodenal Diverticulum

▶ Types
- True diverticulum: Protrusion of the entire duodenal wall
- False diverticula: Mucosal protrusion through muscle gaps
▶ Most commonly located medial descending duodenum, in periampullary region
▶ Often incidental finding, rarely inflammation, bleeding, perforation

Crohn's Disease

▶ Aetiology: Chronic inflammatory bowel disease; transmural inflammation; histologically epithelioid cell granulomas and giant cells
▶ Can affect any part of bowel from mouth to anus
▶ Most commonly small bowel, particularly terminal ileum
▶ Skip lesions with discontinuous segments of bowel affected
▶ Abdominal pain, diarrhoea, rarely bloody, nausea, loss of appetite, weight loss, fever
▶ Smoking a risk factor for development and for more complicated course

▶ **US**
- Mild inflammation: Locally distorted and thickened bowel wall
- Moderate inflammation: Thickened echoic submucosa
- Severe inflammation: All bowel wall layers thickened and hypoechoic
- Skip lesions
- May be asymmetrical involvement of bowel wall
- Prominent mesenteric adipose tissue
- Reactively enlarged lymph nodes
- Local free liquid

▶ **Barium follow through**—now rarely used
- Early stage
  - Disseminated mucosal protrusions
  - Aphthous ulcers
- Acute stage
  - Longitudinal fissures
  - Cobblestone appearance
  - Pseudopolyps
  - Rose thorn ulcers
- Chronic stage
  - Strictures
  - Sinus tracts and fistulae
  - Pseudodiverticulae/pseudosacculation
- Remission stage
  - Smooth mucosa
  - Decreased bowel wall thickening
  - Intestinal wall atony

▶ **MR**
- Acute stage
  - Thickening of the intestinal wall
  - T2 high signal intensity of the intestinal wall
  - Contrast enhancement of the intestinal wall
  - Often inflammatory co-reaction of the mesenteric fat
- Chronic stage
  - No thickening of the intestinal wall
  - Minimal late enhancement of intestinal wall of fibrosed segment

- Circumscribed intestinal lumen stenosis
- Pre-stenotic dilatation of the intestinal lumen

▶ Cobblestone appearance: Extensive mucosal swelling with intervening ulcerations

▶ **Differential Diagnosis**: Diverticulitis, appendicitis, ulcerative colitis, yersiniosis, intestinal tuberculosis

▶ **Diagnosis**: Ileo-colonoscopy with biopsy, upper endoscopy with biopsy, MRI enterography (transmural and extraluminal changes), video capsule endoscopy (intraluminal and mucosal changes)
- Endoscopy: Ulceration, cobblestone appearance of mucosa
- **MRI**: To assess the activity of the disease according to the degree of enhancement

▶ **Complications**: Strictures, ileus, fistulas (gastrocolic, entero-enteral, enterosigmoidal, enterocolic, enterovesical, enteroure-thral, enterovaginal, enterocutaneous, perianal), abscesses, increased risk of malignancy

Inflammatory Changes in the Terminal Ileum

▶ Crohn's disease
▶ Tuberculosis
▶ Shigellosis
▶ Ulcerative colitis (backwash ileitis)
▶ Yersiniosis
▶ Radiation enteritis
▶ Behçet's disease

Small Intestinal Strictures

▶ Aetiology: Surgery, tumour, inflammation, ischaemia, radio-therapy, adhesions
▶ Presentation: Recurrent obstruction, episodic abdominal pain, dyspepsia, vomiting

Small Intestinal Fistula

▶ Aetiology: Surgery, trauma, Crohn's disease, tuberculosis, actinomycosis
▶ Types
  • External fistulae: Enterocutaneous fistula. Cutaneous discharge of bowel contents through fistula with maceration of the abdominal wall skin at the fistula site
  • Internal fistulae: Malabsorption due to intestinal short circuit and blind sac formation with bacterial colonisation/overgrowth

Small Intestine Tumour

▶ Peritoneal carcinomatosis
▶ Lymphoma, gastrointestinal stromal tumour, neuroendocrine tumours, carcinoma, sarcoma, metastases
▶ Syndromes
  • Cronkhite-Canada syndrome: Intestinal polyposis, hypoproteinaemia, alopecia, skin pigmentation, fingernail atrophy
  • Gardner syndrome: Intestinal polyposis, multiple osteomas, dental anomalies, epidermoid cysts
  • Peutz-Jeghers syndrome: Intestinal polyposis, perioral pigmentation
▶ Diagnosis: Video capsule endoscopy, double balloon enteroscopy, MR enterography, CT enterography

TNM Classification Small Intestine Adenocarcinoma

▶ T1a: Lamina propria, muscularis mucosae
▶ T1b: Submucosa
▶ T2: Muscularis propria
▶ T3: Subserosa, non-peritoneal perimuscular tissue (mesentery, retroperitoneum)
▶ T4: Visceral peritoneum, other organs and structures (including mesentery, retroperitoneum, abdominal wall); infiltration of the pancreas only in the duodenum

- ▶ N1: 1 to 2 regional
- ▶ N2: ≥3 regional
- ▶ M1: Distant metastasis

Colon

Gastrointestinal Bleeding

Criteria	Upper gastrointestinal bleeding	Lower gastrointestinal bleeding
Frequency	90%	10%
Bleeding source	Oesophagus, stomach, duodenum	Small intestine, colon, rectum, anus
Symptomatology	Haematemesis, melena, drop in blood pressure, shock	Fresh blood per rectum, iron deficiency anaemia
Gastric tube aspirate	Bloody	Clear
Bowel sounds	Active	Normal
Diagnosis	Upper endoscopy	Colonoscopy, video capsule endoscopy, CT, angiography, scintigraphy

Intestinal Bleeding

- ▶ Aetiology
  - • Coagulopathies: Intestinal wall haematoma
  - • Inflammation, ulcer, diverticulum, trauma: Direct contrast extravasation, increased enhancement of areas of inflammation
  - • Tumour: Atypical vascular architecture, neovascularisation
  - • Angiodysplasia: Arteriovenous shunts, vascular tangles
- ▶ Endoscopic classification for upper GI bleeding—Forrest Classification
  - • I a: Spurting arterial bleed
  - • I b: Oozing bleed
  - • II a: Non-bleeding visible vessel
  - • II b: Adherent clot

- II c: Black ulcer base
- III: Clean ulcer base

▶ Localisation of the source of bleeding in the stomach by upper endoscopy, in the small intestine by video capsule endoscopy, in the large intestine by colonoscopy, and in the entire gastrointestinal tract by CTA

▶ Bleeding detection limit
- With CTA from 0.5 ml/min
- With selective angiography from 0.5–1 ml/min
- With scintigraphy from 0.2 ml/min
  - Detection of intermittent bleeding in the gastrointestinal tract with blood pool scintigraphy (99mTc erythrocytes)

▶ IR: Embolisation of bleeding point (microcoils, cyanoacrylate, particles)

Intestinal Ischaemia

▶ Aetiology
- Acute occlusive
  - Aetiology: Embolism, incarceration of bowel segments (volvulus, hernias), thrombosis
- Acute non-occlusive
  - Aetiology: Shock, hypotension, heart failure
- Chronic
  - Aetiology: Atherosclerosis

▶ Types
- Acute intestinal ischaemia
  - Initial stage: 0–6 hr; sudden abdominal pain, pronounced circulatory collapse
  - Latent stage: 6–12 hr; symptomless interval, dull abdominal pain
  - Final stage: 12–24 hr; paralytic ileus, bloody diarrhoea, increasing symptoms of shock, finally multi-organ failure
  - Often arrhythmia, atrial fibrillation, advanced age
  - Increased lactate, increased CRP, increased leukocytes

- Chronic bowel ischaemia
  - Postprandial abdominal pain
  - Loss of appetite, food intolerance, cachexia
  - Progressive intensity of symptoms
▶ Stages
  - I: Mucosal necrosis
  - II: Submucosal and muscular necrosis
  - III: Transmural necrosis
▶ Arterial occlusion: Superior mesenteric artery (mesenteric infarction), inferior mesenteric artery (watershed splenic flexure, ischaemic colitis), rarely coeliac trunk
▶ Symptoms depend on the collateral circulation (pancreatico-duodenal arcades between the coeliac trunk and the superior mesenteric artery, Riolan anastomosis between the superior mesenteric artery and the inferior mesenteric artery)
▶ **X-ray:**
  - Thumb-printing on the intestinal wall due to submucosal oedema
  - Segmental wall thickening
  - In case of infarction and necrosis—intramural gas accumulation
▶ **CT:**
  - Findings depending on severity, aetiology, pathogenesis, localisation and extension
  - Thickening of the intestinal wall
  - Thinning of the intestinal wall also possible
  - Intestinal dilatation
  - Mesenteric oedema
  - Ascites
  - Pneumatosis intestinalis—air in the bowel wall
▶ **CTA/Angio**
  - Occlusive
    - Arterial embolism: Filling defect within vessel
    - Arterial thrombosis: Irregular complete obstruction, often proximal in vessel
    - Venous thrombosis: Prolonged arterial phase, lack of typical venous course

- Non-occlusive
  - Segmental or diffuse vascular stenosis
  - Main stem/post-stenotic vascular dilatation
  - Limited enhancement in distal vascular branches
▶ **Differential Diagnosis**: Hollow organ perforation, acute pancreatitis, strangulated bowel obstruction
▶ **IR**—therapeutic options
- Acute occlusive bowel ischaemia: Embolectomy, pharmacological measures to improve perfusion or thrombolysis, stenting
- Acute non-occlusive bowel ischaemia: Pharmacological measures to improve perfusion
- Chronic intestinal ischaemia: Stent

Diverticulosis

▶ Aetiology: Acquired change with protrusion of the mucosa and submucosa through the muscularis to form diverticulae
▶ Most frequent locations are sigmoid colon and descending colon
▶ **Barium enema** (rarely now used)
- Barium filled or outlined outpouchings
- 'En face'—contrast pool with meniscus
▶ **CT**: Detection of colonic out-pouches due to diverticula
▶ **Complications**: Diverticulitis, perforation, abscess formation, fistula, obstruction, bleeding

Diverticulitis

▶ Most frequent location sigmoid colon and descending colon
▶ Inflammation from apex via base to surroundings
▶ Secondary processes from pericolic fat tissue via mesenteric fat tissue to peritoneum
▶ Hinchey Classification
- I: Pericolic abscess, limited to mesentery
- II: Paracolic abscess, exceeding the mesocolon
- III: Free perforation with generalised purulent peritonitis
- IV: Free perforation with generalised faecal peritonitis

▶ **US**
- Segmental and circumferential bowel wall thickening
- Diverticulum detection
  - Echo-bright with faecal residue within
  - Echo-poor with fluid within
- Abscesses
  - Encapsulated fluid
  - Often contains gas bubbles
- Echo-bright with faecal residue within peri-diverticulitis

▶ **CT**
- Thickening of the intestinal wall
  - >4 mm with stratification plane perpendicular to the axis of the intestinal segment
  - Circumferential involvement
- Intestinal wall enhancement
- Intestinal lumen narrowing
- Inflammation/streaking of the peri-colic and mesenteric fatty tissue
- Formation of abscesses
  - Pericolic fluid with peripheral enhancement, may contain air bubbles
  - Usually local, pericolic, mesenteric, Pouch of Douglas
- Thickening of the fasciae—eg Gerota fascia
- Air bubbles visible
  - Intramural, paracolic, peritoneal

▶ **Differential Diagnosis:** Colonic carcinoma, appendicitis, Crohn's disease, ulcerative colitis, pelvic inflammatory disease, endometriosis

▶ Occasional co-existence of diverticulitis and colon carcinoma, colonoscopy especially in the inflammation-free interval to exclude tumour

▶ **Complications:** Bleeding, perforation, fistula formation (colovesical, colovaginal, colouterine, colocolic), stenosis, obstruction

▶ **IR:** Abscess drainage, temporising stent for obstruction and haemostasis for bleeding

Ulcerative Colitis

▶ Aetiology: Chronic inflammatory bowel disease; mucosal inflammation; histologically, crypt architecture disorders and crypt abscesses
  - Continuous involvement of large bowel from rectum proximally, no skip lesions
  - In 10%: Backwash ileitis
▶ Abdominal pain (middle lower abdomen), diarrhoea (often bloody), nausea, loss of appetite, weight loss, fever
▶ **Barium enema** (rarely now used)
  - Mucosal erosions
  - Collar-stud ulcers
  - Pseudopolyps
  - Increased distance between sacrum and rectum due to fat proliferation in response to proctitis
  - Loss of haustral markings and normal mucosal detail
  - Lead pipe colon
  - Strictures
▶ **MR**
  - Thickening of the intestinal wall
  - Bowel wall oedema
  - Bowel wall enhancement
  - Loss of mucosal detail
▶ **Differential Diagnosis:** Bacterial colitis, parasitic colitis, antibiotic-induced pseudomembranous colitis, ischaemic colitis, post-radiation colitis
▶ **Diagnosis**: Colonoscopy (ulcerations, pseudopolyps) with biopsy
▶ **Complications**: Toxic megacolon, malignant transformation

Inflammatory Bowel Disease—Extra-Intestinal Associations

Can precede inflammatory bowel disease by many years
▶ Associations include
  - Skin: Erythema nodosum, pyoderma gangraenosum
  - Joints: Polyarthritis, sacroiliitis, ankylosing spondylitis
  - Kidneys: Amyloidosis

- Lungs: Interstitial fibrosis
- Liver: Autoimmune hepatitis
- Bile ducts: Cholelithiasis, primary sclerosing cholangitis, bile duct carcinoma
- Mouth: Aphthous ulcers (Crohn's disease)
- Eyes: Iridocyclitis, uveitis
- Vascular: Anaemia, thrombosis

Infectious Enteritis

▶ Aetiology:
- Proximal small bowel—giardiasis, strongyloides
- Distal small bowel—salmonella, shigella, yersinia,
- Distal ileum +/− caecum—Tuberculosis, typhlitis, amebiasis
▶ Diarrhoea, vomiting, abdominal cramps, fever
▶ CT/ US
- Intestinal wall thickening
- Reduced echogenicity of the intestinal wall on ultrasound/ reduced density with oedema on CT
▶ Barium follow through (Rarely now used)
- Rapid passage of injected contrast
- Fold thickening
- Poor mucosal coating and flocculated contrast medium due to increased liquid
▶ Complications: Dehydration, electrolyte imbalance

Pseudomembranous Colitis

▶ Aetiology: Antibiotics
▶ Occurrence usually about one week (up to eight weeks) after antibiotic therapy
▶ Fever, abdominal pain, diarrhoea
▶ Clostridioides difficile toxin in stool sample
▶ CT/US
- Left-sided predominance but whole colon can be involved
- Long segment of bowel affected

- Marked wall thickening
- Preserved wall stratification
- Significant hypervascularisation
- Thickened mucosa, submucosa

Radiation Colitis

▶ Aetiology: Post radiotherapy exposure
▶ Persistent diarrhoea, may be bloody
▶ US/CT
- Low echogenicity/low density concentric wall thickening
- Slightly thickened wall stratification
- Involvement limited to irradiated sections
▶ Diagnosis: Colonoscopy + pathology + history

Appendicitis

Position of free end of the appendix

▶ Pre-ileal—anterior to the terminal ileum—1 or 2 o'clock
▶ Post-ileal—posterior to the terminal ileum—1 or 2 o'clock
▶ Sub-ileal—parallel with the terminal ileum—3 o'clock
▶ Pelvic—descending over the pelvic brim—5 o'clock
▶ Sub-caecal—below the caecum—6 o'clock
▶ Para-caecal—alongside the lateral border of the caecum—10 o'clock
▶ Retro-caecal—behind the caecum—11 o'clock
▶ Stages of appendicitis
- Early, suppurative, gangrenous, perforated, phlegmonous, spontaneous resolving, recurrent, and chronic
▶ Abdominal pain
- Pain migrates from the epigastric/periumbilical region to the right lower abdomen
▶ Loss of appetite, nausea, pyrexia
▶ Abdominal guarding, maximal tenderness at McBurney point, psoas tension pain
- Characteristic signs
- Rebound tenderness (on releasing hand after deep palpation)

- Rovsing's sign (Pain in right iliac fossa when deep palpate left iliac fossa)
  - Douglas sign (rectal pain)
▶ Leukocytosis, CRP elevation,
  - Normal inflammatory parameters do not exclude acute appendicitis
▶ Scores for estimating the clinical probability of acute appendicitis (Appendicitis Inflammatory Response, Alvarado)
▶ Imaging techniques to reduce the number of negative appendectomies
▶ US
  - Acute appendicitis
    - Tubular structure
    - Non-compressible
    - Blind-ending
    - Thickened appendix wall
      - Appendix diameter greater than 6 mm
      - Appendix wall greater than 2 mm
    - Aperistalsis
    - Bulls-eye appearance—target lesion
    - Adjacent free fluid
    - Increased wall vascularisation
  - Perforated appendicitis
    - Inhomogeneous conglomerate mass
    - Local abscess formation
    - Adjacent or pelvic free liquid
  - Evaluation
    - Negative ultrasound findings do not exclude acute appendicitis
    - Positive ultrasound findings helpful if supporting clinical suspicion
    - More readily diagnosed in children and slim adults
▶ CT
  - Thickened appendix wall
  - Surrounding inflammatory change, fat stranding
  - Regional lymphadenopathy
  - Appendicolith

- Abscess
- Phlegmon

▶ **Differential Diagnosis**
- Right lower abdomen: Crohn's disease, diverticulitis, yersiniosis, ileocecal tuberculosis, intussusception, volvulus, Meckel's diverticulum
- Pelvis: Pelvic inflammatory disease, adnexal torsion, extrauterine pregnancy
- Upper abdomen: Cholecystitis, ulcer perforation, pancreatitis
- Retroperitoneum: Pyelonephritis, urolithiasis, psoas abscess
- Metabolic diseases: Diabetes mellitus, acute intermittent porphyria, sickle cell crisis

Epiploic Appendagitis

▶ Aetiology: Inflammatory change of an epiploic appendix, aseptic ischaemia with consequent necrosis of the pericolic fat tissue, causing torsion with venous thrombosis of the epiploic appendage
▶ Sudden onset of localised abdominal pain in the left or right lower abdomen
▶ Most frequent localisation on the sigmoid colon and descending colon
▶ **CT**
- Pericolic fat density nodule with high attenuation rim (high attenuation ring sign)
- Stranding in the adjacent adipose tissue
- Central hyperdense spot due to thrombosed vein
▶ **Differential Diagnosis:** Diverticulitis, appendicitis

Colon Polyps

▶ Types
- Benign
  - Hyperplastic polyps
  - Tubular adenomas
  - Villous adenomas

- – Tubulovillous adenomas
- – Juvenile polyps
- – Mesenchymal tumours
- Malignant
  - – Carcinoma
  - – Lymphoma (rare)
▶ CT colonography
- Prerequisites: Bowel cleansing, faecal tagging, colonic distension, narrow CT collimation, low-dose protocol
- Both supine and prone sequences acquired
- Diagnostic criteria: Lesion shape, lesion structure, contrast uptake, positional stability
▶ **Diagnosis**: Colonoscopy and biopsy for pathological confirmation

Colorectal Carcinoma

▶ Aetiology: Adenoma-carcinoma sequence
- Tubular adenomas: Common, lower risk of malignant change
- Villous adenomas: Uncommon, higher risk of malignant change
- Risk of malignant change depending on histology and size
▶ Adenocarcinoma, mucinous carcinoma
▶ Most commonly located in rectum, sigmoid colon, descending colon, caecum
▶ Occasionally synchronous carcinomas
▶ Symptoms
- Proximal carcinoma: Occult bleeding, anaemia, weight loss, palpable tumour
  - – May be misdiagnosed as appendicitis
- Distal carcinoma: Bleeding, paradoxical diarrhoea, mucus discharge
  - – May be misdiagnosed as haemorrhoids
▶ US
- Hypoechoic wall thickening
- Lack of wall layering

- Usually localised bowel involvement
- Prestenotic dilatation
- Post-stenotic collapsed lumen

▶ **Barium enema** (rarely now used)
- Ulcerating: Stenosis, overhanging edges (apple-core sign), broad mucosal ulcerations
- Polypoid: Mass, broad base, irregular contour

▶ **CT**
- To identify local eccentric thickening of the bowel wall/ colonic mass
- local staging; identifying complications such as obstruction, invasion or fistulation
- CT also used for identifying and staging distant metastasis
- Consider CT colonography to identify synchronous bowel tumours more proximally, especially if incomplete conventional colonography

▶ **Nuclear medicine**
- No PET-CT within four weeks after administration of systemic chemotherapy or antibody therapy (reduced sensitivity)

▶ **Diagnosis**: Colonoscopy and biopsy

Rectal Cancer

▶ Preserved meso-rectal fascia as a predictor of total meso-rectal excision of the tumour

▶ **MR**
- T-stage
- N-stage
- Minimum distance between the tumour any lymph node metastasis, satellite tumour deposit or extramural vascular tumour infiltration to the plane of resection
  - For tumours of the upper and middle third: The meso-rectal fascia
  - In the case of tumours of the lower third: The meso-rectal fascia, the sphincter apparatus and the levator ani muscle
  - Meso-rectal fascia involvement on MRI predicts positive resection margin

- To identify the presence of involvement of the circumferential resection margin
- To identify the presence of invasion beyond T3
- To identify to presence of extramural vascular infiltration

TNM Classification—Colonic and Rectal Cancer

▶ T1: Submucosa
▶ T2: Muscularis propria
▶ T3: Subserosa, non-peritoneal pericolic/perirectal tissue
▶ T4a: Visceral peritoneum
▶ T4b: Other organs and structures
▶ N1a: 1 regional
▶ N1b: 2 to 3 regional
▶ N1c: Satellites in sub-serosal fat or pericolic/perirectal tissue without regional lymph node metastases
▶ N2a: 4 to 6 regional
▶ N2b: ≥7 regional
▶ M1a: 1 organ
▶ M1b: >1 organ
▶ M1c: Peritoneum

TNM Classification—Cancer of Anal Canal

▶ T1: ≤2 cm
▶ T2: >2 cm to ≤5 cm
▶ T3: >5 cm
▶ T4: Neighbouring organs
▶ N1a: Cancer has spread to the ipsilateral inguinal (groin), perirectal (around the rectum), or internal iliac (pelvic) lymph nodes
▶ N1b: Cancer has spread to the external iliac (pelvic) lymph nodes
▶ N1c: Cancer has spread to the inguinal (groin), perirectal (around the rectum), or internal iliac (pelvic) lymph nodes, and to the external iliac nodes
▶ M1: Distant metastases

Carcinoid

- ► Neuroendocrine tumours
- ► Produce hormones such as serotonin, bradykinin and histamine
- ► Slow growing
- ► Common locations
  - Appendix
  - Small intestine
  - Colon
  - Stomach
  - Duodenum
- ► Carcinoid syndrome—due to hormone production
  - Diarrhoea, flushing, pain, asthma, endocardial fibrosis—hormones broken down in liver but syndrome occurs when metastasis to liver or beyond
- ► CT: Often contain calcifications, often calcified mesenteric nodal metastasis
- ► MR: T1 isointense, T2 hyperintense, strong enhancement
- ► Nuclear medicine: 68Ga-DOTATOC-PET

Bowel Obstruction

- ► Aetiology:
  - Small bowel: Adhesions from previous surgery, hernia, tumour, Crohn's disease, intussusception, abscess, congenital bands
  - Large bowel: Tumours, diverticular disease, volvulus, intussusception, inflammatory bowel disease, hernia
- ► Nausea, vomiting, abdominal cramps, constipation
- ► Active bowel sounds
- ► US
  - Dilated loops of intestine
    - Small intestine diameter >3 cm
    - Large intestine diameter >6 cm
    - Caecum >9 cm
  - Increasing ascites

▶ **X-ray/CT**
- Gas-containing distended intestinal loops with fluid level
- Bowel collapses distal to obstruction

▶ **Complication**: Intestinal necrosis, perforation

Paralytic Ileus

▶ Aetiology: Peritonitis, electrolyte disturbance, protein deficiency, arterial occlusion, venous occlusion, vasculitis, shock, post-surgery

▶ Absence of bowel sounds

▶ **US**
- Small intestine diameter >3 cm
- Large intestine diameter >6 cm
- Caecum >9 cm
- Non-peristaltic bowel

▶ Imaging features very similar to obstructive ileus. Clinical findings and history are key in differentiating the two

Ogilvie Syndrome

▶ Aetiology: Acute pseudo-obstruction of the colon of unknown aetiology, occurring mainly after trauma or surgery and in the presence of inflammation or tumours

▶ Older patients

▶ Initially painless, later painful significant distension of the abdomen, nausea, vomiting

▶ **X-ray**
- Massive dilatation of the colon, especially the caecum and the right-sided colon
- Colonic contrast enema with water-soluble contrast medium for diagnostic and therapeutic indication

▶ **Complications**: Ischaemia, perforation, peritonitis

Abdominal Cavity

Acute Abdomen

▶ Aetiology
- Abdominal
  - Peritonitic: Appendicitis, adnexitis, ulcer perforation, pancreatitis
  - Mechanical: Obstruction, choledocholithiasis, urolithiasis, pseudo-obstruction
  - Vascular: Thromboembolism, aneurysm dissection, sickle cell anaemia
  - Traumatic: Abdominal trauma, intra-abdominal haemorrhage
- Extra-abdominal
  - Thoracic: Myocardial infarction, pulmonary embolism, pneumonia
  - Genital: Testicular and ovarian torsion
- Metabolic
  - Endogenous: Uraemia, ketoacidosis, acute intermittent porphyria, Addison's crisis, haemolysis
  - Exogenous: Poisoning e.g. lead

▶ Severe abdominal pain, peritonitis, acute circulatory collapse, disturbed peristalsis of the intestine, poor general condition

▶ Acute abdomen of the elderly patient occasionally oligosymptomatic or asymptomatic

▶ Subsiding pain after initial severe pain: Mesenteric ischaemia or after perforation (with signs of peritonitis)

▶ Vascular causes of acute abdomen are common, especially in older patients

▶ Diagnosis:
- CT, US
  - Cause of acute abdomen is often diagnosed on CT
  - Free intra-abdominal fluid (pericolic, in Morrison's pouch or Pouch of Douglas)

Ascites

▶ Aetiology: Liver cirrhosis, portal vein thrombosis, peritoneal carcinomatosis, peritonitis, right heart failure, pancreatitis, extrauterine pregnancy, ovarian carcinoma, hypoalbuminaemia, renal failure
▶ Free or loculated
▶ Special types
  • Congenital ascites (newborn)
  • Haemorrhagic ascites (haemoperitoneum)
  • Chylous ascites (chyloperitoneum)
  • Bilious ascites
  • Malignant ascites (peritoneal carcinomatosis)
▶ Localisation
  • Perihepatic
  • Perilienal
  • Pouch of Douglas
  • In the flanks/paracolic
  • Between the intestinal loops
▶ US: Mostly anechoic liquid
▶ X-ray: Centralised and distant intestinal loops
▶ CT: Fluid in abdomen/pelvis

Mesenteritis

▶ Idiopathic process with heterogeneous clinical presentation
▶ Types
  • Mesenteric lipodystrophy
  • Mesenteric panniculitis
  • Retractile mesenteritis
▶ CT
  • Mesenteric lipodystrophy
    – Detection of fat necrosis
  • Mesenteric panniculitis
    – Diffuse increase in density of the affected mesentery (hazy mesentery)

- – Preservation of fat around mesenteric vessels on background of diffuse fat stranding (fat halo sign, or fat ring sign)
- – Enlarged lymph nodes
- – Thin pseudo-capsule around the affected mesentery
- – Space-occupying effect on neighbouring intestinal loops

▶ **Differential Diagnosis**: Lymphoma, liposarcoma

Mesenteric Cysts

▶ Mesenteric lymphangioma
▶ Mesenteric cysts
▶ Mesenteric pseudocysts
▶ Enteric cysts
▶ Omental cysts

Omental Infarct

▶ Causes: Embryological variant of the blood supply of the right-sided omentum
▶ Torsion of the omentum
  - • Primary: Idiopathic
  - • Secondary: Hernias, focal inflammation, tumours, previous laparotomy
▶ **US**: Anechoic, non-compressible, oval mass at site of maximum tenderness
▶ **CT**
  - • Entire spectrum from discrete focal omental fat stranding to larger circumscribed masses
  - • Spherical, whorled, mass around a vascular structure, usually in the right upper quadrant
▶ **Differential Diagnosis**: Epiploic appendagitis—usually in the left lower quadrant

Abscesses

▶ Causes: Surgery, perforation, intestinal inflammation
▶ Location
- Subphrenic
- Subhepatic
- Pouch of Douglas
- Between bowel loops
- Retrocolic

▶ Paralytic ileus, regional peritonitis, leukocytosis
▶ US
- Circumscribed avascular hypoechoic mass which may contain hyperechoic debris
- Occasional bubbles of gas may be present

▶ X-ray (Not usually helpful)
- Soft tissue mass
- Abnormal pockets of gas out with the bowel
- Diaphragmatic elevation
- Pleural effusion
- Basal pneumonia

▶ Diagnosis: US, CT
▶ IR: Drainage
- Indications
  - Unilocular abscess
  - No septa
  - Safe access
  - Demarcated abscess cavity
  - Drainable content
- Drainage is successful when there is resolution of fever, leucocytosis and abscess cavity

Postoperative Fluid Collections

▶ Seroma: Accumulation of peritoneal fluid
▶ Lymphocele: After lymph vessel injury
▶ Bilioma: After Bile duct injury
▶ Urinoma: After ureteral injury

Peritoneum

Pneumoperitoneum

▶ Free gas in the peritoneum
▶ Causes: Surgery, perforation of a hollow viscus laparoscopy
▶ **X-ray**
   • Erect CXR: Air under the diaphragm
   • Decubitus AXR in left lateral position: Air between liver and abdominal wall
▶ Lateral decubitus AXR is more sensitive
▶ **Differential Diagnosis**: Chilaiditi syndrome (mimicker of free gas under diaphragm: Normal gas in colon lying between liver and diaphragm on AXR)
▶ **Diagnosis**: CT is most sensitive imaging test. It may also identify the cause

Peritonitis

▶ Causes
   • Primary (Bacterial) peritonitis
     – Haematogenous spread
     – Risk factors—cirrhosis with ascites, nephrotic syndrome, immunosuppression
   • Secondary peritonitis
     – Perforation
     – Postoperative
     – Post-interventional
     – Post-traumatic
     – Transmigratory (eg via peritoneal dialysis)

▶ Acute abdomen, tenderness and guarding, rigid abdomen
▶ Systemic manifestations and causes
  • Peritoneal oedema → hypovolaemic shock
  • Bacteraemia → septic shock
▶ Organ failure: Lungs, liver, kidney, heart, circulation, adrenal gland
▶ US: Abnormal fluid accumulation in the abdomen
▶ CT
  • Ascites
  • Dilatation of the mesenteric vessels
  • Increase in density of mesenteric fat
  • Enhancement of the peritoneal layers
  • Thickening of the intestinal wall

Peritoneal Carcinomatosis

▶ Causes: Carcinomas of stomach, pancreas, colon, breast, ovary, uterus, bladder
▶ Peritoneal soft tissue deposits
▶ US/CT/MR
  • Imaging findings
    – Nodular thickening of the peritoneum
    – Plaque-like thickening of the viscera
    – Linear or nodular thickening of the mesentery and serosa
    – Nodular thickening of the greater omentum—omental cake
    – Mucinous masses within the abdomen or pelvis
  • Ascites
  • Mesenteric adhesions
  • Often liver metastases
  • Lymph node metastases
  • Specific associations
    – Ovarian carcinoma: Peritoneal deposits may calcify
    – Ovarian cystadenocarcinoma: Pseudomyxoma peritonei possible

Hernias

▶ Protrusion of abdominal viscera (hernial contents) into perito-
  neal outpouching (hernial sac)
▶ Types
  • Indirect inguinal hernia (lateral to the inferior epigastric
    vessels)
  • Direct inguinal hernia (medial to the inferior epigastric ves-
    sels)
  • Femoral hernia—medial to femoral vein—more common
    in females
  • Obturator
  • Spigelian—anterior abdominal wall adjacent to semilunar
    line, at lateral border of rectus abdominis muscle
  • Lumbar hernia—through superior (more common) or infe-
    rior lumbar triangle
  • Richter hernia—contains only one wall of bowel so does
    not obstruct—but can strangulate
  • Internal hernias
    – Rare
    – Closed loop
    – Types include para-duodenal, small bowel mesentery
      related, great omentum related, transverse mesocolon
      related, lesser sac, Roux-en-Y anastomosis related
    – Post surgery (intestinal/mesenteric)
▶ Clinical diagnosis
▶ In the case of mechanical obstruction of uncertain cause, incar-
  cerated internal hernia is a potential cause
▶ US/CT/MRI: Detection of fascial defect and content
  • I: Maximum width of the hernial orifice <1.5 cm
  • II: Maximum width of the hernial orifice 1.5–3 cm
  • III: Maximum width of the hernial orifice >3 cm
  • CT is most helpful in acute presentation

Retroperitoneum

Pneumoretroperitoneum

▶ Free gas in the retroperitoneum
▶ Causes: Duodenal, sigmoid or rectal perforation
▶ **X-ray/CT**:
  • Air along the psoas edges, fascia and vessels
  • In contrast to intraperitoneal air, air in retroperitoneum is static with patient positional change
  • Most reliably detectable when lying down
▶ **Diagnosis**: CT is most helpful

Retroperitoneal Haematoma

▶ Causes
  • Trauma
  • Leaking aortic aneurysm
  • Surgery
  • Clotting disorders
  • Anticoagulation
▶ Non-specific symptoms, back/flank pain, may be in shock
▶ Haemorrhage may enter the peritoneum if dorsal peritoneum is ruptured
▶ **Diagnosis**: CT

Retroperitoneal Fibrosis

▶ Causes: Idiopathic retroperitoneal fibrosis (Ormond's disease); secondary as a result of or in combination with aneurysms, autoimmune diseases, IgG4-related disease, vasculitides, medications
▶ Fibrosis in the retroperitoneal space
▶ Non-specific back and flank pain, feeling of pressure in flanks

▶ **CT/MR**
- Periaortic soft tissue proliferation
- Begins distal to the renal vessels
- Extends to peri-iliac region
- Strong enhancement in active phase
- Features suggestive of malignancy
    - Retro-aortic and supra-renal involvement
    - Enlarged lymph nodes

▶ **CT urography/MR urography**
- Medial deviation of ureters
- Tapered narrowing of ureters
- Prestenotic dilatation of ureters

▶ **Nuclear medicine**: 18F-FDG-PET—usually FDG uptake

▶ **Differential Diagnosis**: Lymphoma, Sarcoma

▶ **Diagnosis**: Percutaneous biopsy

▶ **Complications**: Ureteric obstruction, venous thrombosis, renal failure

Retroperitoneal Tumours

▶ Causes: Lipoma, liposarcoma, leiomyoma, leiomyosarcoma, fibroma, fibrosarcoma, neurofibroma, neuroblastoma and extragonadal germ cell tumours, adrenal tumour

▶ Presentation: Palpable tumour, abdominal pain, loss of appetite, weight loss, constipation, flank pain, neurological deficits

▶ **X-ray**
- Indistinct psoas contour
- Displaced ureters

▶ **CT/MR**: Mass with imaging features suspicious for malignancy: Irregular borders, infiltrative growth, abnormal enhancement

▶ **Diagnosis**: Percutaneous biopsy

Paediatric Radiology: Oesophagus, Stomach, Small Intestine, Colon

Gastrointestinal Atresia

▶ Oesophageal atresia
- Often in combination with VACTERL association or Down syndrome
- Associated malformations of the cardiovascular and gastro-intestinal systems
- Foetal hydramnios, white frothy bubbles in infant's mouth, choking, aspiration
- Immediate regurgitation of feed, coughing when feeding
- **X-ray**
  - Warning: Risk of contrast aspiration
  - Often present in combination with distal tracheoesopha-geal fistula, whereupon air in also seen in the stomach
- **Complications**: Aspiration, pneumonia

▶ Pyloric atresia
- Projectile vomiting soon after feeding
- Spectrum from web to gap between stomach and duodenum
- **X-ray**
  - Gas filled distended stomach
  - Remainder of intestine is gasless

▶ Duodenal atresia
- Bilious vomiting
- **X-ray**
  - Double bubble sign—air-filled stomach and duodenum
  - Distal intestine airless

▶ Small bowel atresia
- Causes: Meconium ileus, ileum atresia, rotational anomaly
- **X-ray**
  - Dilatation and fluid level of the loops of the small intes-tine proximal to the site of atresia
  - No haustrated colon levels
- **Complications**: Obstruction

▶ Imperforate Anus
- May be simultaneously present with fistulas (urinary bladder, urethra, vagina, perineum)
- **X-ray**: Plain radiograph in head-down or prone position with a metal coin at the perineum to demonstrate the distance between rectum and anticipated anal canal to determine level of atresia

VATER Association

▶ Combination of malformations
- Vertebral anomaly
- Anal atresia
- Tracheoesophageal fistula
- Oesophageal atresia
- Renal anomaly

▶ Occurrence also as VACTERL association (vertebral, anal, cardiac, tracheal, oesophageal, renal, limb anomalies)

Hirschsprung's Disease

▶ Cause: Congenital deficiency of enteric ganglion cells in submucosal plexus and myenteric plexus
▶ Congenital megacolon
▶ Large bowel affected in variable degrees extending proximally from anus
- Short-segment and long segment forms
▶ Mostly boys, mostly rectosigmoid
▶ Absence of peristalsis in the aganglionic segment, colonic dilatation proximal to the aganglionic segment, impaired faecal transport in the aganglionic segment
▶ Delayed meconium discharge, distended abdomen, solid intractable constipation, vomiting, ileus, shock
▶ **X-ray**
- Stool-impacted intestinal loops
- Funnel-shaped transition zone into the megacolon
- Often fluid level

► **Diagnosis**: Histological examination of deep biopsies
► **Complications**: Enterocolitis, intestinal perforation, sepsis

Pyloric Stenosis

► Aetiology: Hypertrophy of the pyloric circular muscles
► Presents in the 2nd to 12th week of life
► Especially boys, firstborns, premature babies
► Postprandial pain, projectile vomiting, hypochloraemic alkalosis
► Weight loss, dehydration, pseudo-constipation
► **US**
  • Thickening of the pylorus diameter >4 mm
  • Lengthening of the pyloric canal >14 mm
► **X-ray**
  • Distended stomach
  • Paucity of intestinal air
► **Differential Diagnosis**: Hiatus hernia

Necrotising Enterocolitis

► Causes: Shock, asphyxia, hypoxia
  • Ischaemia → Intestinal wall damage → Bacterial invasion → Inflammation → Necrosis → Perforation → Peritonitis
► Most frequent cause of acute abdomen in the early infant period
► Bilious vomiting, distended abdomen, thin stools, metabolic acidosis
► **US/X-ray**
  • I (early stage): Dilated intestinal loops—lethargy, abdominal distension
  • II (definite NEC): Pneumatosis intestinalis, portal vein gas, mild to moderately ill
  • IIIa (late stage): As above plus ascites, patient shocked
  • IIIb (surgical stage): As above plus pneumoperitoneum due to perforation

Intussusception

▶ Intussusception is a paediatric emergency, usually ileocolic, ileocaecal or ileoileal
▶ 90% of patients between 2 months and 2 years old
▶ Persistent crying, colicky pain, peritonitis and rectal bleeding in the course of 24–48 h
▶ US
  • Rounded mass—concentric rings of bowel wall and internal hyperechoic mesenteric fat
  • Proximal intussusceptum closely surrounded by distal intussuscipiens (bowel-in-bowel appearance)
    – In longitudinal section—pseudokidney sign
    – In cross-section—target sign
  • Peristalsis proximal to the intussusception
  • Free fluid >50%
▶ Fluoroscopic (contrast enema): Claw sign
▶ In the first 6 hours high chance reducing intussusception (hydrostatic or pneumatic)
▶ Contraindications for conservative reduction of intussusception
  • Intestinal perforation
  • Hypovolemic shock
  • Peritonitis
▶ Differential Diagnosis: Food poisoning, gastroenteritis, Henoch-Schönlein purpura

Meckel's Diverticulum

▶ 20–120 cm proximal to the ileocecal valve opposite the mesenteric attachment
▶ Most common cause of massive rectal bleeding in childhood
▶ Other symptoms include periumbilical pain, massive intestinal bleeding
▶ Could be a lead point for intussusception, can result in volvulus or diverticulitis
▶ Nuclear medicine
  • 99mTc pertechnetate
  • Excretion through serous and mucinous glands

- Visualisation of the physiological and ectopic gastric mucosa
- Reasons for false negative Tc Scan
  - Intussusception
  - Arteriovenous malformations
  - Ulcers

▶ **Complications**: Obstruction, intussusception, ulcer, bleeding, perforation

Gluten-Sensitive Enteropathy

▶ Celiac disease, sprue
▶ Aetiology: Remodelling of the mucosa of the small intestine with villous atrophy, crypt elongation and malabsorption
▶ Presentation: Failure to thrive, weight loss, diarrhoea, fatty stools, iron deficiency, anaemia, loss of appetite
▶ Clinical normalisation under gluten-free diet
▶ **Barium follow through/MRI**
- Number and height of jejunal folds reduced (colonisation of the jejunum)
- Increased number and height of ileum folds (jejunisation of the ileum)
- Accelerated bowel transit
▶ **Diagnosis**: Serology (transglutaminase antibodies, endomysium antibodies), small intestine biopsy

Liver, Biliary Tree, Pancreas, Spleen

Anatomy

Liver

▶ Liver segments
- Right liver
  - Anteromedial: Cranial segment VIII, caudal segment V
  - Posterolateral: Cranial segment VII, caudal segment VI
- Left liver
  - Anterior: Segment IV (quadrate lobe), segment III
  - Posterior: Segment II
- Caudate lobe
  - Segment I

▶ Porta hepatis
- Common hepatic duct
- Portal vein
- Common hepatic artery

▶ Arteries
- Common hepatic artery
  - Cystic artery
  - Right branch
  - Left branch

▶ Veins
- Right hepatic vein

© The Author(s), under exclusive license to Springer Nature   177
Switzerland AG 2026
D. Pickuth, J. T. Murchison, *Pocket Guide to Radiology*,
https://doi.org/10.1007/978-3-031-76520-9_5

- Middle hepatic vein
- Left hepatic vein

▶ Topography
- Diaphragm
- Oesophagus
- Stomach
- Gallbladder
- Duodenum
- Colonic flexure
- Transverse colon
- Kidney
- Right adrenal gland

▶ Portosystemic collaterals
- Oesophageal vein and gastric veins (cardia region)—azygos vein and hemiazygos vein
- Oesophageal and gastric veins (cardia region) and left gastric vein—inferior phrenic vein
- Splenic vein—retroperitoneal veins (inferior phrenic vein, renal veins, adrenal vein, abdominal wall veins)
- Left branch of the portal vein—umbilical veins—epigastric veins
- Middle colic vein—left colic vein—testicular/ovarian vein—left renal vein
- Left colic vein—superior rectal vein—middle and inferior rectal veins—internal pudendal vein—iliac veins
- Small mesenteric veins—retroperitoneal veins—inferior vena cava
- Intrahepatic branches of the portal vein—phrenic vein
- Portal vein—lumbar veins, adrenal and renal veins

Biliary Tree

▶ Gallbladder
- Fundus
- Body
- Infundibulum
- Neck

► Bile ducts
  • Right hepatic duct
  • Left hepatic duct
  • Common hepatic duct
  • Cystic duct
  • Common bile duct
► Variants
  • Intrahepatic gallbladder
  • Medial insertion of the cystic duct crossing anterior to the hepatic duct
  • Medial insertion of the cystic duct crossing posterior to the hepatic duct
  • Low insertion of the cystic duct

Pancreas

► Sections
  • Head
  • Body
  • Tail
► Excretory ducts
  • Main pancreatic duct, Wirsung → major papilla
  • Accessory duct (if present), Santorini → minor papilla
► Arterial supply
  • Coeliac trunk
  • Superior mesenteric artery
► Lymph nodes
  • Splenic lymph nodes (tail)
  • Pancreatic lymph nodes (body)
  • Pancreaticoduodenal lymph nodes (head)
► Topography
  • Duodenum
  • Common bile duct
  • Mesenteric vessels
  • Splenic vessels
  • Transverse mesocolon
  • Stomach

- Small intestine
- Left kidney
- Spleen

Spleen

▶ Size
- About 4 cm thick
- About 7 cm wide
- About 11 cm long
- If over 14 cm enlarged
▶ Arteries
- Splenic artery
▶ Veins
- Splenic vein
▶ Topography
- Stomach
- Kidney
- Colon
- Pancreatic tail

Liver

Steatosis

▶ Aetiology: Alcohol, diabetes, hepatitis, ischaemia, obesity, anorexia, medication
▶ Types
- Alcoholic fatty liver disease (AFLD)
- Metabolic dysfunction-associated steatotic liver disease (MASLD)
- Alcoholic steatohepatitis (ASH)
- Metabolic dysfunction-associated steatohepatitis (MASH)
▶ Non-alcoholic fatty liver disease (NAFLD) and non-alcoholic steatohepatitis (NASH) as hepatic manifestations of the metabolic syndrome, association with obesity

► Classification of steatosis
  • Grade I: <33% of hepatocytes with fatty degeneration
  • Grade II: 33–66% of hepatocytes with fatty degeneration
  • Grade III: >66% of hepatocytes with fatty degeneration
► Asymptomatic or feeling of fullness, weakness, lethargy
► Imaging manifestation as diffuse or focal steatosis or focal fatty sparing
► Focal steatosis or focal fatty sparing
  • Especially in the regions of the gallbladder fundus, branching portal veins, falciform ligament, vena cava, liver dome
  • Geographic borders
  • Absent mass effect
► US
  • Enlarged liver
  • Convex rounded contours
  • Obtuse-angled rim
  • Hyper-reflectivity
► CT
  • Hypoattenuating
► MR
  • T1 Signal increase
  • T2 Signal increase
  • Signal drop on opposed-phase (in/out-of-phase) imaging
  • Quantification of fat concentration with the proton density fat fraction and MRS
► Diagnosis: Liver biopsy to assess the extent of pure steatosis, the combination of steatosis and inflammatory activity, and the presence of fibrosis
► Complications: Liver cirrhosis

Viral Hepatitis

► Aetiology: Hepatitis viruses
  • A: Faecal-oral transmission, acute course, good prognosis; foreign travel
  • B: Parenteral transmission, chronic course, poor prognosis; drug abuse, foreign travel, health-care professionals

- C: Parenteral transmission, gradual progression, poor prognosis; drug abuse, health-care professionals
- D: Parenteral transmission, chronic course, poor prognosis; haemophiliacs
- E: Faecal-oral transmission, acute course, good prognosis; foreign travel

▶ Jaundice, fatigue, loss of appetite
▶ US/CT/MR
- Hepatomegaly
- Gallbladder wall thickening
- Periportal lymphoedema
- Lymph node enlargement
- Regenerative nodules
▶ Exclusion of biliary obstruction by MRCP

Liver Cirrhosis

▶ Aetiology
- Viral: Hepatitis B, hepatitis C, hepatitis D
- Toxic: Alcohol
- Autoimmune: Primary biliary cirrhosis, autoimmune hepatitis
- Bacterial: Secondary biliary cirrhosis
- Metabolic: Haemochromatosis, Wilson's disease
- Functional: Hepatic vena cava syndrome, constrictive pericarditis
▶ Liver skin signs: Spider naevi, fissured tongue, gynaecomastia, body hair loss, striae, collateral veins, palmar erythema, Dupuytren's contracture, white nails, finger clubbing, jaundice, ascites, collateral circulation
▶ US/CT/MR
- Hepatomegaly in early stages, shrunken liver in late stage
- Hypertrophied left lobe and caudate lobe
- Rounded rim, plump shape
- Irregular contours

- Heterogeneous, coarsened echotexture
- Thin hepatic veins with irregular calibre
- Widening of the fissures and the porta hepatis, regenerative nodules
- Additional findings
  - Splenomegaly
  - Portosystemic collaterals
  - Ascites
  - Pericaval fat deposits
- ► **Colour Doppler US:** Portal venous flow may be hepatofugal
- ► **US or MR elastography** for identification and quantification of liver fibrosis and cirrhosis
- ► Classification of lesions in the cirrhotic liver according to LIRADS criteria
- ► **Complications:** Ascites, oesophageal variceal haemorrhage, hepatic encephalopathy, hepatocellular carcinoma

Haemochromatosis and Haemosiderosis

- ► Types
  - Primary: Haemochromatosis (iron deposition in hepatocytes)
  - Secondary: Haemosiderosis (iron deposition in Kupffer cells of the liver, spleen and bone marrow)
- ► Men > women
- ► Hepatomegaly, liver cirrhosis, splenomegaly, arthropathy, cardiomyopathy, pancreatic fibrosis, hyperpigmentation, diabetes, testicular atrophy, impotence
- ► **CT:** Increased liver attenuation
- ► **MR:** T1 low signal, T2 low signal, in haemosiderosis also low signal spleen
  - Quantification of the iron concentration with the signal intensity ratio method and the relaxometry method with determination of R2 and R2* values
- ► **Complication:** Hepatocellular carcinoma

Cystic Liver Disease

► Congenital liver cysts
  • Asymptomatic
  • **US:** Anechoic, round or oval shape, smooth wall, posterior acoustic enhancement
  • **CT:** Fluid density lesions, no enhancement
  • **MR:** T1 very low signal, T2 very high signal, no enhancement
  • **Differential Diagnosis:** Post-traumatic cyst, Hydatid disease (Echinococcus)
► Von Meyenburg complexes
  • Biliary hamartomas
    – Proliferated bile ducts with cystic dilatations
    – No connection to the biliary system
    – Associated with polycystic liver disease
    – Asymptomatic
    – Multiple
  • **MR**
    – Multiple 1 mm to 1 cm diameter foci
    – Subcapsular or intraparenchymal localisation
    – T2 hyperintense
  • **Differential Diagnosis:** Caroli disease (cystic dilatation of the intrahepatic bile ducts)
► Hydatid disease (echinococcosis)
  • Aetiology: Echinococcus granulosus, dog tapeworm, end host dog
  • Natural cycle: Dog—sheep—dog
  • Structure
    – Endocyst consisting of inner germinative membrane and outer laminar membrane
    – Germinative membrane forms vesicles (brood capsules) by budding, which contain protoscolices (larval form)
    – Pericyst forms (outer layer) as a reaction of the host to the infection
  • Stages
    – Group 1: Active stage; growing cysts, vital protoscolices safe

- Group 2: Involvement stage; degenerating cysts, vital protoscolices still probable
    - Group 3: Inactive stage; calcified cysts, vital protoscolices unlikely
- Symptoms of a space occupying process
- **US/CT:** Cysts, daughter cysts, septa, calcifications
- **Complication**: In case of ruptured hydatid anaphylactic reaction

▶ Alveolar liver echinococcosis
- Aetiology: Echinococcus multilocularis, fox tapeworm, end host fox
- Natural cycle: Fox—rodent—fox
- Symptoms of a space occupying process
- Lymphatic or haematogenous spread possible
- **US/CT:** Solid mass, cystic parts, infiltrative growth, amorphous calcifications, perifocal enhancement, hilar lymph nodes
- **Complication**: Cyst rupture, anaphylaxis

▶ Pyogenic liver abscess
- Aetiology
    - Bile ducts: Ascending cholangitis (mostly multiple abscesses)
    - Septicaemia: Via portal vein from abdominal sepsis or hepatic artery, from systemic infection eg SBE
    - Local spread: Perforated gastric ulcer, perforated duodenal ulcer, lobar pneumonia, pyelonephritis
    - Trauma: From accident, biopsy, surgery
- Fever, pain, nausea, loss of appetite, weight loss
- **X-ray:** Diaphragmatic elevation, pleural effusion, atelectasis
- **US:** Echo-poor mass, gas inclusions, fluid level
- **CT:** Hypodense mass, rim enhancement, double target sign (abscess cavity—hyperdense inner ring (abscess membrane)—outer hypodense, oedematous parenchymal ring), gas inclusions, segmental liver enhancement
- **Differential Diagnosis:** Amoebic abscess, secondary infected necrotic liver metastases, echinococcus cysts
- **IR:** Drainage

► Non-pyogenic liver abscess
  • Amoebic abscess
    – **US**: Often solitary occurrence, often right liver lobe, partly infiltrative growth
    – **Complication**: Rupture of abscess
  • Mycotic abscess
    – Candida, Aspergillus, Cryptococcus
    – **US**: Multilocular occurrence
  • Schistosomal abscess
    – **US**: Ligamentous periportal fibrosis

Liver Haemangioma

► Women more often than men
► Solitary or multiple
► **US**
  • Typically hyperechoic, sharply circumscribed mass
  • Change in echogenicity due to thrombosis, fibrosis, calcification, haemorrhage and necrosis
    – In dynamic contrast-enhanced sonography—centripetal filling
    – **Differential Diagnosis**: Hyperechoic metastasis, hepatocellular carcinoma if there is known liver cirrhosis
► **CT**
  • Hypodense mass
  • Iris sign (centripetal, from peripheral to central)
  • Early discontinuous, peripheral nodular enhancement with progressive 'filling-in'
► **MR**
  • T1 low signal
  • T2 very high signal-rich and smoothly circumscribed
  • Light bulb sign (signal increasing with increasing T2 weighting)
  • On early images—iris diaphragm sign (centripetal, enhancement from peripheral to central), on late images—pooling sign (complete homogeneous enhancement)
  • On SPIO T2—slight enhancement

▶ **Nuclear medicine**
- Colloid scintigraphy (99mTc colloid): Storage defect
- Blood pool scintigraphy (99mTc erythrocytes): Perfusion phase low storage, blood pool phase high storage
- 18F-FDG-PET: Negative FDG uptake

Focal Nodular Hyperplasia

▶ Women, young to middle age
▶ Mostly solitary
▶ US: Isoechoic, often subtle, rarely pedunculated
- In dynamic contrast-enhanced sonography, arterial hyper-vascularisation, centrifugal filling (from inside out) and sometimes central scarring
▶ CT
- Hypodense mass
- Early arterial enhancement
- Early washout
- Central scar in 60% >3 cm, enhances late
▶ MR
- T1 isointense
- T2 isointense with hyperintense scar
- Early arterial enhancement, early washout, central scarring
- Scar with enhancement on late images
- With hepatobiliary contrast agents, enhancement persists to be hyperintense to the background liver
- On SPIO T2—enhancement with prominent hyperintense scar
▶ **Nuclear medicine**
- Colloid scintigraphy (99mTc colloid): Increased or normal uptake
- Liver function scintigraphy (99mTc—HIDA): Perfusion phase increased uptake, parenchymal phase foci similar to normal tissue, excretion phase prolonged enhancement

Hepatic Adenoma

▶ Classification—Bordeaux (2006)
  • Type I: Inflammatory (I-HCA) most common, highest bleed rate
  • Type II: Hepatocellular adenoma inactivated for HNF-1alpha (H-HCA), least common, women, oral contraceptives, often multiple, contain fat
  • Type III: Beta catenin activated hepatocellular adenoma (beta-HCA), least common, highest men, anabolic steroids, glycogen storage disease, FAP
  • Type IV: Unclassified
  • Type V: Newly classified, Sonic hedgehog-activated hepatocellular adenoma (sh-HCA)
▶ Often not possible to diagnose with certainty
  • Hepatic adenoma most frequent hepatic tumour in young women on the oral contraceptive pill
▶ US: Solitary well demarcated heterogeneous mass, variable echogenicity
▶ CT
  • Generally isodense mass
  • Variable and hyperdense if haemorrhage components or hypodense if higher fat content
  • Calcification can be seen in old haemorrhage
  • Ruptures
▶ MR
  • T1 iso- to hyperintense signal (fat content), signal decrease with fat suppression sequences in H-HCA subtype
    – Fat detection important criterion in differential diagnosis to other liver lesions
  • T2 iso to mildly hyper intense, I-HCA have hyperintense rim (atoll sign)
  • Strong enhancement in the arterial phase, isodense by portal venous phase, usually hypointense late phase with hepatobiliary contrast agents cf. FNH
  • Following SPIO T2 slight enhancement
▶ Complications: Hepatocellular carcinoma, risk of haemorrhage (27%) with larger adenomas and subcapsular location

Nodular Regenerative Liver Hyperplasia

▶ Aetiology: Seen in idiopathic/non cirrhotic portal hypertension, systemic diseases, steroids, chemotherapeutic agents, IBD, coeliac disease
▶ Nodular liver remodelling with numerous regenerative foci (normal hepatocytes) without fibrotic component
▶ Nodule size—a few millimetres to a few centimetres
▶ **Diagnosis:** Difficult, non hyper-enhancing, biopsy often required
▶ **Differential Diagnosis:** Regenerative nodules of liver cirrhosis, liver metastases

Hepatocellular Carcinoma

▶ Aetiology: Liver cirrhosis, chronic hepatitis, steatohepatitis, haemochromatosis, aflatoxin
▶ Types
  • Solitary hepatocellular carcinoma (50%)
  • Multifocal hepatocellular carcinoma (40%)
  • Diffuse hepatocellular carcinoma (10%)
▶ Men, Asian and African ethnicity
▶ Nonspecific symptoms, occasionally palpable mass, progressive liver insufficiency
▶ AFP often raised (75%)
▶ **US:** Hypoechoic (early stage) to hyperechoic mass with hypoechoic rim focal fat sparing (late stage)
  • Imaging of liver tumour microvascularisation with dynamic contrast-enhanced sonography
    – Arterial phase: Hypervascular
    – Portal venous phase: Normalises to background
    – Late venous phase: Wash-out
    – **Differential Diagnosis:** Liver metastases (rapid washout), intrahepatic cholangiocarcinoma (later enhancement, less enhancement, faster washout)
  • Washout in late-stage in liver tumours is suspicious of malignancy

► **CT**
- Hypodense
- In the case of strongly vascularised tumours, hyper-enhancing in the early phase and hypo-enhancing in the late phase
- Protracted enhancement in weakly vascularised tumours
- **Differential Diagnosis**: Transient hepatic attenuation differences (THADs), cirrhosis of the liver with regenerative nodules

► **MR**
- T1 variable, hypointense, isointense or hyperintense (intra-tumoural fat)
- T2 moderately hyperintense
  - "Nodule in nodule"
- Diffusion restriction
- Arterial hyperenhancement
- Portal venous washout
- Tumoural capsules
- Size progression
- On SPIO T2, depending on the degree of differentiation, little or no enhancement
  - Classification according to LIRADS
- **Differential Diagnosis**: Transient hepatic intensity differences (THID), liver cirrhosis with regenerative nodules

► **Angio**
- Hypervascularisation
- Blush pattern
- Irregular vessels
- Arteriovenous shunts

► **IR management**
- Local ablative procedures
  - Thermal ablation (microwave ablation, radiofrequency ablation)
  - Hepatic intra-arterial chemotherapy (HAI)
  - Transarterial chemoembolisation (TACE)
  - Selective intra-arterial radiotherapy (SIRT)

▶ Microwave ablation
- Principle: Oscillation of polar water molecules by electro-magnetic waves
- Mode of action: Coagulation necrosis due to heat
- Ablation time: About 5 min
- Ablation defect: Greater than radiofrequency ablation
- Ablation limit: Very sharp
- Heat sink effect: Present

▶ Radiofrequency ablation
- Principle: Ion agitation through high-frequency current flow
- Mode of action: Coagulation necrosis due to heat
- Ablation time: About 15 min
- Ablation defect: <5 cm
- Ablation boundary: Rather blurred
- Heat sink effect: Pronounced

Fibrolamellar Carcinoma

▶ Young adults, non cirrhotic
▶ Better prognosis than hepatocellular carcinoma
▶ US: Variable echogenicity, smooth border, central calcifications
▶ CT: Isodense, heterogeneous enhancement, calcifications
▶ MR
- T1 iso- to hypointense
- T2 hyperintense
- Early arterial heterogeneous enhancement and iso/hypointense on portal venous and delayed phases
- Central scar, septa
- Scar with or without enhancement on late images
▶ Differential Diagnosis: Focal nodular liver hyperplasia (more homogeneous and T2 hyperintense scar)

TNM Classification Liver Cancer

▶ Hepatocellular carcinomas
  • T1a: Solitary ≤2 cm with/without vascular invasion
  • T1b: Solitary >2 cm without vascular invasion
  • T2: Solitary >2 cm with vascular invasion, multiple ≤5 cm
  • T3: Multiple >5 cm
  • T4: Larger branches of the portal vein, hepatic veins, neighbouring organs (except gallbladder), visceral peritoneum
  • N1: Regional
  • M1: Distant metastases

Liver Metastases

▶ Aetiology: Colon carcinoma, stomach carcinoma, pancreatic carcinoma, breast carcinoma, bronchial carcinoma
▶ Solitary or multiple, focal or diffuse, expansive or infiltrative
▶ Preoperative determination of number, size and segment localisation
▶ US: Hypoechoic, hyperechoic lesions, hypoechoic halo—bull's eye or target lesions
▶ CT
  • Hypodense mass pre and post contrast administration
  • In hypervascular metastases (carcinoid, islet cell tumour, phaeochromocytoma, renal cell carcinoma)—early phase hyper-enhancing, late phase iso-enhancing
▶ MR
  • T1 hypointense
  • T2 slightly hyperintense, but less so than haemangiomas, hyperintense rim
  • Hypo-vascular metastases: After contrast enhancement-hypointense or isointense, on late images peripheral washout with hypointense rim
  • Hyper-vascularised metastases: Arterial enhancement after contrast agent application
  • On SPIO T2—no enhancement

▶ **IR**

- Local ablative procedures
  - Thermal ablation (microwave ablation, radiofrequency ablation)
- Locally effective procedures
  - Hepatic intra-arterial chemotherapy (HAI)
  - Transarterial chemoembolisation (TACE)
  - Selective intra-arterial radiotherapy (SIRT)

Chemoembolisation of Liver Tumours

▶ Principle
- Slowed capillary passage time of therapeutically active agents
- Tumour hypoxia

▶ Procedure
- Aortography
  - Visualisation of all hepatic arteries
- Splenoportography
  - Patency of the portal vein
- Selective visualisation of all existing hepatic arteries
- Selective catheterisation of the hepatic arteries supplying the tumour
- Chemoembolisation
  - cTACE: Occlusion of the capillaries by lipiodol, Chemotherapeutic agent, Occlusion of the arterioles by particles
  - DEB-TACE: Drug eluting beads
  - DSM-TACE: Soluble starch microspheres
- Checks on completion
  - Visualisation of reduced arterial inflow to the target area
  - Display of the opacification of the tumour
  - Preserved arterial supply to the non-treated area

▶ Variations
- Combination of chemoembolisation with thermoablation
- Use of 90Y instead of chemotherapeutic agents
- Combination of 90Y with immune checkpoint inhibitors

▶ Treatment response in hepatocellular carcinoma depends on tumour type, tumour size and stage of cirrhosis

▶ **Complications**: Non-target embolisation of other organs, post embolisation syndrome, access site haematoma, arterial dissection, abscess formation of the liver, deterioration of liver function

Liver Circulation Disorders

▶ Arterial
- Aneurysm of the hepatic artery
  - Polyarteritis, atherosclerosis, congenital, post-traumatic, pancreatitis, cholecystitis
- Infarct
  - Rare—due to dual vascularity
- Intrahepatic portal venous gas (often peripheral v biliary tree more central)
  - Intestinal infarction, inflammatory bowel disease, haemorrhagic pancreatitis, portal vein intervention

▶ Hepatic veins
- Congestion
  - Chronic heart failure, constrictive pericarditis
- Budd-Chiari syndrome
  - Aetiology: Coagulopathies, neoplasms, trauma, pregnancy, web
  - Primary or secondary occlusion of the intrahepatic or supra-hepatic veins
  - Hepatomegaly, ascites
  - **Complications**: Liver cirrhosis

▶ Portal venous
- portal hypertension when portal vein pressure is elevated above 8 mm Hg
- Types
  - Prehepatic: Portal vein thrombosis
  - Intrahepatic presinusoidal: Primary biliary cirrhosis
  - Intrahepatic intrasinusoidal: Steatohepatitis, liver cirrhosis

- Intrahepatic postsinusoidal: Veno-occlusive disease
- Posthepatic: Chronic heart failure, Budd-Chiari syndrome, constrictive pericarditis

- **US/CT/MR**
  - Hepatofugal collaterals (gastro-oesophageal, paraumbilical, retroperitoneal, mesenteric, gastrorenal, splenorenal)
  - Hepatopetal collaterals (periportal veins with cavernous transformation)
  - Hepatosplenomegaly
  - Ascites
  - Oesophageal varices
  - Fundal varices
  - T1 Gandy gamna bodies (haemosiderin deposits) as hypointense foci of a few millimetres in size in the liver and spleen
- **Splenoportography**
  - Patency and flow direction of the portal vein
  - Type of collaterals
  - Course and size of the splenic vein and the left renal
  - Closing pressure of the hepatic veins

Transjugular Intrahepatic Portosystemic Shunt

▶ TIPSS
▶ Connection between hepatic vein and portal vein for portal pressure reduction
▶ Indications
  - Elective insertion after recurrent variceal bleeding despite adequate therapy
  - Elective insertion for uncontrollable ascites
  - Elective or emergency insertion for Budd-Chiari syndrome
  - Emergency insertion for bleeding uncontrollable by endoscopic or pharmacological management
▶ Contraindications
  - Absolute: Liver failure, chronic mesenteric occlusion, advanced hepatocellular carcinoma, severe pulmonary hypertension, cardiac failure
  - Relative: Sepsis, arterial stenosis, severe obstructive lung disease

▶ **Complications**: Shunt dysfunction, encephalopathy, hepatic failure, coma, haemorrhage

Liver Trauma

▶ Aetiology: Blunt or penetrating liver trauma
▶ Types
  • Capsule injury
  • Parenchyma tear
  • Subcapsular haematoma
  • Active bleeding
▶ Liver most frequently injured organ after spleen and kidneys
▶ Most commonly right lobe of the liver
▶ **Diagnosis**: US, CT
▶ **Complications**: Bleeding, bile duct injuries
▶ **IR**: Embolisation

Paediatric Radiology: Liver

Liver Tumours

▶ Infantile hepatic haemangioma (Haemangioendothelioma)
  • Most common benign liver tumour in childhood
▶ Hepatoblastoma
  • Most frequent liver tumour in childhood
  • <4 years, boys
  • Mass effect, AFP elevation, thrombocytosis
  • Association with hemihypertrophy, familial adenomatous polyposis, renal anomalies
  • **CT/MR**: Heterogeneous mass with necrosis, haemorrhages, calcifications, septae

Metastasis

▶ **Differential Diagnosis**: Neuroblastoma, Wilms tumour, lymphoma

Biliary Tree

Bile Duct Cysts

▶ Todani classification
- I: Segmental dilatation of the common bile duct (choledochal cyst)
- II: Diverticular, saccular dilatation of the common bile duct (choledochal diverticulum)
- III: Saccular herniation of the common bile duct into the duodenum (choledochocele)
- IV: Multiple intra- and extrahepatic bile duct cysts
- V: Intrahepatic bile duct cysts (Caroli disease)

Cholelithiasis

▶ Aetiology: Fat, female, fertile, forty, parity
▶ Preliminary stages
- Sludge formation
- Cholesterol polyps
▶ More commonly cholesterol rather than pigment stones
▶ Symptom-free or biliary colic

Mirizzi Syndrome

▶ Compression of the common hepatic duct by a hydropic gallbladder or calculus in the gallbladder neck
▶ US
- Echogenic focus
- Posterior acoustic shadowing
- Mobile
- Differential Diagnosis: Polyp, tumour (non-mobile)
▶ Complications: Gallbladder hydrops, cholecystitis, gallbladder empyema, choledocholithiasis, cholangitis, pancreatitis, gallstone ileus

Gallstone Ileus

▶ Aetiology: Stone migration through cholecyst-enteric fistula resulting in small bowel obstruction
▶ US/X-ray: Pneumobilia and small bowel dilatation

Cholestasis

▶ Types
  • Extrahepatic cholestasis
  • Intrahepatic cholestasis
▶ Pale stools, dark urine, pruritus, jaundice
▶ US: Dilated common bile duct >6 mm (>10 mm after cholecystectomy)

Choledocholithiasis

▶ Biliary colic, icterus, concomitant pancreatitis
▶ US
  • Echogenic focus, acoustic shadowing
  • Cholestasis
▶ MRCP: Signal void in CBD
  • Differential Diagnosis: Vascular impression, sphincter contraction, mucosal fold, pneumobilia, polyp, sludge
▶ Complications: Cholangitis, pancreatitis

Acute Cholecystitis

▶ Types
  • Acalculous cholecystitis
  • Calculous cholecystitis
  • Emphysematous cholecystitis
▶ Upper abdominal pain, fever, leukocytosis
▶ US
  • Gallbladder dilatation
  • Thickened gallbladder wall
  • Oedematous gallbladder wall
  • Pericholecystic fluid
  • Usually gallstones

- Often sludge
- Tender on palpation
  - Murphy sign positive
▶ **Differential Diagnosis**: Appendicitis, pancreatitis, myocardial infarction, renal colic, gastric ulcer, mesenteric ischaemia, pulmonary embolism, pleurisy
▶ **Complications**: Gallbladder empyema, haemorrhagic cholecystitis, emphysematous cholecystitis, gallbladder perforation

Gallbladder Empyema

▶ **US**
- Similar appearance to acute cholecystitis, sometimes with increased luminal content
- Echogenic material in the gallbladder (cell detritus, pus, cholesterol crystals)

Chronic Cholecystitis

▶ Non-specific upper abdominal pain
▶ **US**
- Small volume gallbladder
- Thickened gallbladder wall
- Gallbladder wall calcification (porcelain gallbladder)
- Large volume gallstones
- Poor gallbladder contractility

Pneumobilia

▶ Aetiology: Gallstone perforation with cholecyst-enteric fistula, emphysematous cholecystitis, hepaticojejunostomy, sphincterotomy
▶ **Complications:** Gallstone ileus if due to gallbladder perforation and cholecyst-enteric fistula

Primary Sclerosing Cholangitis

▶ Aetiology: Chronic disease of the bile ducts with diffuse inflammation and fibrosis

▶ Both intra- and extrahepatic bile ducts affected
▶ Associated with Crohn's disease, ulcerative colitis, retroperitoneal fibrosis, mediastinal fibrosis and various autoimmune diseases
▶ Fatigue, signs of cholestasis, upper abdominal discomfort, febrile episodes
▶ **MR/MRCP**
  • Calibre irregularities of the bile ducts
  • Beading/stricturing bile duct wall
  • Wall thickening of the bile ducts
  • Enhancement of the bile duct wall
  • Enlargement of the caudate lobe
  • Lymphadenopathy at the porta hepatis
▶ **Differential Diagnosis**: Cholestatic liver diseases, secondary sclerosing cholangitis
▶ **Diagnosis**: Biopsy
▶ **Complications**: Cholangitis, choledocholithiasis, liver cirrhosis, liver failure, gallbladder carcinoma, bile duct carcinoma

Biliary Stricture

▶ Aetiology: Mostly iatrogenic following cholecystectomy
▶ Intermittent episodes of jaundice and cholangitis
▶ **Diagnosis**: MRCP
▶ **Complications**: Secondary biliary cirrhosis of the liver, portal hypertension

Sphincter of Oddi Stenosis

▶ Aetiology: Duodenitis, stone passage, sphincterotomy, Sphincter of Oddi dilatation
▶ **Complications**: Biliary duct dilatation, chronic obstructive pancreatitis, secondary sclerosing cholangitis

Gallbladder and Bile Duct Tumours

▶ Gallbladder wall thickening
  • Benign: Cholesterolosis, adenomyomatosis (deep Rokitansky-Aschoff sinus associated with marked tunica muscularis hyperplasia), gallbladder polyps

- Malignant: Gallbladder carcinoma,
  - Adenocarcinoma >90%, squamous ~3%
  - Most common in elderly females, gallstones usually present
  - Increased risk with porcelain gallbladder
  - Aggressive form with irregular margins, less aggressive lobular form

▶ Bile duct
  - Aetiology: Chronic cholangitis, parasitic liver disease, congenital biliary tract anomalies
  - Painless occlusive jaundice, Courvoisier's sign, no history of gallstones
  - Benign: Adenoma, papilloma, lipoma
  - Malignant: Cholangiocarcinoma (intrahepatic, Klatskin tumour, extrahepatic)
    - Classification of Klatskin tumours according to Bismuth
    - I: Common hepatic duct
    - II: Hepatic bifurcation
    - III: Up to the segmental outlets, infiltration of the right hepatic branch (III a), infiltration of the left hepatic branch (III b)
    - IV: Both branches of the common hepatic duct (IV a), beyond the segmental branches and common bile duct (IV b)
  - **MR/MRCP**
    - Lobulated mass
    - No capsule
    - T1 hypointense
    - T2 sometimes hypointense (high fibrous stroma)
    - Low enhancement
    - Intrahepatic biliary dilatation, retracted liver capsule
  - **Differential Diagnosis**: Primary sclerosing cholangitis, bile duct gallbladder debris
  - **Diagnosis**: ERCP, endoscopic ultrasound, SpyGlass cholangioscopy, brushings for cytology, endoscopic biopsy
  - **IR**: Percutaneous transhepatic tumour recanalisation, percutaneous transhepatic stent implantation, percutaneous biliary drainage

TNM Classification Gallbladder and Bile Duct Tumours

▶ Gallbladder and cystic duct
- T1a: Mucosa
- T1b: Muscular wall layer
- T2a: Perimuscular connective tissue on the peritoneal side
- T2b: Perimuscular connective tissue on the liver side
- T3: Serosa, liver, neighbouring organs
- T4: Portal vein, common hepatic artery, ≥2 neighbouring organs
- N1: 1 to 3 regional
- N2: ≥4 regional
- M1: Distant metastases

▶ Intrahepatic bile ducts
- T1a: Solitary ≤5 cm without vascular invasion
- T1b: Solitary >5 cm without vascular invasion
- T2: Solitary with vascular invasion, multiple with/without vascular invasion
- T3: Visceral peritoneum
- T4: Extrahepatic structures
- N1: Regional
- M1: Distant metastases

▶ Perihilar bile ducts
- T1: Bile duct wall
- T2a: Beyond the bile duct wall
- T2b: Liver
- T3: Unilateral branches of the portal vein or hepatic artery
- T4: Main branch of the portal vein or bilateral branches, main branch of the common hepatic artery or bilateral branches, unilateral second order bile ducts with infiltration of contralateral branches of the portal vein or hepatic artery
- N1: 1 to 3 regional
- N2: ≥4 regional
- M1: Distant metastases

▶ Distal extrahepatic bile ducts
- T1: Bile duct wall ≤5 mm
- T2: Bile duct wall >5 mm to ≤12 mm
- T3: Bile duct wall >12 mm

- T4: Coeliac trunk, superior mesenteric artery, common hepatic artery
- N1: 1 to 3 regional
- N2: ≥4 regional
- M1: Distant metastases

► Ampulla of Vater
- T1a: Only ampulla Vateri or sphincter Oddi
- T1b: Beyond the sphincter Oddi, submucosa of the duodenum
- T2: Muscularis propria of the duodenum
- T3a: Pancreas up to ≤5 mm
- T3b: Pancreas >5 mm, peripancreatic tissue
- T4: Coeliac trunk, superior mesenteric artery, common hepatic artery
- N1: 1 to 2 regional
- N2: ≥3 regional
- M1: Distant metastases

MRCP of the Extrahepatic Bile Ducts

► Anatomical representation
- MRCP allows reliable imaging of all sections of the extrahepatic bile ducts, including Calot's triangle; the normal calibre and prepapillary common bile duct are also adequately imaged
- Main advantages of MRCP are lack of contrast agent application, lack of radiation exposure, short examination time, lack of invasiveness and lack of complications

► Lumen width
- The bile duct width determined during MRCP corresponds to the measurements made during sonography, intraoperative cholangiography and CT
- With MRCP, the bile ducts are imaged in their physiological state

► Normal variants
- With MRCP, normal variants of the bile duct anatomy are already reliably recorded preoperatively, so that exact surgical planning is possible

- MRCP has the potential to reduce the rate of intraoperative cholangiography and iatrogenic bile duct injury

▶ Choledocholithiasis
  - MRCP is the gold standard in the diagnosis of choledocholithiasis
  - MRCP detects bile duct stones with a similarly high sensitivity and specificity as sonography detects gallbladder stones
  - MRCP enables an immediate decision on therapy if a stone is detected, without the need for further procedures to confirm the diagnosis
  - If choledocholithiasis is suspected, there is no longer an indication for diagnostic ERCP or intraoperative cholangiography after stone exclusion by MRCP
  - If a diagnosis of choledocholithiasis has already been made sonographically, MRCP is unnecessary, as sonography has a high specificity
  - Interventions on the bile ducts remain reserved for ERCP

▶ Cholangitis
  - MRCP is suitable for checking the success of therapy in acute bacterial cholangitis
  - In primary sclerosing cholangitis, MRCP and conventional MR reveal very characteristic findings up to the third-order intrahepatic bile ducts
  - MRCP is suitable for primary diagnostics and progress monitoring

▶ Bile duct tumours
  - MRCP is indicated in patients with suspected bile duct tumours; both proximal and distal masses can be reliably detected and characterised
  - If a tumour is detected, conventional contrast-enhanced MR with MRA should be followed to clarify tumour stage and resectability
  - The indication for diagnostic ERCP remains, if necessary for biopsy

▶ Bile duct cysts
  - Bile duct cysts of all types can be safely visualised with MRCP; this also applies to the strictures of the common hepatic duct often associated with the cysts

- MRCP is also suitable for the visualisation of neonatal bile duct anatomy and the diagnosis of neonatal jaundice
▶ Postcholecystectomy syndrome
  - The biliary causes of a postcholecystectomy syndrome are easily detectable with MRCP; the most common finding is a long cystic stump
  - Iatrogenic bile duct injuries and hepaticojejunostomy anastomoses can be reliably clarified or assessed with MRCP

Paediatric Radiology: Biliary Tree

Biliary Atresia

▶ Absence of, or significant deficiency of the extrahepatic biliary tree
▶ From the 3rd week of life, increasing jaundice, dark brown urine, pale stools, severe hepatomegaly, increasing failure to thrive
▶ US: Gallbladder not visible even when fasting
▶ Nuclear Medicine: Absence of excretion of radionuclides into the intestine at 24hrs
▶ Differential Diagnosis: Neonatal hepatitis (sonographically identifiable functional gallbladder with excretion of radionuclides into the intestine)
▶ Complications: Biliary cirrhosis of the liver

Pancreas

Malformations of the Pancreas

▶ Pancreas divisum
  - Fusion anomaly with lack of fusion of the ventral and dorsal anlages so that there is no connection between duct of Wirsung (ventral pancreatic duct) and duct of Santorini (dorsal pancreatic duct)
  - Higher incidence of acute pancreatitis

- **MRCP**: Horizontal crossing of the middle or distal bile duct by the dorsal pancreatic duct to drain into the minor papilla
▶ Annular pancreas
  - Circular course of the pancreatic parenchyma and duct around the duodenum
  - Duodenal stenosis, bilious vomiting, concomitant pancreatitis
▶ Partial pancreatic agenesis

Pancreatic Changes with Age

▶ Pancreatic lipomatosis
▶ Pancreatic fibrosis
▶ Pancreatic atrophy

Pancreatic Cysts

▶ Pseudocysts
▶ Retention cysts
▶ Parasitic cysts
▶ Dysontogenetic cysts
▶ Cystic pancreatic tumours

Acute Pancreatitis

▶ Aetiology: Cholelithiasis, alcohol, medication, hyperlipidaemia, hypercalcaemia, mumps, vasculitis, trauma, ERCP
▶ Types
  - Interstitial oedematous pancreatitis
  - Necrotising pancreatitis
  - Haemorrhagic pancreatitis
▶ Spread of the peripancreatic fluid in the anterior pararenal space cranially and caudally, also into the omental bursa and the transverse mesocolon
▶ Upper abdominal pain radiating to the back

▶ Vomiting, feeling sick, meteorism, ileus, fever, shock
▶ **US**
- Enlarged pancreas
- Hypo-echo areas internally (oedematous)
- Anechoic shadows
- Blurred outline
- Peripancreatic fluid

▶ **CT/MR**
- Enlarged pancreas with indistinct contours
- Hypodense (exudate), isodense (parenchyma) and hyperdense (haemorrhages) areas
- Non-enhancing parts, necrotic areas
- CT grading of severity based on Balthazar score
  - Grade A: Normal pancreas
  - Grade B: Swollen, enlarged pancreas
  - Grade C: Inflammatory changes of the pancreas and peripancreatic fat
  - Grade D: Solitary, poorly defined single peripancreatic fluid collection
  - Grade E: Two or more poorly defined peripancreatic fluid collections

▶ **Complications**
- Abscess
  - especially in the case of extensive parenchymal necrosis
  - **CT**: Hypodense collection, foci of gas
- Pseudocyst
  - 10–20% of all patients
  - In acute necrotising pancreatitis, there is usually no connection to the pancreatic duct
  - After an acute episode of chronic pancreatitis often connection to the pancreatic duct
  - Expansion of the pancreatic fluid via ligaments of the upper abdomen, atypical location in liver, spleen and large gastric curvature possible
  - **Complications**: Biliary duodenal obstruction, pancreatico-enteric fistulae
  - **IR**: Percutaneous, endoscopic via the stomach or surgical drainage

- • Haemorrhage
    - – Aetiology: Splenic artery erosion, splenic artery pseudoaneurysm, splenic vein thrombosis
- • Spleen
    - – Perisplenic fluid
    - – Splenic vein thrombosis
    - – Splenic infarction
    - – Subcapsular haemorrhage
- ▶ Fat necrosis
- ▶ Sepsis
- ▶ Multi-organ failure

Chronic Pancreatitis

- ▶ Aetiology: Alcohol, gallstones, autoimmune, radiotherapy
- ▶ Upper abdominal pain, mid-abdominal pain, weight loss, nausea, vomiting, steatorrhoea
- ▶ In the final stage, irreversible damage to the exocrine and endocrine pancreatic function
- ▶ US/CT/MR
    - • Strictures and calibre variations of the pancreatic duct
    - • Calcifications, usually multiple and small
    - • Parenchymal atrophy
    - • Cambridge classification by means of MRCP or ERCP
        - – Stage I: Normal main duct, <3 pathological side branches
        - – Stage II: Normal main duct, ≥3 pathological side branches
        - – Stage III: Pathological main duct, ≥3 pathological side branches
        - – Stage IV: Pathological main duct, ≥3 pathological side branches, cysts, duct stones, strictures, neighbouring organs involved
- ▶ Differential Diagnosis: Pancreatic carcinoma
- ▶ Complications
    - • Pseudocysts
        - – 30% of all patients
        - – Egg-shell wall calcification possible

– Retention cysts in chronic pancreatitis with internal connection to the pancreatic duct
- Pancreatic carcinoma
- Biliary strictures
- Duodenal stenosis
- Gastrointestinal bleeding
- Splenic vein thrombosis
- Fistulae

Cystic Pancreatic Tumours

▶ Serous cystic neoplasia (SCN)
- Mostly women, about 60 years
- Types
  - Microcystic: Pancreatic body, pancreatic tail; no ductal connection; innumerable microcysts; radial fibrous septa; enhancement in the late phase; central scar with or without central calcification; sponge-like (cysts peripherally larger than centrally), honeycomb-like (cysts peripherally and centrally the same size)
  - Oligocystic: Pancreatic head; no duct connection; few macrocysts
- Cyst content after FNA: Amylase normal, mucin ↓, CEA normal
- Almost always benign
- Management: Monitoring
▶ Mucinous cystic neoplasia (MCN)
- Almost exclusively women, about 50 years
- Preference for pancreatic tail
- No duct connection, macrocystic or unilocular, few single cysts
- Cyst content according to FNA: Amylase normal, mucin ↑, CEA normal or ↑
- Often malignant
- Suspected malignancy
  - Cyst size >3 cm
  - Mural tumour nodules
  - Peripheral eggshell calcifications
- Management: Resection

▶ Intraductal papillary mucinous neoplasia (IPMN)
  • Mostly men, about 60 years
  • Cystic, mucus-forming tumour originating from the ductal epithelium
  • In contrast to serous and mucinous cystic neoplasms where there is no connection to the ductal system
  • Can lead to the development of pancreatic fibrosis and pancreatic atrophy
  • Types
    – Main duct type: Pancreatic head > body > tail; duct connection; macrocystic; cystic main duct dilatation
    – Side-branch type: Head and uncinate process; ductal connection; microcystic; 'bunch of grapes' like cyst formations
    – Mixed type: Appears as advanced side branch lesion with main duct dilatation >5mm
  • Cyst content according to FNA: Amylase ↑, mucin ↑, CEA ↑ or ↑↑
  • Main branch type often malignant, side branch type variable
  • Suspected malignancy
    – Main duct type
    – Duct expansion >5 mm
    – Cyst size >2 cm
    – Contrast enhancing solid nodules
    – Mass around the pancreatic duct
    – Dilated common bile duct
    – Intraluminal calcifications
    – Lymphadenopathy
  • Management
    – Main duct type: Resection
    – Side branch type: Differentiated (risk factors, malignancy signs)
  • **Differential Diagnosis**: Pseudocyst (cyst contents after FNA: amylase ↑↑, mucin ↓, CEA normal)
▶ Solid pseudopapillary neoplasia (SPN)
  • Almost exclusively women, ~30 years
  • Found in all pancreatic sections

- No ductal connection, mixed solid-cystic mass lesion
- Cyst content after FNA: Amylase normal, mucin normal, CEA normal
- Mostly benign
- Management: Resection

Pancreatic Carcinoma

▶ Aetiology: Ductal Adenocarcinoma
▶ Especially pancreatic head
▶ Papillary tumours with slower growth, metastasis later and better prognosis
▶ Weight loss, jaundice, abdominal pain, indigestion
▶ **Endoscopic US**: Sensitive method for detecting small pancreatic tumours, locoregional staging
▶ **US**
  - Bulging contour
  - Low-echo internal structure
  - Dilated pancreatic duct
  - Vascular infiltration
▶ **CT**
  - Hypodense mass after IV contrast enhancement
  - Loss of pancreatic lobulation
  - Deformity of the pancreatic contour
  - Distal pancreatic atrophy
  - Dilatation of the pancreatic duct
  - Dilatation of the bile duct
  - Doughnut sign due to vessel encasement
▶ **MR**
  - T1 hypointense, T2 variable
  - In the early phase mild enhancement, in the late phase moderate enhancement
  - Ill-defined organ contour
  - Peripancreatic oedema
▶ **MRCP**
  - Blunt cut-off of the pancreatic duct
  - Double duct sign in pancreatic head carcinoma (obstruction of pancreatic duct and bile duct at tumour level)

▶ **MRA**
- Vascular involvement
- Calibre variations and intraluminal tumour thrombus to diagnose vascular infiltration
- Vascular encasement measured in degrees (0°, 90°, 180°, 270°, 360°)

▶ Lymph node metastases, liver metastases, peritoneal carcinomatosis, ascites

▶ Inoperability in case of distant metastases (liver, distant lymph nodes, peritoneum), infiltration of neighbouring organs (stomach, transverse colon, spleen) and vascular infiltration (coeliac trunk, hepatic artery, mesenteric artery, mesenteric vein, portal vein)

▶ **IR**: Coeliac nerve block for analgesia

TNM Classification Pancreatic Malignancy

▶ T1a: ≤0.5 cm
▶ T1b: >0.5 cm to ≤1 cm
▶ T1c: >1 cm to ≤2 cm
▶ T2: >2 cm to ≤4 cm
▶ T3: >4 cm
▶ T4: Involvement of coeliac axis, superior mesenteric artery or common hepatic artery
▶ N1: 1 to 3 regional
▶ N2: ≥4 regional
▶ M1: Distant metastases

Pancreatic Endocrine Tumours

▶ Carcinoid syndrome
- Serotonin as the active hormone
- Diarrhoea, flushing, pain, asthma, endocardial fibrosis
▶ Insulinoma
- Insulin as the active hormone
- Hypoglycaemic symptoms, central nervous disorders, reduced performance, long-term weight gain

- **Endoscopic US**: Sensitive method for detecting small pancreatic tumours
- **CT**: Hyper-enhancing mass in the arterial phase
- **MR**: T1 hypointense, T2 hyperintense, complete enhancement in smaller tumours, peripheral enhancement in larger tumours
- **Diagnosis**
  - Intra-arterial calcium stimulation test
  - Transhepatic peripancreatic venous blood sampling

▶ Gastrinoma
  - Zollinger-Ellison syndrome
  - Gastrin as the active hormone
  - Pain, ulcers, diarrhoea, steatorrhea, reflux oesophagitis
    - Atypically located, multiple, therapy-resistant, often recurrent ulcers

▶ VIPoma
  - Aka Verner-Morrison syndrome
  - Vasoactive intestinal polypeptide as the active hormone
  - Hypokalaemia, watery diarrhoea, dehydration

▶ Glucagonoma
  - Glucagon as the active hormone
  - Diabetes, necrolytic migratory erythema, weight loss

▶ Somatostatinoma
  - Somatostatin as the active hormone
  - Cholelithiasis, diarrhoea, steatorrhoea, diabetes

▶ **Nuclear Medicine**: 68Ga-DOTATOC-PET, 18F-FDG-PET

Pancreatic Trauma

▶ Aetiology: Commonly steering wheel contusion with bruising or compression of the organ between the steering wheel and the spinal column

▶ Types
  - Parenchymal contusion, indistinct region of oedema
  - Parenchyma laceration, discrete linear tear
  - Parenchymal transection, full-thickness tear
  - Parenchymal comminution (fracture), shattered pancreas,

▶ Often initially asymptomatic
▶ **Complications**: Pancreatitis, necrosis, pseudocysts, ductal strictures, aneurysms, fistulae

---

Spleen

Splenic Variants

▶ Asplenia
▶ Polysplenia
▶ Splenunculus
  • Localisation commonly in the region of the spleno-pancreatic or gastro-splenic ligaments
  • Blood supply via branches of the splenic artery
  • After splenectomy, increase in size up to the original spleen size possible
  • **US/CT/MR**
    – Iso-echoic, isoattenuating or isointense to the spleen
    – Spherical, smooth-edged, homogeneous mass
  • **Nuclear medicine**: Detection of splenunculi with blood pool scintigraphy (99mTc erythrocytes)
  • **Differential Diagnosis**: Splenosis
▶ Wandering spleen

Splenomegaly

▶ Congestive
  • Splenic vein thrombosis
  • Portal hypertension
  • Right heart failure
▶ Neoplasia
  • Sarcoma
  • Leukaemia
  • Lymphomas
  • Metastases

▶ Infection
  • Viral: Infectious mononucleosis, hepatitis
  • Bacterial: Sepsis, endocarditis
  • Parasitic: Malaria, histoplasmosis
▶ Haematological
  • Hereditary spherocytosis
  • Sickle cell disease
  • Thalassaemia
▶ Connective tissue disease
▶ Sarcoidosis
▶ Amyloidosis
▶ Storage diseases

Splenic Changes in Haematological Diseases

▶ Leukaemia: Splenomegaly
▶ Myelofibrosis: Splenomegaly
▶ Polycythaemia: Splenomegaly, splenic infarcts
▶ Sickle cell disease: Splenomegaly initially, splenic infarcts, later small, calcified spleen
▶ Thalassaemia: Splenomegaly, iron deposits
▶ Paroxysmal nocturnal haemoglobinuria: Iron deposits
▶ Idiopathic thrombocytopenic purpura: Splenomegaly

Splenic Changes in Systemic Diseases

▶ Rheumatoid arthritis: Splenomegaly
▶ Amyloidosis: Splenomegaly, splenic rupture
▶ Wegener's granulomatosis: Splenic infarctions
▶ Polyarteritis nodosa: Splenic artery aneurysms, splenic rupture, splenic abscesses
▶ Gaucher's disease: Splenomegaly, splenic infarcts, splenic fibrosis
▶ Haemosiderosis: Iron deposits
▶ Systemic lupus: Splenomegaly, splenic atrophy, splenic calcifications

Splenic Calcification

► Infarction, haematoma, vascular calcification
► Cysts
► Post-infectious "starry sky"
► Hamartoma
► Tuberculosis, histoplasmosis, brucellosis

Splenic Infarction

► Aetiology
  • Endocarditis
  • Atrial fibrillation
  • Sickle cell disease
  • Leukaemia
  • Pancreatitis
  • Vasculitis
► Branches of the splenic artery are end arteries, so that occlusion results in ischaemia/infarction
► Enlargement of the infarct due to simultaneous occlusion of the splenic vein
► US/CT/MR
  • Wedge-shaped area
  • Extends to the capsule
  • Well-demarcated
► Complications: Abscess, rupture, bleeding

Splenic Abscess

► Solitary
  • Endocarditis, sepsis, trauma
► Multiple
  • Candidiasis, aspergillosis, cryptococcosis
► Multiple abscesses in immunocompromised patients

Splenic Tumours

▶ Benign
- Haemangioma
  - Solitary, multiple, haemangiomatosis
  - Complications: Rupture
- Lymphangioma
- Cyst
- Hamartoma

▶ Malignant
- Lymphomas
  - Solitary, multiple, diffuse
- Metastases
  - Melanoma, breast carcinoma, bronchial carcinoma
- Sarcomas

Splenic Trauma

▶ Types
- Subcapsular haematoma
- Intraparenchymal haematoma
- Capsule tear
- Splenic rupture
- Vascular pedicle injury

▶ Spleen most frequently injured in blunt trauma to the upper abdomen

▶ Pain, breathlessness, signs/symptoms of shock

▶ Two-stage splenic rupture—parenchymal laceration with haematoma, under whose increasing pressure the capsule ruptures

▶ CT: Contour defect best demonstrated after contrast administration, typically on lateral splenic surface due to rib fracture

▶ IR: Embolisation

Kidneys, Adrenal Glands, Urinary Tract, Prostate, Testes

Anatomy

Kidneys

▶ Components
  - Cortex, medulla
  - Kidneys longer in craniocaudal direction
  - Functional unit of the kidney is the nephron with its secretory (glomeruli, tubules) and excretory (collecting tubules) parts
  - Collecting tubules → papillae → calyces → renal pelvis (ampullary, dendritic)
▶ Size
  - About 4 cm AP
  - About 7 cm transverse
  - About 11 cm craniocaudal
▶ Retroperitoneal location surrounded by
  - Fibrous Capsule
  - Perirenal fat
  - Renal Fascia (Gerota's fascia)
  - Pararenal fat

© The Author(s), under exclusive license to Springer Nature Switzerland AG 2026
D. Pickuth, J. T. Murchison, *Pocket Guide to Radiology*,
https://doi.org/10.1007/978-3-031-76520-9_6

▶ Arteries
- Renal Artery branches
  - Segmental renal arteries (renal hilum)
  - Interlobar Arteries (corticomedullary junction)
  - Arcuate branches (base of renal pyramid)
  - Interlobular arteries (renal cortex)
  - Afferent arterioles
- Vascular supply 75% single renal artery, 25% two or more renal arteries
- Accessory arteries most common at the poles, polar arteries occasionally arise from the iliac artery
- Renal arteries are end arteries

▶ Veins
- Renal vein
- Renal veins usually anterior, renal arteries middle, ureter posterior
- Retroaortic left renal vein—about 2% of cases

▶ Adjacent Structures
- Right kidney: Right adrenal gland, right liver lobe, hepatic flexure, duodenum, diaphragm, quadratus lumborum muscle, psoas muscle
- Left kidney: Left adrenal gland, stomach, spleen, tail of pancreas, omental bursa, splenic flexure, diaphragm, quadratus lumborum muscle, psoas muscle

Adrenal Glands

▶ Sections
- Adrenal cortex
  - Zona glomerulosa: Aldosterone
  - Zona fasciculata: Cortisol
  - Zona reticularis: Androgens, Oestrogens, Progestogen
- Adrenal medulla
  - Adrenalin
  - Noradrenaline

▶ Size
- About 1 cm AP
- About 3 cm transverse
- About 5 cm craniocaudal

▶ Arteries
- Superior adrenal artery (from inferior phrenic artery)
- Middle adrenal artery (from aorta)
- Inferior adrenal artery (from renal artery)

▶ Veins
- Adrenal vein
  - Right drains to inferior vena cava
  - Left drains to renal vein

▶ Adjacent structures
- Right adrenal gland
  - Anterior: Liver
  - Posterior: Diaphragm
  - Caudal and lateral: Right kidney
  - Medial: Inferior vena cava, abdominal aortic plexus, thoracic vertebral bodies 11 and 12, right diaphragmatic muscle
- Left adrenal gland
  - Anterior: Stomach
  - Posterior: Diaphragm
  - Caudal and lateral: Left kidney
  - Medial: Aorta, abdominal aortic plexus, 11th and 12th thoracic vertebral bodies, left diaphragmatic muscle

Ureters

▶ Sections
- Abdominal, pelvic
- Ureters cross anterior to the iliac arteries
- Vesicoureteric junctions—slit-like openings in the upper lateral angle of the bladder trigone

▶ External indentations or narrowings of ureter:
- Pelviureteric junction (PUJ)

- As the ureter enters the pelvis and crosses over the common iliac bifurcation
- At the vesicoureteric junction (VUJ) as the ureter enters the bladder wall

Urinary Bladder

▶ Anatomy
- Neck, base, body, apex
- Trigone—the space between both ureteral orifices and the internal urethral ostium

▶ Capacity
- about 250–500 ml

▶ Residual urine measurement
- Ultrasound
- Length × width × depth/2
- Limited accuracy in neurogenic urinary bladder if marked prostate enlargement

▶ Detrusor muscle
- Medial longitudinal muscle layer
- Middle circular muscle layer
- Outer longitudinal muscle layer

▶ Lymph nodes
- Upper bladder lymphatic vessels drain to external iliac lymph nodes
- Lower bladder lymphatic vessels drain to internal iliac lymph nodes

▶ Adjacent structures
- Male
  - Prostate
  - Seminal vesicles
  - Vas deferens
  - Rectum
- Female
  - Vagina
  - Uterus
  - Peritoneal reflection

- Male and female
  - Pelvic side wall
  - Abdominal wall
  - Sigmoid colon
  - Small intestine

Urethra

▶ Male urethra
  - About 20 cm long
  - Sections
    - Posterior urethra comprising membranous and prostatic portions
    - Anterior urethra comprising penile and bulbar portions
  - Narrowings
    - Urethral crest
    - Urethral sphincter
    - External urethral orifice
▶ Female urethra
  - About 4 cm long

Penis

▶ Anatomy
  - Bulb
  - Body
    - Corpora cavernosa
    - Corpus spongiosum
  - Glans

Prostate

▶ Anatomy
  - Inferior apex
  - Superior base
▶ Zones
  - Peripheral zone

- 75%
- Caudal and peripheral
- Location of most prostate carcinomas
- Transitional zone (pre-prostatic segment)
  - 5%
  - Between the neck of the urinary bladder and the seminal vesicle, proximal to the urethral curvature
  - Location of benign prostatic hyperplasia
- Central zone
  - 20%

▶ Adjacent structures
- Urinary bladder
- Seminal vesicles
- Urethra
- Rectum
- Pelvic connective tissue

Seminal Vesicles

▶ Adjacent structures
- Urinary bladder base
- Vas deferens
- Prostate
- Rectum

Testes

▶ Testes
- Ovoid, 4 cm long
- Volume—18 ml on average (12–30 ml)

▶ Epididymis
- Head
- Body
- Tail

▶ Spermatic cord
- Vas deferens
- Testicular arteries (from aorta)

- Artery to the ductus deferens (arises from the internal iliac artery via the umbilical artery)
- Cremasteric artery (arises from inferior epigastric artery which arises from the external iliac artery)
- Cremaster muscle
- Spermatic nerve
- fascia
▶ Arteries
- Testicular artery (branch of the aorta)
▶ Lymph nodes
- Drainage of testes to para-aortic nodes

Pelvic Floor

▶ Pelvic diaphragm
- Levator ani muscle
- Ischiococcygeus muscle
▶ Urogenital Diaphragm
- Superficial transverse perineal muscle
- Deep transverse perineal muscle
▶ Sphincter and erectile tissue muscles
- External anal sphincter
- Bulbospongiosus muscle
- Ischiocavernosus muscle

Kidneys

Renal Cysts

▶ Inherited renal cystic disease
- Autosomal recessive hereditary polycystic kidney disease (Potter type 1)
  - Infantile form
- Autosomal-dominant hereditary polycystic kidney disease (Potter type 3)
  - Adult form

- Pain, haematuria, proteinuria, hypertension, urinary tract infections, nephrolithiasis
- Bilateral renal cysts, often liver cysts, palpably enlarged kidneys, intracranial aneurysms, positive family history
- Von Hippel-Lindau syndrome
    - Association with renal cell carcinoma and phaeochromocytoma
- Tuberous sclerosis
    - Association with angiomyolipoma

▶ Congenital cystic kidney disease
- Obstructive cystic renal dysplasia (Potter type 4)
    - Results from distal renal tract obstructive pathology, eg posterior urethral valve, urethral agenesis, obstructing ureterocele, congenital vesicoureteric junction obstruction
- Segmental and focal renal dysplasia
- Medullary sponge kidney
    - Cystic expansion of the collecting tubes in the pyramids with small calcifications
    - Impaired kidney function, kidney stones, haematuria, recurrent urinary tract infections
- Multilocular cysts
- Calyceal diverticulum

▶ Acquired cystic kidney disease
- Renal cysts
    - Bosniak type I: Simple cyst
    - Bosniak type II: Benign cyst with fine septa, with fine calcifications, without enhancement
    - Bosniak type II F as Bosniak type II, but multiple septa, (4 or more), smooth minimally enhancing wall or smooth minimally thickened (3mm) septal enhancement; follow-up indicated
    - Bosniak type III: Cystic mass with thickened septa, with irregular wall, with enhancement
    - Bosniak type IV: Malignant mass with solid component, with irregular wall, with enhancement
- Multicystic dysplastic kidney (Potter type 2)
    - Normal renal tissue replaced by multiple cysts

- – Usually unilateral, often picked up on routine scan in utero, or shortly after birth
- – May be large but often shrinks with time. At increased risk of UTIs and hypertension in later life
- – **Differential Diagnosis**: Hydronephrosis, Wilms tumour, neuroblastoma
- Dialysis cystic disease

Hydronephrosis

▶ Causes: Obstructive urinary tract disorders due to calculi, tumours, lymphomas, haematomas, abscesses, strictures, vascular variants, retroperitoneal fibrosis

▶ **US**
  - Stage I: Anechoic dilatation of the renal pelvis; preserved renal cortex; marked sinus echogenicity
  - Stage II: Anechoic dilatation of renal pelvis, calyx neck and renal calices; preserved renal cortex; reduced sinus reflex
  - Stage III: Anechoic dilatation of renal pelvis, calyx neck and renal calices into the periphery; marked parenchymal thinning; reduced renal sinus echogenicity
  - Stage IV: Anechoic dilatation of the renal pelvis, calyx and renal calices into the periphery; moderate cortical thinning; absent sinus echogenicity

▶ **CT/MR**: Demonstrate level and possible cause of renal tract obstruction

▶ **Nuclear Medicine**
  - 99mTc-MAG3: Combined renal function scintigraphy and excretion scintigraphy
    - – Evaluation of relative function and excretion of both kidneys
    - – Functional assessment of obstruction
  - 99mTc-DMSA: Static renal scintigraphy
    - – Assessment of cortical function
  - 99mTc-DTPA: Renal perfusion scintigraphy
    - – Determination of the glomerular filtration rate

▶ **Differential Diagnosis**: Parapelvic cysts, low echo sinus lipomatosis, ampullary renal pelvis, subpelvic ureteral stenosis

Urinary Tract Infection

▶ Causes: Escherichia coli, Proteus mirabilis, Pseudomonas aeruginosa, Klebsiella, Enterococci, Staphylococci
▶ Types
- Primary, uncomplicated inflammation
- Secondary, complicated inflammation
- Lower urinary tract infection (cystitis)
  - Dysuria
  - Frequency
  - Haematuria
  - Strong smelling urine
  - Lower abdominal pain
- Upper urinary tract infection (pyelonephritis)
  - High fever
  - Toxic
  - Renal angle pain
  - Concomitant cystitis
  - Uremic symptoms

Acute Pyelonephritis

▶ Associations: Pregnancy, diabetes, gout, prostatic hyperplasia, immunosuppression, reflux, paraplegia
▶ Interstitial, bacterial, destructive inflammation of the renal interstitium and renal pelvicalyceal system
▶ Mostly ascending from bladder, rarely haematogenous or lymphatic route of infection
▶ More common in females
▶ US
- Occasional increased renal size
- Widened hypoechoic renal parenchyma
- Occasionally ill-defined renal margin
▶ MR
- Renal parenchyma T1 hypointense, T2 hyperintense
- Loss of corticomedullary differentiation
▶ **Complications**: Chronic pyelonephritis, renal abscess, pyonephrosis, renal failure

Chronic Pyelonephritis

▶ Chronic interstitial nephritis
▶ Fatigability, headache, loss of appetite, thirst, polyuria
▶ **US**
  - Reduced renal size
  - Cortical thinning
  - Calyceal dilatation
  - Calyceal distortion
▶ **Complications**: Renal scarring, hypertension, renal failure, uraemia

Xanthogranulomatous Pyelonephritis

▶ Cause: Chronic, purulent, destructive inflammation of the renal parenchyma and renal pelvis with lymphocytic infiltrates (pseudoxanthoma cells)
▶ Middle-aged women
▶ Flank pain, malaise, fever
▶ **US:** Mass, distorted renal outline, usually a centrally located calculus
▶ **CT:** Staghorn calculus, enlarged kidney, areas of reduced attenuation, bear paw sign (renal cortex thinned out, renal pelvis dilated)
▶ **MR**
  - Fatty changes in the renal parenchyma with marked enhancement in the late phase
  - Bear paw sign
▶ **Differential Diagnosis:** Renal cell carcinoma, renal tuberculosis, malakoplakia
▶ **Complication**: Fistulas

Papillary Necrosis

▶ Causes: Analgesic nephropathy, liver cirrhosis, diabetes mellitus, pyelonephritis, sickle cell anaemia
▶ Papillary destruction with deposition of a brown lipofuscin-like pigment in the papilla

▶ Shrinkage of the renal parenchyma
▶ Symptoms of urinary tract infection, haematuria, colics
▶ **CT urography/MR urography**
- Sloughed papillae with clubbed calyx
- Ball on tee sign
- Lobster claw sign
- Calcification when chronic
▶ **Complications**: Urinary obstruction due to sloughed papillae in ureter

Pyonephrosis

▶ Causes: Urinary retention disorder, diabetes mellitus
▶ Pus accumulation in the renal pelvicalyceal system
▶ Dull flank pain, subfebrile temperatures
▶ **US:** Dilated renal pelvis with echogenic debris
▶ **CT:** Increased density of the dilated renal pelvis
▶ **Differential Diagnosis:** Abscess, pyelonephritis, paranephritic abscess
▶ **Diagnosis:** Fine needle aspiration followed by percutaneous nephrostomy and drainage

Urogenital Tuberculosis

▶ Particularly involves kidneys, urinary bladder, prostate and epididymis
▶ Stages
- Early-Parenchymal stage, papillary necrosis single or multiple,
- Progressive—multifocal strictures and hydronephrosis
- End stage—Destructive stage
  - Pyonephrosis
  - Amorphous dystrophic calcification (Putty kidney)
▶ **CT urography/MR urography**
- Papillary destruction
- Calyx neck stricturing

- Cystic areas
- Parenchymal calcifications
- Ureteral strictures

Benign Kidney Tumours

▶ Angiomyolipoma
- Benign renal tumour consisting of blood vessels, smooth muscle cells and fat
- May be multiple in tuberous sclerosis
- Round, well-defined, smooth bordered
- **US**
  - Echogenic mass
  - Homogeneous internal structure
  - Spherical shape
  - No acoustic shadow
  - Solitary appearance
- **CT**: Fat containing mass
- **MR**: T1 hyperintense, T2 hyperintense, signal decrease in fat suppression sequences
  - Fat detection particularly supports the diagnosis
- **Complication**: Haemorrhage, higher risk with larger size
▶ Renal adenoma
- Tumour originating from the epithelial tissue of endocrine and exocrine glands
- Size mostly under 2 cm
- Imaging does not allow reliable differentiation from renal cell carcinoma
▶ Oncocytoma
- Rare type of adenoma in older age
- **CT**: Smoothly confined mass with central scar and homogeneous enhancement
- **MR**: T1 hypo- to isointense, T2 hyperintense, often capsule, star-shaped scar
  - Imaging not always able to differentiate from renal cell carcinoma

Renal Cell Carcinoma

▶ Associations: Nicotine, obesity, hypertension
▶ 90% of all primary renal neoplasms
▶ Subtypes
  • Clear-cell
  • Papillary
  • Chromophobic
  • Sarcomatous
▶ Most common in older men
▶ Haematuria, flank pain, weight loss, pyrexia
▶ Occasional symptomatic varicocele
▶ Lung metastases, bone metastases (expansile, lytic)
▶ Metabolic, haematological, endocrine, neuromuscular paraneoplasia
▶ Often incidental discovery
▶ **US**
  • Exophytic mass
  • Internal structure isoechoic or hypoechoic
  • Renal pelvis distortion
    – Imaging of renal tumour microvascularisation with dynamic contrast-enhanced sonography
  • **Differential Diagnosis:** Foetal lobulation, inflammatory pseudo-tumours, xanthogranulomatous pyelonephritis
▶ **CT**
  • Early arterial phase enhancement, parenchymatous phase low density
  • Tumour thrombus in the renal vein and inferior vena cava with enhancement, secondary thrombus without enhancement
▶ **MR**
  • T1 inhomogeneous, T2 inhomogeneous
  • T2 hypointense pseudocapsule
  • Enhancement is the main criterion
  • Malignancy criteria for complicated cyst
    – Inhomogeneous signal intensity
    – Enhancement in thickened septa and solid parts
    – Irregular wall border

▶ **IR**
- Thermal ablation (microwave ablation, radiofrequency ablation, cryoablation)
  – Feasible if: Tumour small, unifocal, spherical, peripheral; histology
- Transarterial chemoembolisation
  – Application: For tumour bleeding, before thermal ablation

TNM Classification Renal Cell Carcinoma

▶ T1: Confined to kidney ≤7 cm
- T1a: ≤4 cm
- T1b: >4 cm to ≤7 cm

▶ T2: Confined to kidney >7 cm
- T2a: >7 cm to ≤10 cm
- T2b: >10 cm

▶ T3: Involves major veins or perirenal tissue within Gerota's fascia
- T3a: Renal vein, perirenal tissue
- T3b: IVC below the diaphragm
- T3c: IVC above the diaphragm or invades wall of IVC

▶ T4: Extends beyond Gerota fascia or involves ipsilateral adrenal gland

▶ N1: Regional

▶ M1: Distant metastases

Renal Pelvic Carcinoma

▶ 10% of all primary renal neoplasms

▶ Mostly transitional cell carcinoma, rarely squamous cell carcinoma

▶ Usually older men

▶ Haematuria, colic

▶ **CT/MR**
- Renal pelvic mass with enhancement lower than renal parenchyma
- Excretory phase, filling defect evident

▶ **CT urography/MR urography**
- Filling defects in collecting system
- Collecting system contour irregularities

TNM Classification Renal Pelvic Carcinoma

▶ T1: Subepithelial connective tissue
▶ T2: Muscularis
▶ T3: Beyond the muscularis, peripelvic tissue, renal parenchyma
▶ T4: Directly involves neighbouring organs, perirenal tissue
▶ N1: Solitary ≤2 cm
▶ N2: Solitary >2 cm, multiple
▶ M1: Distant metastases

Renal Artery Occlusion

▶ Acute ischaemia syndrome
▶ Causes
- Global: Cardiac embolism, traumatic intimal dissection, sudden renal vein thrombosis
- Segmental: Cardiac embolism
- Subsegmental: Vasculitis
▶ Development of a renal infarction
▶ Sudden onset of flank pain, haematuria
▶ **CT**
- Wedge-shaped hypodense area or partially hypodense kidney
- Cortical rim sign (collaterals from capsular arteries)
- Parenchymal atrophy and scarring
▶ **MRA**: Occlusion of the vessel
▶ **Complications**: Renal function impairment, renal insufficiency, infection, abscess formation
▶ **IR**
- Thrombolysis, stenting
- **Complications**: Re-occlusion, haemorrhage, embolism, renal failure

Renal Artery Stenosis

▶ Chronic ischaemia syndrome
▶ Causes
  • Renal atherosclerosis (90%)
    – Most common in older men
    – Renal artery origin, proximal third of renal artery
    – Eccentric stenoses, wall irregularities, plaques, calcifica-
      tions, collaterals, post-stenotic dilatation
    – Aorta mostly involved
  • Fibromuscular dysplasia (10%)
    – mainly women, low age
    – most commonly middle third of renal artery,
    – Pearl, cord-like and ring-shaped constrictions
    – Aorta rarely involved
  • Rare: Anastomotic stenoses, aneurysms, vasculitides,
    haemolytic-uraemic syndrome, malignancies, cysts,
    hydronephrosis
▶ In renal artery stenosis, first reduced renal blood flow and then
  renovascular hypertension via the Goldblatt effect (activation
  of the renin-angiotensin-aldosterone system)
▶ Hypertension, ischaemic nephropathy, renal failure
▶ **Colour Doppler US**
  • Peak systolic velocity (PSV)
    – PSV > 180–200 cm/s highly sensitive and specific for
      >50% stenosis
    – Increased accuracy with contrast-enhanced sonography
  • Renal aortic ratio (RAR)
  • Resistance index (RI)
  • Acceleration time (AT)
▶ **MRA**: Determination of the degree of stenosis
▶ **Nuclear Medicine**: 99mTc-MAG3 captopril renal scintigra-
  phy to assess the functional relevance of renal artery stenosis
▶ **IR**: PTA (stenting for ostial, calcified, eccentric and dis-
  sected renal artery stenoses, no stenting for fibromuscular
  dysplasia)

Renal Artery Aneurysm

▶ Cause: Atherosclerosis
▶ Usually in the proximal third of the renal artery or at the site of division into the ventral and dorsal branches

Renal Vein Thrombosis

▶ Causes: In children due to dehydration, in adults due to tumour or glomerulonephritis
▶ Left renal vein significantly more often than right renal vein
▶ Flank pain, haematuria, thrombocytopenia
▶ Types
  • Acute occlusion: Haemorrhagic infarction
  • Subacute/chronic occlusion: Nephrotic syndrome
▶ MR
  • T2 Signal loss of the renal cortex as an early sign
  • Swelling of the kidney in the early stage, shrinking kidney in the late stage
▶ CT: Tumour thrombus with enhancement, bland thrombus without enhancement
▶ Complications: Kidney function impairment, kidney loss, infection, abscess formation

Nephrosclerosis

▶ Cause: Hypertension
▶ Types
  • Benign form: Lumen narrowing of the arterioles
  • Malignant form: Calibre increase of the interlobar arteries at the medullary border, vascular occlusion with infarcts, shrunken kidney with renal insufficiency

Nephrocalcinosis

▶ Causes: Hyperparathyroidism, osteoporosis, skeletal metastases, hypervitaminosis D, plasmacytoma, cystinuria, oxalosis
▶ Diffuse intrarenal calcifications

▶ US: Punctate calcifications in the renal cortex or papillae area
▶ **Complications**: Renal insufficiency

Acute Tubular Necrosis

▶ Causes: Hypotension, sepsis, drugs, nephrotoxins
▶ Azotaemia (elevated creatinine, urea and other nitrogen-rich compounds)
▶ Reversible renal insufficiency with or without oliguria
▶ US: Renal enlargement

Renal Insufficiency

▶ Causes
  • Acute: Shock, renal infarction, renal vein thrombosis, acute glomerulonephritis, acute urinary retention
  • Chronic: Numerous renal diseases, especially diabetic nephropathy, chronic glomerulonephritis, vascular nephropathies, interstitial nephritis, hereditary kidney diseases
▶ CKD stages
  • 1: Normal GFR, but haematuria/proteinuria, GFR > 89 ml/min
  • 2: Mild renal impairment, GFR 60–89 ml/min
  • 3: Moderate renal impairment, GFR 30–59 ml/min
  • 4: Severe renal impairment, GFR 15–29 ml/min
  • 5: Dialysis requirement, GFR < 15 ml/min
▶ US/CT/MR
  • Acute: Normal or increased renal size—may be reduced cortico-medullary differentiation
  • Chronic: Reduced renal size, reduced cortico-medullary differentiation
▶ **Nuclear Medicine**: Renal function scintigraphy for quantification of right/left relative renal function

Renal Trauma

▶ Causes: Blunt trauma (e.g. road traffic accident, falls), iatrogenic trauma (e.g. percutaneous biopsy, surgery, nephrostomy)
▶ Spectrum of injuries
▶ Grade I
  • Subcapsular haematoma or contusion
▶ Grade II
  • Superficial laceration <1 cm depth, not including the collecting system
▶ Grade III
  • Laceration >1 cm not involving the collecting system
  • Vascular injury or bleeding not extending beyond the Gerota fascia
▶ Grade IV
  • Laceration involving the collecting system with urinary extravasation
  • Laceration of renal pelvis and/or complete ureteropelvic disruption
  • Vascular injury to segmental renal artery or vein
  • Active bleeding extending beyond the Gerota fascia
  • Segmental infarcts without associated active bleeding (due to vascular thrombosis)
▶ Grade V
  • Avulsion of renal hilum or laceration of main renal artery or vein
  • Devascularised kidney with active bleeding
  • Shattered kidney
  • Haematuria, localised pain, localised fluctuant mass, shock
▶ US: Haematomas initially hypoechoic, then increasingly hyperechoic during resorption
▶ Colour Doppler US: Perfusion defect
▶ CT
  • Pre-contrast: Blood, renal disruption, perinephric/retroperitoneal stranding and free fluid
  • Early arterial: Renal artery thrombosis, perfusion deficits
  • Excretory phase: Renal pelvis, ureter

- **CTA:** Detection of vascular lesions
- **Complications**
  - Hydronephrosis
  - Renal hypertension
  - Nephrolithiasis
  - Chronic pyelonephritis
  - Urinoma
  - Arteriovenous fistula

Renal Transplant

▶ Complications
  - Renal: Rejection, acute tubular necrosis
  - Extrarenal: Renal artery stenosis, renal vein thrombosis, ureteral leakage, ureteral stricture, haematoma, abscess, lymphocele, urinoma
▶ Regular monitoring of urine volume, body weight, retention parameters, electrolytes, immunosuppressant levels
▶ **US**
  - Parenchymal oedema
  - Loss of corticomedullary differentiation
  - Urinary outflow obstruction
▶ **Colour Doppler US**
  - Analysis of the Doppler spectrum of the interlobar arteries
  - Preserved systolic flow
  - Reduced diastolic flow

Paediatric Radiology: Kidneys

Kidney Malformations

▶ Anomalies of number
  - Renal agenesis
  - Duplex kidney—has two draining ureters
  - Supernumerary kidney—may or may not be fused

▶ Anomalies of size
- Renal hypoplasia/hyperplasia

▶ Anomalies of position
- Isolated renal malrotation
  - pelvic ectopic kidney
  - intrathoracic ectopic kidney -rare
- Crossed fused renal ectopia

▶ Anomalies of fusion
- Horseshoe kidney
  - Partial fusion of the kidneys at the upper or lower pole
  - Associated with reflux, ureteral duplication, cryptorchidism, urethral anomalies PUJ obstruction, calculi, increased risk of trauma, infection, and malignancy
- Pancake kidney
  - Complete fusion of the upper and lower poles of the kidneys, usually lie anterior to aortic bifurcation

▶ Cystic anomalies

Nephroblastoma

▶ Wilms tumour
▶ Peak onset usually at the age of 3–4 years
▶ Occasionally bilateral
▶ Stages
- I: Intrarenal
- II: Intra/extracapsular
- III: Intra-abdominal spread
- IV: Haematogenous metastases
- V: Bilateral

▶ Palpable mass, rapid growth
▶ Abdominal pain is uncommon, haematuria, loss of appetite, hypertension
▶ Lymph node metastases, lung metastases
▶ US
- Solid mass, heterogeneous echogenicity
- Expansive growth, typical pseudocapsule
- Cysts, necrosis, haemorrhage, calcifications

▶ **MRI**
- Complex heterogeneous mass
  - Volumetry of the tumour by slice-by-slice planimetry
  - Simplification of volumetrics through deep learning algorithms

▶ **Differential Diagnosis**
- Benign: Polycystic kidneys, hydronephrosis, adrenal haemorrhage, renal abscess, pyonephrosis, xanthogranulomatous pyelonephritis
- Malignant: Neuroblastoma, rhabdomyosarcoma, hepatoblastoma, teratoma, ganglioneuroma, lymphoma

▶ Larger solid component and intratumoral haemorrhage can be adverse imaging features

▶ No biopsy for nephroblastoma (risk of tumour seeding)

Adrenal Glands

Hyperfunction of the Adrenal Cortex

▶ Cushing's syndrome
- Causes: Elevated cortisol; mostly unilateral adenoma, rarely carcinoma
- Plethora, moon face, truncal obesity, diabetes, hypertension, hypogonadism, osteoporosis, striae
- Differentiating adenoma from carcinoma
- Most (70%) adrenal adenomas are lipid rich
- Lipid poor adenomas typically have rapid contrast wash-out rate
- **CT**
  - Non-contrast examination: Density of lipid-rich adenomas <10 HU
  - Contrast medium examination: Lipid poor adenomas—absolute washout >60% or relative washout >40% 15 min after contrast medium administration; density of the lesion <30 HU 30 min after contrast medium administration

- Absolute washout calculation: [(density portal venous—density after 15 min)/(density portal venous—density native)] × 100
- Relative washout calculation: [(density portal venous—density after 15 min)/density portal venous] × 100
- **MR**
  - T2 carcinomas higher signal than adenomas
  - Fatty lesions such as lipid rich adenomas—signal loss with out of phase imaging
  - Chemical shift MRI detects the fat in lipid rich adenomas
- Detection of hypercortisolism by means of dexamethasone suppression test, cortisol excretion in the collected urine and cortisol diurnal rhythm; detection of suppressed adrenocorticotropic hormone (ACTH) in adrenal Cushing's syndrome

▶ Conn syndrome
- Causes: Aldosterone; mostly bilateral hyperplasia, rarely unilateral adenoma, very rarely carcinoma
- Hypertension, hypokalaemia, proteinuria, muscle weakness, polyuria, hypernatraemia
- Determination of the aldosterone-renin quotient

▶ Congenital adrenal hyperplasia
- Cause: Sex hormones; mostly bilateral hyperplasia
- Impaired sexual development
- Beyond infancy, hirsutism, virilisation and amenorrhoea in girls and women, pseudopubertas praecox in boys, often unnoticed in adult males

TNM Classification Adrenal Carcinoma

▶ T1: ≤5 cm without extraadrenal infiltration
▶ T2: >5 cm without extraadrenal infiltration
▶ T3: Local infiltration
▶ T4: Direct involvement of neighbouring organs
▶ N1: Regional
▶ M1: Distant metastases

Hyperfunction of the Adrenal Medulla

▶ Phaeochromocytoma
- Sporadic or in the context of multiple endocrine neoplasia as well as phacomatosis (neurofibromatosis, von Hippel-Lindau syndrome)
- 10% bilateral, 10% extraadrenal, 10% malignant, 10% familial
- Usually larger than 5 cm at the time of diagnosis
- Hypertension, headache, sweating, tachycardia
- **CT/MR**
  - Strong enhancement and slow contrast agent elimination
  - Necrosis
  - Haemorrhage
  - Calcifications
  - Cysts
- **MR**: No signal loss in out-of-phase-GE sequences compared to in-phase-GE sequences
- **Nuclear Medicine**
  - Search for extra-adrenal or metastatic manifestations
  - Conventional: 123I-MIBG
  - PET: 68Ga-DOTATOC, 18F-DOPA
  - Determination of plasma metanephrines, determination of catecholamines and metanephrines in 24 hour collected urine, performance of the clonidine test

▶ Neuroblastoma
- Infants
- Tumour of the sympathetic nervous system (adrenal gland, abdomen, neck, mediastinum)
- Progression
  - Spontaneous regression
  - Maturation to ganglioneuroma
  - Progressive growth
- Symptoms
  - Non-specific: Fever, pain, weight loss
  - Metabolic: Flush, sweating, diarrhoea
  - Characteristic: Paraplegic syndrome, Opsoclonus myoclonus syndrome, Horner's syndrome

- Early metastasis to lymph nodes, bones, liver and skin
- Tumour markers are catecholamines and NSEs
- **US/CT/MR**: Staging
- **Nuclear medicine**
  - Conventional: 123I-MIBG
  - PET: 68Ga-DOTATOC, 18F-DOPA

Adrenal Incidentaloma

▶ Mostly incidental finding
- Most common= endocrine inactive adrenal adenoma
▶ Probability of carcinoma increases with increasing size
▶ Dedicated sequence protocol in MR for targeted clarification and with regard to the clinical procedure
- Adenoma-typical versus adenoma-atypical imaging
- Follow-up versus adrenalectomy

Adrenal Metastases

▶ Common origins: Bronchial carcinoma, breast carcinoma, melanoma, renal cell carcinoma
▶ **MR**
- T1 usually low signal, T2 usually high signal
- With gadolinium—progressive enhancement
- Lack of signal loss in out of phase imaging

Adrenal Haemorrhage

▶ Causes: Anticoagulants, trauma, stress, sepsis, renal vein thrombosis, asphyxia
▶ **US**: Hyperechoic
▶ **CT**: High attenuation and enlarged, calcification later

Adrenal Calcification

▶ Haematoma
▶ Abscess
▶ Addison's disease

▶ Tuberculosis
▶ Hamartoma

Ureters

Urolithiasis

▶ Causes: Crystallisation of salts; prerenal causes (nutrition, immobilisation, hyperparathyroidism, hyperuricaemia), renal causes (hypercalciuria, renal tubular acidosis, cystinuria), postrenal causes (urinary outflow disorders, urinary tract infections)
▶ Types of stone with relation to cause
  • Urinary stones due to an acquired metabolic disorder: Calcium oxalate stones, urate stones, brushite stones, carbonate apatite stones
  • Urinary stones due to urinary tract infection: Struvite stones, carbonate apatite stones
  • Urinary stones due to a congenital metabolic disorder: Cystine stones, xanthine stones
▶ Radiodensity of stones according to type
  • Radiopaque stones (90%): Calcium oxalate stones, brushite stones, carbonate apatite stones, struvite stones, cystine stones
  • Radiolucent stones (10%): Urate stones, xanthine stones
▶ Men more often than women
▶ Colicky flank pain radiating to groin, nausea, vomiting
▶ Common sites of obstruction, pelviureteric junction, pelvic brim and vesicoureteric junction
▶ 80% stones pass spontaneously, but less than 50% when stones measuring >8 mm
▶ Prone to recurrent episodes
▶ US
  • Direct evidence of calculi (shadowing)
  • Hydronephrosis
  • Absence of urine jet seen in bladder

▶ **CT**
- Direct evidence of calculi
- Dilated ureter
- Thickening of the ureteral wall
- Stranding of the fatty tissue

▶ **CT urography**: Filling defect

▶ **Differential Diagnosis**
- Blood clots, papillary necrosis, polyps, tumours
- Cholelithiasis, appendicitis, tubo-ovarian abscess, adnexal torsion, extrauterine pregnancy, diverticulitis

▶ **Diagnosis:** Non-contrast CT KUB, CT urography

Ureteritis Cystica

▶ Multiple small benign submucosal cysts

▶ Typically seen in diabetics with recurrent urinary tract infections

▶ **CT urography/MR urography**: Multiple, evenly distributed, small filling defects

▶ **Differential Diagnosis**: Vascular impressions, tumours

Ureteral Polyp

▶ Younger adults

▶ **CT urography/MR urography**: Narrow-based pedunculated, smoothly contoured, position-dependent variable-shaped mass

Ureteral Carcinoma

▶ Mostly transitional cell carcinoma, rarely squamous cell carcinoma

▶ Multifocal occurrence in one third

▶ Especially older men

▶ Haematuria, colic

▶ **CT urography/MR urography**
- Irregularly configured filling defect
- Wall irregularities
- Ureteral stenosis

► **Differential Diagnosis:** Post-inflammatory, external or post-traumatic stenosis
► **Diagnosis:** CT urography, MR urography, retrograde pyelography, ureteroscopy

TNM Classification Ureteral Carcinoma

► T1: Subepithelial connective tissue
► T2: Muscularis
► T3: Beyond the muscularis, periureteral tissue
► T4: Neighbouring organs
► N1: Solitary ≤2 cm
► N2: Solitary >2 cm, multiple
► M1: Distant metastases

Paediatric Radiology: Ureters

Pyeloureteral Stenosis

► Congenital causes include idiopathic e.g. pyeloureteral kinking, or extrinsic ureter compression/encasement by a crossing vessel
► Most common cause of antenatal hydronephrosis
► Permanent, temporary or intermittent
► **Differential Diagnosis:** Congenital megacaliectasis
► **Diagnosis:** MR Urography, renal scintigraphy
► **Complication:** Hydronephrosis

Ectopic Ureter

► Abnormal migration of the ureteric bud caudal to the normal trigonal insertion site
  • In males, the ureter may insert into the lower urinary bladder, posterior urethra, seminal vesicle, ductus deferens, ejaculatory duct or rectum

- In women, the ureter may insert into the bladder neck/upper urethra, vaginal vestibule or vagina, cervix and uterus
- Associated with duplex kidneys in 80%

▶ Can present with recurrent urinary tract infections and pyelo-nephritis, epididymo-orchitis in men, urinary incontinence in women

▶ **US:** Dilatation of the upper pole moiety collecting system of a duplex kidney

▶ **Diagnosis:** MR Urography

Ureterocele

▶ Abnormal congenital cystic dilatation of the distal ureter

▶ Types
- Ectopic ureterocele (childhood) more common
- Intravesical ureterocele (usually in adults)

▶ Ectopic ureteroceles are almost always associated with a duplex collecting system and can present with urinary tract infections and obstruction. Intravesical ureterocele is far less common and in adults may be asymptomatic

▶ **US**
- Cystic structure projecting into the bladder close to the vesicoureteric junction
- If associated duplex kidney may see obstructed dilated upper moiety with ectopic ureterocele

▶ **MR urography:** Cobra head sign of an uncomplicated ureterocele

Ureteral Duplication

▶ Unilateral, bilateral, partial or complete

▶ Complete ureteral duplication
- Two ureteric orifices in the urinary bladder

▶ Ureter fissus (incomplete duplication)
- One distal ureteric orifice in the urinary bladder

▶ Meyer-Weigert rule: With a duplex kidney and complete ureteral duplication, the insertion of the upper moiety ureter into

the urinary bladder is medial and caudal to the insertion of the lower moiety ureter
► Variable clinical symptoms including infection, reflux and obstruction
► Voiding urosonography or micturating cystourethrography (MCU) for reflux evaluation (yo-yo sign with back and forth oscillation of the urine)
► Diagnosis: MR Urography

Megaureter

► Types
  • Refluxing megaureter
    – Primary: Congenital reflux
    – Secondary: Infravesical obstruction, neurogenic urinary bladder
  • obstructing megaureter
    – Primary: Distal adynamic ureteric segment
    – Secondary: Infra-vesical obstruction, neurogenic urinary bladder
  • Non-refluxive-non-obstructive megaureter
    – Primary: Idiopathic
    – Secondary: Residual condition after surgical correction, can be associated with diabetes insipidus
► Can present with febrile urinary tract infections, colicky pain, haematuria, urolithiasis if urinary stasis
► A non-refluxing, non-obstructive megaureter can be managed conservatively
► Diagnosis: MR urography, voiding urosonography, micturating cystourethrography (MCU)

Vesicorenal Reflux

► Types
  • Primary: Shortened submucosal ureteral tunnel in the urinary bladder so that the ureteral orifice is not adequately closed by the bladder muscles when intravesical pressure rises

- Secondary: Infravesical obstruction, consequence of cystitis, neurogenic urinary bladder
- Low-pressure reflux: Urine reflux during the filling phase of the urinary bladder
- High-pressure reflux: Urine reflux only during the emptying phase of the urinary bladder

▶ Classification
- I: Reflux into the ureter
- II: Reflux up to the renal pelvis, no dilatation
- III: Reflux into the kidney with mild dilatation of ureter and pelvicalyceal system
- IV: Reflux into the kidney with ureteric tortuosity and moderate dilatation
- V: Severe dilatation with ureteral tortuosity, loss of fornices and papillary impressions, sacculated kidney

▶ Recurrent urinary tract infections, enuresis, pollakiuria, dysuria, hypertension, renal insufficiency, renal growth failure

▶ **Diagnosis**: Voiding urosonography, micturating cysturethrography, reflux scintigraphy

▶ **Cystoscopy**
- Ureteral position: A (trigonal) to D (lateralised)
- Ureteral morphology: Normal shape, stadium shape, horseshoe shape, golf hole shape

▶ **Complications**: Parenchymal scarring, pyelonephritis, renal insufficiency, hypertension

---

Urinary Bladder

Cystitis

▶ Causes: Escherichia coli, indwelling catheter, urethral stricture, urinary bladder neck, prostatic hyperplasia, prostatic carcinoma, radiotherapy, cytostatic therapy, pregnancy, gynaecological diseases

▶ In children, urinary tract infections may be associated with congenital urinary tract abnormalities

▶ **US/CT/MR**
- Thickening of the urinary bladder wall
- Stranding of the perivesical fatty tissue
- Reduced urinary bladder capacity

Schistosomiasis

▶ Cause: Infection with Schistosoma haematobium, intercalatum and mansoni
▶ Dependence on the presence of certain snails in stagnant waters
▶ Prognosis depends on the stage of the disease at the start of therapy
▶ Stages
- I: Invasive stage
- II: Acute stage
  - II a: Toxaemia
  - II b: Oviposition (haematuria, pollakiuria, dysuria)
- III: Chronic stage (urinary flow disturbance, urinary bladder capacity restriction, urinary bladder carcinoma)
▶ **US**
- Urinary bladder stones
- Shell-like calcium deposits in the urinary bladder wall
- Reduced volume of urinary bladder
▶ **Differential Diagnosis:** Carcinoma of the urinary bladder, tuberculosis
▶ **Complications:** Stone formation, stenosis, bladder carcinoma (squamous cell)

Urinary Bladder Carcinoma

▶ Causes: Amines, nitrosamines, chronic inflammation, nicotine, schistosomiasis
▶ Mostly urothelial carcinoma, rarely squamous cell carcinoma, adenocarcinoma
▶ Most commonly trigone area, rear wall and side wall
▶ Often multifocal, high recurrence rate

► Most common in older men
► Painless haematuria
► **CT**
  • Papillary, solid or flat lesion
    – Assessment of involvement of the perivesical fat tissue
    – Assessment of the whole urinary tract with CT urography or MR urography
► **MR**
  • Early phase enhancement
  • Tumour typically enhances more than urinary bladder wall
  • Assessment of muscle invasion
    – Multiparametric MR for local tumour staging with classification according to VIRADS
► **Diagnosis**: Urine cytology, cystoscopy with photodynamic diagnostics, biopsy

TNM Classification Urinary Bladder Cancer

► T1: Subepithelial connective tissue
► T2: Musculature
► T2a: Superficial musculature (inner half)
► T2b: Deep musculature (outer half)
► T3: Perivesical tissue
► T3a: Microscopic
► T3b: Macroscopic (extravesical tumour)
► T4: Prostate, seminal vesicles, uterus, vagina, pelvic wall, abdominal wall
► T4a: Prostate, seminal vesicles, uterus, vagina
► T4b: Pelvic wall, abdominal wall
► N1: Solitary
► N2: Multiple
► N3: Common iliac artery
► M1a: Non-regional lymph node metastases
► M1b: Other distant metastases

Urachal Carcinoma

▶ Urachus as tubular structure between urinary bladder roof and umbilicus
▶ Usually adenocarcinoma
▶ MR: Visualisation of the mass best seen in the sagittal plane

Neurogenic Urinary Bladder

▶ Causes: Spinal cord injuries, myelodysplasias
▶ Urinary bladder dysfunction of various degrees
  • Spinal shock: Atonic overflow urinary bladder; absence of urge to urinate; retention with urinary bladder distension, urinary dribbling
  • Complete paraplegia: Spinal uninhibited urinary bladder, reflex urinary bladder; lack of urge to urinate, sweating and increase in blood pressure; involuntary reflex micturition with low urinary bladder filling
  • Conus medullaris syndrome: Denervation of the urinary bladder, autonomous urinary bladder; lack of urge to urinate; spontaneous emptying of small amounts of urine, large residual amount of urine
▶ US: Thickened trabeculated urinary bladder with pseudodiverticula
▶ Complications: Urinary bladder emptying disorder, vesicoureteral reflux, distal ureteral obstruction, stone formation

Urinary Bladder Trauma

▶ Causes: Extraperitoneal rupture (e.g. symphysis rupture, pubic bone fracture), intraperitoneal rupture (e.g. blunt trauma with full bladder)
▶ Classification
  • Type I: Urinary bladder contusion
  • Type II: Intraperitoneal rupture
  • Type III: Interstitial injury
  • Type IV: Extraperitoneal rupture
  • Type V: Combination injury

▶ Lower abdominal bleeding, pain, urinary ascites, peritonitis
▶ **Cystourethrography**
  • Contrast leaks
  • Urethral injuries

Paediatric Radiology: Urinary Bladder

Urinary Bladder Exstrophy

▶ Cleavage formations of varying severity
  • From sole symphyseal dehiscence to glandular epispadias and cloacal exstrophy
▶ Urinary bladder exstrophy always combined with epispadias of the penis or clitoris
▶ Partial absence of the anterior abdominal wall, everted urinary bladder, visible ureteric orifices
▶ Urinary incontinence, infections, superinfections, skin irritations
▶ Can be accompanied by inguinal hernias, cryptorchidism, imperforate anus, spinal anomalies

Urinary Bladder Diverticulum

▶ Types
  • Primary: Congenital
  • Secondary: Infra-vesical obstruction, neurogenic urinary bladder
▶ Outpouching of the urinary bladder wall
▶ most often near the ureteral orifices
▶ Enuresis, feeling of incomplete emptying of the bladder, urinary tract infection
▶ **US**:
  • Diverticula of the urinary bladder wall
  • Detection of the diverticular neck
▶ **Complications**: Urinary retention, inflammation, stone formation

Patent Urachus

▶ Other types of congenital urachal remnant anomalies include urachal sinus, urachal cysts, vesicourachal diverticula
▶ secondary infections
▶ **MRI:** Fistula filling from the umbilicus

Urethra

Urethra Inflammation

▶ Infectious
  • Gonococcal urethritis
  • Condylomata acuminata
  • Tuberculosis
▶ Non-infectious
  • Reiter's syndrome
  • Granulomatosis with polyangiitis
  • Malakoplakia

Urethral Strictures

▶ Causes: Iatrogenic, bacterial, idiopathic
▶ Most commonly involves the anterior urethra
▶ Obstructive micturition problems
▶ **Diagnosis:** Uroflowmetry, cystourethrography (ascending and descending)

Paediatric Radiology: Urethra

Urethra Malformations

▶ Epispadias
▶ Hypospadias
▶ Urethral valves

▶ Urethral diverticulum
▶ Urethral prolapse
▶ Urethral duplications

Prostate

Prostatitis

▶ Types
  • I: Acute bacterial prostatitis
  • II: Chronic bacterial prostatitis
  • III: Chronic abacterial pelvic pain syndrome
    – III a: Chronic abacterial pelvic inflammatory pain syndrome
    – III b: Non-inflammatory chronic abacterial pain syndrome of the pelvis
  • IV: Asymptomatic prostatitis
▶ Often associated with cystitis, urethritis and epididymitis
▶ Acute dysuria, urinary urgency, fever, chills, perineal pain, urge to defecate
▶ Chronic perineal pain, radiation to testicles and groin, low back pain
▶ US
  • Acute prostatitis: Oedematous swelling of the organ, focal hypoechoic region
  • Prostate abscess: Abolished zonal structure, discrete fluid collection, ill-defined margin, scattered internal echoes
  • Chronic prostatitis: Inhomogeneous areas, may be areas of calcification
▶ MR
  • Diffusely enlarged with inflammatory change in the periprostatic fat
  • T2 hyperintense, T1 diffusely enhancing with gadolinium

Prostate Cysts

▶ Types
- Congenital
  - Intraprostatic: Utriculus cysts (midline, no sperm), ductus ejaculatorius cysts (midline, sperm)
  - Paraprostatic: Müllerian duct cysts
- Acquired
  - Retention cysts (lateral, prostatic secretion, no sperm)

▶ US
- Anechoic space
- Round-oval shape
- Smooth wall
- Dorsal acoustic amplification
- Lateral acoustic shadow

Benign Prostatic Hyperplasia

▶ Enlargement of the glandular and fibromuscular parts of the transitional zone
▶ Most frequent cause of male urinary bladder voiding dysfunction
▶ Micturition symptoms
- Obstructive symptoms
  - Weak urine stream
  - Prolonged micturition
  - Difficulty initiating micturition
  - Nocturia
  - Urinary retention
- Irritative symptoms
  - Increased micturition frequency
  - Painful micturition
  - Urgency

▶ US
- Prostate enlargement (volume >30 ml)
  - Intravesical prostatic protrusion as an important indication of urinary bladder outlet obstruction

- Post voiding bladder residue
- Urinary bladder trabeculations
- Urinary bladder pseudodiverticulum

▶ **Transrectal US**
- Symmetrical enlargement
- Enlarged transitional zone, heterogeneous, nodular
- May be prostatic calculi
- May be cystic degeneration of BPH nodules

▶ **MR**
- With glandular hyperplasia—T2 hyperintense
- With fibromuscular hyperplasia—T2 hypointense
- Peripheral intact low signal pseudocapsule
- Well-defined nodules

▶ **Differential Diagnosis:** Prostate carcinoma, especially with pronounced fibromuscular components

▶ **Complication:** Urinary tract infections, urinary retention, residual urine formation, urinary bladder trabeculation, urinary retention, renal insufficiency

▶ **IR:** Prostate artery embolisation (particles)

Prostate Carcinoma

▶ Adenocarcinoma
▶ 75% in the peripheral zone, 25% in the transitional zone
▶ Usually multifocal growth
▶ Asymptomatic or symptoms as in benign prostatic hyperplasia
▶ Low back pain, dragging pelvic pain and sciatic pain with bone metastases
▶ PSA 4-10 ng/ml with a positive predictive value of 41% for prostate carcinoma, PSA > 10 ng/ml with a positive predictive value of 69% for prostate carcinoma. Up to 10% may not be PSA secreting
▶ Infiltration of urinary bladder, seminal vesicles, neurovascular bundles, rectum, pelvic wall
▶ Lymph node metastases, bone metastases

▶ **Transrectal US**
- Asymmetric prostatic enlargement

- Irregular usually hypoechoic (60–70%) lesion most commonly in the peripheral zone
- Infiltrative growth
  - Breaching the prostate capsule
  - seminal vesicle invasion
▶ Combination of transrectal sonography (B-TRUS) with colour Doppler sonography (D-TRUS), contrast-enhanced sonography (CE-TRUS) and elastography (USE) in the sense of a multiparametric sonography
▶ **MR**
  - T2 hypointense
    - Assessment of extraprostatic extension with T2
    - Poorly defined, blurring of edges
  - Restricted diffusion
    - High DWI signal at high b-value and low ADC signal at the same time
  - Early arterial enhancement
  - Quick washout
  - Invasion through capsule
    - Tumour extension through the capsule
    - Signal alteration of the periprostatic fat tissue
    - Asymmetry or infiltration of the neurovascular bundles
    - Distorted rectoprostatic angle
    - Capsule thickening
▶ **MRS**: Markedly increased choline signal
▶ Combination of MR with DWI, DCE and MRS in multiparametric MR
▶ Limited detection of e.g. small, ventral or apical carcinomas in sonography compared to MR
▶ Classification according to PIRADS
  - Scoring of T2, DWI and DCE
    - T2 dominant sequence for the transitional zone
    - DWI dominant sequence for the peripheral zone
▶ **Diagnosis**
  - Biopsy
    - Multiparametric MR plus ultrasound-targeted transrectal biopsy, transperineal biopsy
    - Multiple non-guided but ultrasound directed biopsies

- • **Complications**: Haematuria, haemospermia, prostatitis, prostate abscess
- ▶ Staging of prostate carcinoma
  - • Radiological—CT, MRI
  - • **Nuclear medicine**
    - – 68Ga-PSMA-PET/18F-PSMA-PET: PSMA ligand
    - – 11C-choline PET: Membrane metabolism
    - – 18F-FDG-PET: Glucose analogue
    - – Tc99m: Bone metastases
- ▶ Recurrence diagnosis with multiparametric MR in combination with 68Ga-PSMA-PET/18F-PSMA-PET

TNM Classification Prostate Cancer

- ▶ T1: Neither palpable nor visible
- ▶ T1a: ≤5%
- ▶ T1b: >5%
- ▶ T1c: Needle biopsy
- ▶ T2: Limited to prostate
- ▶ T2a: ≤ half of a lobe
- ▶ T2b: > half of a lobe
- ▶ T2c: Both lobes
- ▶ T3: Capsule involved
- ▶ T3a: Extracapsular
- ▶ T3b: Seminal vesicle
- ▶ T4: Fixed, neighbouring structure invasion other than seminal vesicles (sphincter externus, rectum, levator muscle, pelvic wall)
- ▶ N1: Regional
- ▶ M1a: Non-regional
- ▶ M1b: Bones
- ▶ M1c: Other localisations

Testes

Hydrocele

▶ Types
  • Primary: Congenital hydrocele, infantile hydrocele, spermatic cord hydrocele
  • Secondary: Inflammation, trauma, torsion, tumour
▶ US: Fluid collection between visceral and parietal sheets of the tunica vaginalis, septations
▶ Differential Diagnosis: Testicular tumour, hernia

Spermatocele

▶ Retention cyst of the small tubules in the epididymis
▶ Mostly in the epididymal head
▶ Asymptomatic
▶ US: Cystic structure on the epididymis
▶ Differential Diagnosis: Epididymal tumour

Varicocele

▶ Aetiology: Idiopathic (insufficient venous valves, congenital vascular wall weakness), secondary (extraperitoneal tumours, retroperitoneal lymphomas)
▶ Abnormal dilatation and tortuosity of the pampiniform plexus veins
▶ 15% of men, 98% left
▶ Right-sided varicoceles can be associated with obstruction due to renal malignancy with venous involvement
▶ Complication: Oligoasthenoteratozoospermia
▶ IR: Embolisation

Orchitis

▶ Causes: In adults mumps, gonorrhoea, tuberculosis, trauma
▶ Mostly aged 9–16

▶ Gradual onset
▶ Swelling, pain, fever, signs of inflammation
▶ US: Enlarged, inhomogeneous, hypoechoic testis
▶ **Complications**: Epididymitis, hydrocele, azoospermia, testicular atrophy, infertility

Epididymitis

▶ Causes: In adults gonococcal urethritis, cystitis, prostatic hyperplasia, urethral stricture, catheterisation, cystoscopy
▶ Mostly aged 9–16
▶ Gradual onset
▶ Swelling, pain, fever, signs of inflammation
▶ Radiation of pain along the spermatic cord into the groin region and the lower abdomen
▶ Prehn's sign: Decrease in pain with testicular elevation
▶ US
  • Enlarged epididymis
  • Reduced echogenicity of the epididymis
  • Often accompanying hydrocele
▶ Colour Doppler US
  • Increased perfusion of testis and epididymis
  • **Differential Diagnosis**: Reduced perfusion in testicular torsion
▶ **Complications**: Orchitis, hydrocele, necrosis, abscesses, infertility

Testicular Torsion

▶ Partial or total pedicle rotation of the testis, extravaginal (outside the tunica vaginalis) in infancy, intravaginal (inside the tunica vaginalis) in adolescence
▶ Usually clockwise rotation of the right testicle, counterclockwise rotation of the left testicle
▶ Usually aged 12–18
▶ Acute onset
▶ Most severe pain, pressure, painful spermatic cord, absent cremasteric reflex, abdominal symptoms, no fever

▶ Retraction of the testis
▶ **Colour Doppler US**
- Centrally no arterial and venous perfusion: Torsion
- Central arterial perfusion but no venous perfusion: Partial torsion
- Central hyperperfusion: Spontaneous detorquing, intermittent torsion
- **Differential Diagnosis**: Increased perfusion of testis and epididymis in epididymitis
▶ **Complications**: Testicular infarction, testicular atrophy, testicular fibrosis

Torsion of the Appendix Testis (Torsion of the Hydatid of Morgagni)

▶ Usually around 6–12 years of age
▶ Subacute onset
▶ Less pronounced pain, no pressure, painful spermatic cord, no abdominal symptoms, blue dot sign
▶ Normal testis
▶ **US:** Small spherical nodule (~6mm) between the head of the epididymis and the upper pole of the testis, hyperechoic after torsion
▶ **Colour Doppler US:** No internal vascularity, surrounding hypervascularity

Idiopathic Scrotal Oedema

▶ Usually under the age of 3
▶ Gradual onset, self limiting
▶ Thickening and oedema of the scrotal wall
▶ Normal testis
▶ **US:** Thickening and oedema of scrotal wall, normal testis and epididymis
▶ **Colour Doppler US:** Hypervascular wall thickening

Testicular Tumours

▶ Histological types
- Germ cell
  - Seminomatous
  - Non-seminomatous
    - Embryonal cell carcinoma
    - Teratocarcinoma
    - Choriocarcinoma
- Lymphomas
- Leukaemia infiltrates
- Metastases

▶ 5% contralateral synchronous tumour

▶ Often affects younger men

▶ Testicular tumour most frequent malignant tumour in 20–35 year-olds

▶ Malignant lymphoma most common testicular tumour in over 50s

▶ Painless development of unilateral testicular swelling

▶ Feeling of heaviness, tension, back pain, gynaecomastia

▶ US
- Seminoma: Rather homogeneous texture and sharply demarcated
- Non-seminomatous: Rather inhomogeneous texture and irregular margins
  - Imaging of testicular tumour microvascularisation with dynamic contrast-enhanced sonography
  - Strong enhancement, rapid washout

TNM Classification Testicular Cancer

▶ T1: Testis and epididymis without lymphovascular invasion

▶ T2: Testis and epididymis with lymphovascular invasion or involvement of the tunica vaginalis

▶ T3: Involves spermatic cord

▶ T4: Involves scrotum

▶ N1: ≤2 cm and less than 5 involved nodes

► N2: >2 cm to ≤5 cm or more than 5 nodes involved
► N3: >5 cm
► M1a: Non-regional lymph node or lung metastases
► M1b: Other distant metastases

Paediatric Radiology: Testes

Testicular Malformations

► Cryptorchidism
  • Absent testis or testes in the scrotal sac
  • Includes undescended, ectopic, atrophic or absent
► Ectopic testis
  • Congenitally abnormally located testis descended away from the normal path of descent including lying within the inguinal, perineal, or femoral regions or contralateral scrotum
► Pendulum testicles
► Sliding testicles
► US: Differentiation from lymph nodes occasionally difficult
► Complications: Infertility, risk of developing testicular germ cell tumour

Pelvis

Pelvic Calcifications

► Phleboliths
► Urinary bladder and ureteric stones
► Prostate calcifications
► Seminal vesicle calcifications
► Teratomas
► Uterine fibroids

Pelvic Fistulae

▶ Vesicovaginal fistula
- After vaginal delivery, gynaecological operations, bladder carcinoma, cervical carcinoma

▶ Enterovesical fistula
- Causes—Diverticulitis, Crohn's disease, malignancy

▶ Perianal fistula
- In Crohn's disease
- May be combination of fistulas (intersphincteric, trans-sphincteric, supra sphincteric, extrasphincteric) with abscesses (perianal, ischiorectal, supralevatoric, intramuscular)

Pelvic Floor Disorders

▶ Cystocele
- Urinary bladder neck below the pubococcygeal line
- Most common
- Posterior vaginal vault below the pubococcygeal line

▶ Rectocele
- Protrusion of the anterior wall of the rectum in relation to the rectovaginal septum by more than 1 cm
- Extension ventral, perineal, dorsal and lateral
- Impossible or incomplete emptying of the rectum while bearing down
- **Diagnosis**: Defaecography, MR Defaecography

▶ Enterocele
- Pouch of Douglas space below the pubococcygeal line
- **Diagnosis**: Defaecating proctogram, MR Defaecography

▶ Uterine prolapse
- Stage 1—uterus descends to the upper vagina
- Stage 2—uterus descends to the introitus
- Stage 3—uterus extends outside the introitus
- Stage 4—both cervix and uterus descend outside the introitus

Uterus, Ovaries

Anatomy

Vulva

▶ Parts
- Mons pubis
- Labia majora
- Labia minora
- Vaginal vestibule
- Clitoris

Uterus

▶ Parts
- Cervix, 2–3 cm long
  - Ectocervix (bordering vagina)
  - Endocervix, contains endocervical canal
- Isthmus
- Body
  - Endometrium
  - Inner myometrium (junctional zone)
  - Outer myometrium
▶ MR
- T1 Body, cervix, vagina isointense
- T2 Body

© The Author(s), under exclusive license to Springer Nature Switzerland AG 2026
D. Pickuth, J. T. Murchison, *Pocket Guide to Radiology*,
https://doi.org/10.1007/978-3-031-76520-9_7

- – Inner hyperintense:Endometrium, mucus
- – Immediately around endometrium—hypointense myometrium: Junctional zone—not seen on US
- – Outer isointense: Myometrium
- T2 Cervix, vagina
  - – Inside hyperintense: Epithelium, mucus
  - – Outside hypointense: Stroma
- Thickness of the endometrium greatest during the secretory phase, least just after menstruation—the proliferative phase—best timed to show polyps
- Different thickness of the junctional zone depending on the uterine contractions
- Adenomyosis—junctional zone thickness greater than 12 mm—85% accuracy, 96% specificity
- Some fluid in the Pouch of Douglas is normal, especially in the second half of the cycle

▶ Arteries
  - Uterine artery (branches from internal iliac artery)

▶ Lymph nodes
  - Parauterine
  - Paravesical
  - Paravaginal
  - Pararectal
  - Iliac

Fallopian Tube

▶ Parts
  - Interstitial
  - Isthmus
  - Ampulla
  - Infundibulum

▶ Arteries
  - Supplied by anastomosis of tubal branches of the ovarian artery and ascending branches of the uterine artery

▶ Lymph nodes drainage—mirrors ovary—see below

Ovary

▶ Functional states
- Follicle maturation (primordial follicle, primary follicle, secondary follicle, tertiary follicle)
- Ovulation
- Corpus luteum formation
- Corpus albicans formation

▶ Arteries
- Ovarian artery (laterally from aorta): Via the suspensory ligament of the ovary and the ovarian branch of the uterine artery from medially within the ovarian ligament

▶ Lymph node drainage
- Via the suspensory ligament of the ovary, the ovarian ligament, and the round ligament of the uterus
    - Para-aortic
    - Aorto-caval
    - Obturator
    - Internal iliac
    - Superficial inguinal

Ligaments

▶ Ligaments other than 'suspensory' (ovarian vessels run alongside the suspensory ligament)
- Round (teres) ligament—traverses inguinal canal
- Broad ligament
    - Mesosalpinx
    - Mesovarium
    - Mesometrium
- Parametrial, paracervical supports
    - Pubocervical ligament
    - Recto-uterine ligament—immediately posterior
    - Sacro-uterine ligament—posteriorly and superiorly to the sacrum
    - Cardinal (transverse) ligament—the uterine vessels run along between its parametrial and paracervical components

Uterus

Nabothian Cysts/Follicles

- ▶ Superficial retention cysts of the endocervical glands
- ▶ Benign, rarely larger than 4 cm, asymptomatic
- ▶ Colposcopically smooth, yellowish

Bartholin Cysts

- ▶ Secretion in the glands of the vagina or vulva with varying protein content
- ▶ In bartholinitis, pain and usually unilateral inflammatory redness and swelling of the large and small labia

Congenital Uterine Abnormalities

- ▶ Agenesis, hypoplasia
- ▶ Unicornuate uterus
- ▶ Uterus didelphys
- ▶ Bicornuate uterus (unicollis/bicollis)
- ▶ Septate/subseptate uterus
  - • Urinary tract malformations
- ▶ **Diagnosis**: Ultrasound optimal if performed in the late secretory phase, MRI, hysterosalpingo-contrast sonography, hysterosalpingography, laparoscopy

Causes of Abnormal Uterine Bleeding

- ▶ Endometriosis
- ▶ Adenomyosis
- ▶ Endometrial polyps
- ▶ Uterine fibroid (uterine leiomyoma)
- ▶ Uterine malignancy

Endometriosis

► Non-neoplastic endometrial tissue residing outside the uterine cavity and myometrium
► Responds to hormonal stimulation with cyclical haemorrhage, inflammation, adhesions and fibrosis
► Usually women of childbearing age
► Dysmenorrhoea, dyspareunia, dyschezia (functional constipation), dysuria, sterility
► Often delayed diagnosis
► Most commonly pelvic and intraperitoneal
► **Transvaginal US**:
► Diagnosis of ovarian endometrioma—this may be an indication to further evaluate for deep endometriosis
  • Bowel-Colonic layers—if there is 5 mm invasion of muscularis propria, the submucosal layer is usually displaced
  • Evaluate motion of the ovary on compression, also against bowel on cervix serosa, including integrity of serosal layer and evaluate the torus from the posterior fornix—torus is the posterior collar around the cervical-uterine body junction—examine behind cervix for irregularly marginated (due to desmoplastic response) hypoechoic lesions
  • Bladder and ureters should also be evaluated
  • AP dimension >4 cm is key in adenomyosis (and fibroids), global or asymmetric thickening of the uterine wall with radial striated, heterogeneously hypoechoic structures or anechoic areas in the myometrium. Be aware that contractions can last for 25 min and beyond
► **MR**
  • Uterine
    – Adenomyosis: Irregularly thickened junctional zone, indistinctly delineated space in the myometrium, punctate hyperintense foci-may co-exist with endometriosis
    – Endometrioma—most common in ovary (cystic ovarian endometriosis): T1 hyperintense (very marked hyperintense blood breakdown products), T2 hypointense with heterogeneity, Shading sign (blood breakdown products

at various stages), kissing ovaries sign (bilateral involvement of adherent ovaries in near midline), T2 dark spot sign (discrete markedly hypointense foci within the cyst with or without T2 shading)
- T1 C+ (Gd) may have wall enhancement. Enhancing mural nodule suggestive of malignant transformation
- Encapsulated fluid collections
- Haematosalpinx
- Hydrosalpinx
- Peritoneal endometriosis
  - Flat plaques
  - Distortion of peritoneal reflections
▶ **Diagnosis**: Laparoscopy

Endometrial Polyps

▶ No symptoms, or irregular bleeding
▶ **Transvaginal US** examination in the proliferative phase assists focal lesion detection
- Mostly oval, can be multiple, sessile, pedunculated, echogenic, may be isoechoic with the endometrium
- Colour Doppler ultrasound detection of the single pedicle artery sign is typical of endometrial polyp

Uterine Fibroid (Uterine Leiomyoma)

▶ Benign tumour consisting of smooth muscle and connective tissue (fibroleiomyoma)
▶ Types
- Submucosal (menometrorrhagia)
- Intramural (menorrhagia)
- Subserous (symptom-free)
- Intraligamentary (compression symptoms)
▶ Most frequent benign neoplasia in women with multiple manifestations
▶ Growth linked to ovarian function
▶ No development and no growth of fibroids after menopause

▶ **US**
- Round, sharply circumscribed, hypoechoic neoplasm
- Expansive growth
- Circular vascularisation

▶ **CT**
- Hypodense mass
- Often calcifications

▶ **MR**
- T1 isointense
- T2 hypointense
- Well-defined
- Reduced enhancement
- Pseudocapsule, cysts, necrosis, calcifications

▶ **Differential Diagnosis:** Adenomyosis, endometrial polyp, leiomyosarcoma-rapid growth, very vascular often

▶ **IR:** Uterine artery embolisation (particles)

▶ **MRI**—guided percutaneous laser ablation

▶ **MRI**—guided transcutaneous focus high-intensity focused ultrasound

Vulvar Carcinoma

▶ Aetiology: Often infection with human papilloma viruses
▶ Squamous cell carcinoma
▶ Rare-usually elderly women
▶ Pruritus, induration, ulceration
▶ Metastatic spread to inguinal, then iliac lymph nodes
▶ **MR/CT:** Staging (assess tumour depth, local infiltration, distant metastases)

Vaginal Carcinoma

▶ Squamous cell carcinoma
▶ Rare—usually elderly women
▶ Vagina often site of secondary tumour spread from vulva or cervix
▶ Lymph node metastases

- from the lower third of the vagina-inguinal
- from the middle and upper third of the vagina-iliac

▶ **MR/CT**: Staging (assess tumour depth, local infiltration, distant metastases)

▶ **Complications**: Fistula formation between vagina, urinary bladder and rectum

Cervical Carcinoma

▶ Aetiology: Human papillomavirus infection. promiscuity, immunosuppression, herpes, poor genital hygiene;

▶ Squamous cell carcinoma, adenocarcinoma 5–10%

▶ Exophytic or endophytic growth

▶ Peak ages between 35 and 45 and between 65 and 75 years old

▶ Menorrhagia, contact bleeding

▶ Lymph node metastases

▶ **MR**
- T2 hyperintense
- In the case of parametrial infiltration, hypointense stroma is disrupted by hyperintense space occupying lesion and obliterated fat planes
- Differentiation from scar/recurrence
  - Difficult in the first 6 months after surgery/radiotherapy
  - Misinterpretation due to repair processes, oedema or inflammatory changes
  - Recurrence most common in vaginal stump
  - T2 after 12 months—scar hypointense, recurrence hyperintense
  - IV contrast—rapid enhancement with recurrence

▶ **MR/CT**: Staging (depth extension, surrounding infiltration, distant metastases)

Endometrial Carcinoma

▶ Aetiology: Older age, obesity, nulliparous, unopposed oestrogen therapy, late menopause, chronic anovulation

▶ Adenocarcinoma, sarcoma

► Most frequent malignant neoplasm of the female genital tract
► Peak age between 65 and 75 years
► Postmenopausal bleeding, intermenstrual bleeding,
► In case of obstruction of the cervical canal—hydrometra, haematometra or pyometra
► **Transvaginal US**—check local guidelines on cut-off values which may vary
  • Endometrial thickness (ET) >5.0 mm in a symptomatic patient. >10 mm if asymptomatic and endometrium not fully demonstrated requires gynaecological opinion
  • Indistinct boundary
► Assessment of the endometrio-myometric transition zone
► **MR**
  • T1 isointense, T2 variable
  • Enlarged uterus
  • Dilated uterine cavity
  • Interrupted junctional zone as a criterion for deep myometrial infiltration
► **MR/CT**: Staging (depth extension, surrounding infiltration, distant metastases)
► **Diagnosis**: Hysteroscopy, fractionated curettage, surgery

TNM Classification Cancer of Vulva, Vagina, Cervix and Endometrium

► Vulva
  • T1: Limited to vulva/perineum
  • T1a: ≤2 cm, stromal infiltration ≤1 mm
  • T1b: >2 cm, stromal infiltration >1 mm
  • T2: Lower third urethra/vagina, anus
  • T3: Upper two-thirds urethra/vagina, urinary bladder mucosa, rectal mucosa, fixed to pelvic bone
  • N1a: 1 to 2 < 5 mm
  • N1b: 1 ≥ 5 mm
  • N2a: ≥ 3 < 5 mm
  • N2b: ≥ 2 ≥ 5 mm

- N2c: Extracapsular
- N3: Fixed/ulcerated
- M1: Distant metastases

▶ Vagina
- T1: Vagina
- T2: Paravaginal tissue
- T3: Pelvic wall
- T4: Urinary bladder mucosa, rectal mucosa, beyond pelvis
- N1: Regional
- M1: Distant metastases

▶ Cervix
- T1: Limited to uterus
- T1a: Only microscopic
- T1a1: Depth ≤3 mm, horizontal spread ≤7 mm
- T1a2: Depth >3 mm to ≤5 mm, horizontal spread ≤7 mm
- T1b: Clinically visible or only microscopically >T1a2
- T1b1: ≤4 cm
- T1b2: >4 cm
- T2: Beyond the uterus
- T2a: Without parametrium invasion
- T2a1: ≤4 cm
- T2a2: >4 cm
- T2b: With parametrium invasion
- T3: Lower vaginal third, pelvic wall, hydronephrosis, non-functioning kidney
- T3a: Lower third of the vagina
- T3b: Pelvic wall, hydronephrosis, non-functioning kidney
- T4: Urinary bladder mucosa, rectal mucosa, beyond the pelvis
- N1: Regional
- M1: Distant metastases

▶ Endometrium
- T1: Limited to corpus uteri
- T1a: Endometrium, < half myometrium invaded
- T1b: ≥ half myometrium invaded
- T2: Cervix
- T3: Local and/or regional

- T3a: Serosa, adnexa
- T3b: Vagina, parametrium
- T4: Urinary bladder mucosa, rectal mucosa
- N1: Regional
- M1: Distant metastases

Interventional Radiological Therapy for Pelvic Bleeding

▶ Types
  - Temporary embolisation
    – Post-traumatic, puerperal, postoperative
    – Embolisation coils/Gelfoam
    – Temporary balloon occlusion in case of massive haemorrhage
  - Permanent embolisation
    – Neoplastic
    – e.g. cyanoacrylate/lipiodol
▶ Vasoconstrictive response can mimic successful embolisation
▶ **Complications**: Ischaemia pain, fever, leucocytosis, necrosis

Ovaries, Adnexa

Ovarian Cysts

▶ Physiological cysts
  - Types
    – Follicular cyst
    – Simple cyst
    – Corpus luteal cyst
  - **Differential Diagnosis**: Para-ovarian cysts, peritoneal cysts, hydrosalpinx, extrauterine pregnancy, ovarian cancer
▶ Polycystic ovarian syndrome
  - Amenorrhoea, infertility, obesity, hirsutism
  - Ultrasound: 'String of pearls' appearance due to peripheral uniform-sized cysts

Pelvic Inflammatory Disease

▶ Inflammation of the adnexa usually caused by a bacterial infection spreading up from the vagina or cervix into the uterus, fallopian tubes and ovaries
▶ Predisposing factors
  • Sexual activity
  • Birth
  • Postpartum
  • Menstruation
  • Surgery
▶ Often initial dysuria, vaginosis and cervicitis
▶ In the acute phase, pain, tenderness and guarding in the lower abdomen
▶ After the acute phase, pressure pain, tugging pain and stretching pain in the lower abdomen
▶ US
  • Fallopian tube thickening
  • Pyosalpinx
  • Tubo-ovarian mass
  • Free fluid
  • Ovarian abscess
  • Pouch of Douglas abscess
▶ Differential Diagnosis: Appendicitis, peritonitis, degenerated fibroids, tubo-ovarian abscess, adnexal torsion, extrauterine pregnancy, endometriosis, endometritis, ruptured ovarian cyst, ovarian carcinoma, diverticulitis
▶ Complications: Infertility

Benign Ovarian Tumours

▶ Serous cystadenoma
  • Predominantly cystic, usually unilocular
  • Occasionally septated
  • Peak 4th–5th decades
  • May have mural calcification
▶ Mucinous cystadenoma

- Less common than serous cystadenoma
- Multi-loculated
- Mural calcification more common than with serous cystadenoma
- Generally larger than serous cystadenoma

▶ Dermoid cyst
  - Childhood ovarian tumour
  - Layering phenomenon with cystic and solid parts
  - Fat content and calcifications

▶ Ovarian fibroma
  - Predominantly stromal parts
  - Meigs syndrome: Ovarian fibroma, ascites, pleural effusion

Malignant Ovarian Tumours

▶ Ovarian cancer
  - Aetiology: Older age, obesity, few pregnancies, polycystic ovarian syndrome; association with breast carcinoma; protective factors—hormonal contraceptives and long breast-feeding
  - Most frequently serous cystadenocarcinoma
  - Gynaecological neoplasia with the highest mortality rate
  - Older women
  - Often late presentation with abdominal symptoms
  - Early lymph node, peritoneal, mesenteric, omental and pleural metastases
  - Often delayed diagnosis
  - US
    - Irregular solid components
    - Lobular
    - Irregular septa
    - Free fluid
    - Typical central vascularisation
  - MR
    - Size >5 cm premenopausal, size >1 cm postmenopausal
    - Wall thickness >3 mm
    - Septa >3 mm
    - Solid

- Diffusion restriction
- Enhancing
- Infiltration
- Necrosis
- Ascites
- Pleural effusion
- Lymph nodes
- Metastases
- **MR/CT:** Staging (surrounding infiltration, distant metastases)
- **Differential Diagnosis:** Benign ovarian tumours, periovulatory ovary, endometriosis, ovarian metastasis
- **Complications:** Fistula formation, infection, ileus, urinary retention, ascites, protein loss syndrome

▶ Ovarian metastases
- Aetiology: Carcinomas of the breast, gastrointestinal tract (Krukenberg tumour) and endometrium

TNM Classification Ovarian Cancer

▶ T1: Limited to ovaries
- T1a: 1 ovary, capsule intact
- T1b: Both ovaries, capsule intact
- T1c1: Tumour cell dissemination during surgery
- T1c2: Capsular rupture before surgery, tumour on ovarian surface
- T1c3: Malignant cells in ascites or in peritoneal lavage

▶ T2: Spreading in the pelvis
- T2a: Uterus, tubes
- T2b: Other pelvic tissues

▶ T3: Peritoneal metastases beyond the pelvis and/or regional lymph node metastases
- T3a: Microscopic peritoneal metastases with/without retroperitoneal lymph node metastases
- T3b: Macroscopic peritoneal metastases ≤2 cm
- T3c: Macroscopic peritoneal metastases >2 cm and/or regional lymph node metastases including spread to the liver capsule and splenic capsule without parenchymal involvement of the organs

▶ N1a: Retroperitoneal ≤10 mm
▶ N1b: Retroperitoneal >10 mm
▶ M1: Distant metastases

Infertility Investigation

▶ **Hysterosalpingo contrast US**
- Visualisation of uterine cavity and tubes
- Detection of uterine malformations, adhesions, tubal occlusions
- Perturbation to check tube patency

▶ **Hysterosalpingography**

Ovarian Vein Thrombosis

▶ Aetiology: Stasis in ovarian veins due to sudden drop in flow velocity after delivery
▶ 80–90% right ovarian vein
▶ **MR:** Dilated thrombosed vein with wall enhancement
▶ **Differential Diagnosis**
- Endometritis
- Tubo-ovarian abscess
- Adnexal torsion
- Appendicitis
- Pyelonephritis

Breast

Anatomy

Breast

▶ Structure
- Inhomogeneous structure
- 15–25 glandular lobes converging towards the nipple
- Glandular lobe consists of glandular lobules and milk ducts
- Glandular lobules made up of acini and tubules, which drain into lactiferous tubules. These converge into lactiferous ducts and sinuses
- Glandular lobules superimpose mammographically to form composite shadows
- Glandular lobules may decrease with age, a process known as involution
- Surrounding connective supporting tissue, including Cooper's ligaments and adipose tissue intervening between glandular lobules
- Cooper's ligaments anchor the breast volume to the chest wall

▶ Lymph nodes
- Axillary lymph nodes—dominant pathway >75%. 3 surgical levels divided by pectoralis minor and the clavicle
- Internal mammary/thoracic lymph nodes
- Supraclavicular lymph nodes

© The Author(s), under exclusive license to Springer Nature
Switzerland AG 2026
D. Pickuth, J. T. Murchison, *Pocket Guide to Radiology*,
https://doi.org/10.1007/978-3-031-76520-9_8

Pathology

Mammography

▶ Standard projections
  • Craniocaudal (CC)
  • Mediolateral oblique (MLO)
▶ Additional projections
  • Lateral: Further assessment of focal findings, exclusion of composite effects
  • Magnification: Analysis of microcalcifications
  • Compression: Reduction of composite effects
  • Rolled: Reduction of composite effects
  • Tangential: Visualisation of dermal lesions including cutaneous microcalcifications
  • Axillary tail view: Visualisation of axillary focal findings
  • Cleavage view
  • Eklund/Pushback: Visualisation of the breast tissue overlying the implant after augmentation
▶ Additional techniques
  • Tomosynthesis—sectional images through the breast to obtain a more 3D-like image
  • Contrast mammography—evolving technique which presents a physiological alternative to breast MRI

Breast Ultrasound

▶ Layers of the breast from superficial to deep
  • Skin
  • Subcutaneous fat
  • Cooper ligaments
  • Superficial fascia
  • Mammary gland
    – Glandular lobules
    – Milk ducts
    – Connective tissue
    – Fatty tissue
  • Deep fascia

- Retromammary adipose tissue
- Muscle fascia
- Pectoralis major and pectoralis minor muscles
- Ribs and intercostal muscles
- Pleura

Structural Changes of the Breast

▶ **Mammogram**
- Juvenile breast: Radiopaque, homogeneous. Mammography generally not indicated or informative in the evaluation of symptoms in younger women due to tissue density, unless there are clinically suspicious findings
- Breast of the sexually mature female: Can be heterogeneous and variable in density
- Involuted breast: Radiolucent, homogeneous

▶ **US**
- Skin: Hyperechoic
- Connective tissue: Hyperechoic
- Adipose tissue: Hypoechoic
- Glandular tissue:
  - Younger women: Parenchyma homogeneously hyperechoic due to dense glandular tissue
  - Older women: Parenchyma may become more heterogeneously hypoechoic with age with involution of the glandular tissue
- Nipple: Hypoechoic, can cause acoustic shadowing
- Milk ducts: Tubular tortuous anechoic structures
- Cooper ligaments: Hyperechoic, can cause posterior acoustic shadowing

▶ **MR**
- Normal glandular parenchyma shows variable background enhancement. This tends to be gradual and similar in both breasts, depending on anatomical composition. Correlation with glandular distribution mammographically is informative
- Degree of enhancement is hormone dependent and scans timed to day 6–16 of the menstrual cycle can minimise hormonal influence

Normal Variants of the Breast

▶ Polymastia, Polythelia
▶ Amastia, Athelia
▶ Anisomastia
▶ Micromastia, macromastia
▶ Inverted nipple, cleft nipple

Calcifications in Mammography

▶ Skin calcifications
  • **Mammo**: Deposits with typical transparent centre at cutaneous level
▶ Atherosclerosis
  • **Mammo**: Track-like often discontinuous linear macrocalcifications at the site of blood vessels which accumulate over time
▶ Fat necrosis
  • **Mammo**: Progressive curvilinear and dystrophic macrocalcifications at site of previous operations or after trauma
▶ Oil cyst
  • **Mammo**: Rounded, curvilinear calcification with smooth wall and fat-density centre
▶ Scarring
  • **Mammo**: Irregular macrocalcifications in the area of surgical scars
▶ Fibroadenoma
  • **Mammo**: Coarse to popcorn-like calcification. Eventually complete calcification
▶ Plasma cell mastitis
  • **Mammo**: Mostly coarse needle-shaped calcifications directed towards the nipple, can show branching
▶ Adenosis
  • **Mammo**
    – Blunt duct adenosis: Roundish microcalcifications in the lobule area
    – Microcystic adenosis: Typical sedimentation of calcareous milk-like cysts (teacup sign)

Fibrocystic Mastopathy

▶ Components of mastopathy
- Cysts: Microcysts, macrocysts
- Epitheliosis: Hyperplasia of intraductal structures
- Adenosis: Hyperplasia of extraductal structures
  - Simple adenosis: Increasing lobules in terms of number and size
  - Blunt duct adenosis: Dilatation of the lobule up to about 2 mm
  - Microcystic adenosis: Formation of cysts up to about 5 mm
  - Sclerosing adenosis: Periductal sclerosis with constriction of the lobulus lumina
- Radial scar: Adenosis with central sclerosis

▶ Degree of mastopathy
- I (70%): Connective tissue proliferation, cysts, ductasia, glandular tissue proliferation
- II (25%): Intraductal/intralobular cell proliferation
- III (5%): Strong proliferation, cell atypia
- Grade cannot be determined mammographically

▶ Histopathological changes within the ductal system (ductal)
- Ductal hyperplasia
- Atypical ductal hyperplasia
- Ductal carcinoma in situ
- Invasive ductal carcinoma

▶ Histopathological changes within the lobules (lobular)
- Lobular hyperplasia
- Atypical lobular hyperplasia
- Lobular carcinoma in situ
- Invasive lobular carcinoma

▶ Swelling of the glandular tissue and painfulness about one week before the onset of menstruation with dominant oestrogen and low progestogen levels

▶ Tension, heaviness, pain, hardening, nodularity

▶ **Mammogram**
- Increased radiodensity
- Cystic changes

- Benign opacities
- Benign microcalcifications
  - Scattered, punctiform, monomorphic
  - Lobular arrangement
  - Intracystic calcification (teacup sign curvilinear layering in the lateral projection)

▶ **US**
- Anechoic or mixed echogenicity areas
- Variable but predominantly hypoechoic echotexture
- Posterior acoustic enhancement may be observed
- Mostly cysts, these may be microcystic

▶ **MR**
- Mostly diffuse or patchy enhancement
- Mostly slow and continuous signal increase (benign enhancement curve)
  - **Differential Diagnosis:** Ductal carcinoma in situ (DCIS)

Breast Cysts

▶ Microcysts ≤3 mm, macrocysts >3 mm
▶ **Mammo**
- Round or oval, well-defined, solitary or multiple
- May be better demonstrated by tomography, particularly amongst dense tissue

▶ **US**
- Anechoic
- Round-oval shape
- Smooth wall
- Posterior acoustic enhancement
- Lateral acoustic shadowing (edge shadowing)

▶ **MR**
- T2 homogeneously high signal
- Possible rim enhancement/compression of normal tissue

▶ In case of atypical cyst (haemorrhage, infection, mass) further clarification is required with ultrasound and/or biopsy
▶ **IR:** Fine needle aspiration for symptomatic cysts

Radial Scar

▶ Adenosis with central sclerosis, variant fibrocystic mastopathy
▶ Can be associated with atypia and malignancy
▶ **Mammo**
  • Architectural distortion in the absence of a surgical history
  • Star-shaped configuration, no central density
  • Longer, more gracile spicules when compared to carcinoma, with translucent/low density centre (black star)
  • If visible ultrasonically, may be identified as a subtle alteration in tissue texture or distortion

Papilloma

▶ Solitary or multiple benign tumours with intraductal and intracystic forms. Intraductal forms may be branching
▶ Associated with bloody secretion from the nipple
▶ Multiple papillomas can present a management challenge requiring multidisciplinary planning and surveillance
▶ **Mammo:** Peripheral focal finding, usually benign looking mass or cluster of calcifications or focal dilated duct
▶ **US:** Hypoechoic focal finding, may be associated with a cyst or visible duct. May be branching
▶ **MR:** T1/T2 smooth, hypointense, variable enhancement
▶ juvenile papillomatosis
  • Presents in younger women
  • Papillary epithelial hyperplasia associated with multiple duct ectasias and cysts
  • **MR:** T2 multiple small internal cysts
▶ **Differential Diagnosis:** Papillary carcinoma

Fibroadenoma

▶ Fibroepithelial mixed tumour with mesenchymal (connective tissue) and epithelial (milk ducts, acini) elements
▶ Any age, peaks before the age of 40
▶ Growth possible under hormone medication

▶ **Mammo**
- Round, oval or lobulated, smoothly bordered, homogeneous
- Halo as an indication of benignity
- Associated with coarse to popcorn-like, and finally complete calcification

▶ **US**
- Homogeneously isoechoic mass with thin, well-defined border (can be hyperechoic)
- May be associated with posterior acoustic enhancement
- Displaces rather than infiltrative into adjacent structures
- Mobile and compressible

▶ **MR**
- Moderate enhancement, continuous signal increase (benign enhancement curve)
- Stronger enhancement possible in young women and under hormone medication

▶ **Differential Diagnosis**: Cyst, medullary carcinoma, mucinous carcinoma

Phyllodes Tumour

▶ Stromal/connective tissue, categorised as benign, borderline or rarely malignant

▶ **Mammo**: May mimic fibroadenoma, though are less commonly calcified

▶ **US**: More heterogeneous than fibroadenoma, though with an organised ultrasonic appearance. Can present as cystic/solid lesions or have cystic elements and internal vascular channels

▶ **MR**: T2 hyperintense. Can appear heterogeneous due to cystic cavities. Variable enhancement

▶ **Differential Diagnosis**: Fibroadenoma

Lipoma

▶ **Mammo**: Radiolucent mass with delicate capsule and no associated calcification

▶ **US**: Hyperechoic, compressible mass

Adenofibrolipoma/Hamartoma

▶ Mammo: Inhomogeneous mass consisting of variable elements of dense glandular and lucent adipose or ductal tissue. May have a fine, defined pseudocapsule
▶ US: Inhomogeneous, usually defined lesion, composed of elements of echogenicity matching those elsewhere within the same breast
▶ Classically described as a 'breast within the breast'

Lymph Nodes

▶ Intramammary (especially upper outer quadrant) or axillary
▶ Mammo: Oval or kidney-shaped, smoothly marginated mass with central lucency (lymph node hilum)
▶ US: Well-defined hypoechoic and uniform periphery, with hyperechoic lymph node hilum. Hilum can show blood flow
▶ MR: T1 low signal periphery with increased/fat signal hilum. Rapid enhancement

Bleeding

▶ Mammo
- Diffuse haemorrhage: Generalised ill-defined increased density/increased echogenicity at the site of haemorrhage
- Postoperative haematoma: Rounded density that can contain lucencies (air)

Scar

▶ Mammo
- Linear opacities with associated architectural distortion
- Different appearance in different projections, persists on compression views
- Occasional cicatricial calcification

▶ **US**
- Linear hypoechoic area. Can be associated with dense posterior acoustic shadowing
- Occasional connection to the skin scar

▶ **MR**
- New or recent surgical sites/scars may enhance
- No enhancement in older scars (from 6 months after surgery or 12 months after radiotherapy)

▶ **Differential Diagnosis**: Carcinoma, radial scar

Radiotherapy Changes

▶ Spectrum of radiological appearances which may be apparent following breast-conserving therapy

▶ **Mammo**
- Asymmetry
- Skin thickening
- Reticular thickening, breast oedema

Acute Mastitis

▶ Types
- Puerperal mastitis
- Non-puerperal mastitis

▶ Mostly staphylococci, rarely anaerobes

▶ High fever, chills, local signs of inflammation, lump formation

▶ **Mammo**
- Skin thickening
- Increased density of the glandular parenchyma due to oedema
- Mammography is of limited value during breastfeeding due to lactational density of the glandular tissue
- Ultrasound may show subtle lack of definition of parenchymal structures due to oedema. Increased vascularity may also be present
- Ultrasound may identify associated abscess formation, and permit percutaneous drainage

▶ **MR**
- T2 diffuse hyperintense
- Skin thickening
- Increased enhancement of the entire breast

▶ **Differential Diagnosis**: Inflammatory breast carcinoma

▶ **Diagnosis**: In the absence of response to antibiotic therapy to exclude carcinoma. Punch biopsy or clinical biopsy of the affected tissue if no radiological focal target

▶ **Complications**: Abscess (subcutaneous, subareolar, intramammary, retromammary), fistula formation after spontaneous perforation or iatrogenic drainage

Chronic Mastitis

▶ Plasma cell mastitis
▶ Chronic granulomatous mastitis
▶ Tends to be bilateral
▶ **Mammo:** Mostly coarse needle-shaped calcifications directed towards the nipple, partly centrally more lucent

Breast Carcinoma

▶ Risk factors: Early menarche, late menopause, high oestrogen levels, obesity, alcohol, high breast density, genetic changes, positive family history
  - Particularly high risk in women with a proven pathogenic mutation in one of the known highly penetrant breast cancer risk genes

▶ Types
  - 70% invasive ductal carcinoma
  - 10% Invasive lobular carcinoma
  - 5% medullary, mucinous, tubular, papillary carcinoma
  - 15% non-invasive carcinomas
    – 95% ductal carcinoma in situ
    – 5% lobular carcinoma in situ

▶ Palpable mass, indentation/skin or nipple indrawing, ulceration, bloody secretion. May be asymptomatic

▶ About 50% of carcinomas in the upper outer quadrant
  • Multifocality: Other foci related to the main tumour, in one quadrant
  • Multicentricity/multisite: Other foci unrelated to the main tumour, in different quadrants/sites
  • Bilaterality: Both breasts affected, published rates between 2% and 10%
▶ Lymphatic metastasis mainly to the axilla, haematological metastasis to bone, lung, liver, brain most frequently
▶ If the breasts are dense malignant disease may be obscured and therefore occult. If there are clinically suspicious findings where breast tissue is dense, cancer cannot be excluded mammographically
▶ Mammography screening
  • Mammography is currently the only screening method with proven reduction in breast cancer mortality
  • National screening programmes offer invitation to attend for mammography at nationally agreed intervals, with recall assessment at specialist units when a mammographic abnormality is found
  • In future, artificial intelligence may assist with screening programmes, this is a field of active research
  • High risk patients/specific gene carriers identified by genetic screening are eligible for annual MR screening
▶ Features suspicious for malignancy
▶ **Mammo**
  • Focal grouping of microcalcifications in two planes
    – Mostly pleomorphic, rarely monomorphic
    – Clustered, segmental, haphazard, chaotic and irregular
  • Other suspicious features (particularly when a mammographic finding is new):
    – Irregular lesion
    – Ill-defined, microlobulated or angular border
    – Associated increased density
    – Associated architectural distortion
    – Dilated mammary ducts
    – Asymmetry

- Calcification may be intralesional or extend out with an invasive focus
- Ancillary findings such as skin thickening/retraction or dense, enlarged axillary nodes
- Improving the sensitivity and specificity of mammograms
  - Tomosynthesis
  - Contrast enhancement

▶ **US**

- The ultrasonic appearance of breast cancer varies widely, influenced by the histological type and grade
- The echogenicity of a tumour varies widely, and will reflect the underlying histology of the disease
- Irregular border, angular margins and microlobulation all positively predict a lesion is malignant. The greater the percentage irregularity of a lesion, the greater the probability of malignancy
- An ill-defined perilesional margin is a suspicious feature, which may indicate peritumoural oedema or compressed tumour spicules
- Acoustic shadowing may be present, though some tumour subtypes (mucinous for example) may demonstrate acoustic enhancement
- Taller rather than wider (vertical orientation) parameters can indicate a malignant lesion, although most positively predictive when lesions are very small, less than 1.5 cm
- Distortion of architecture surrounding a lesion is predictive of malignancy
- Fixed to surrounding structures, or visibly infiltrating into them
- Malignant lesions may be incompressible or immobile

▶ **Colour Doppler US**

- Asymmetry to the opposite side
- Increased vascularity
- Radial vascular course
- Branched vessels
- High total blood flow
- High flow rate

- High flow resistance
- Variability of the flow profiles

▶ **3D US:** Retraction pattern
▶ **MR**
  - Lesion types
    - Mass like enhancement, asymmetrical, localised, correlating with known disease sites
    - Non mass like enhancement: discontinuous distribution pattern, may be segmental, no space-occupying component
    - Motion artefact will cause disruption of subtraction and limit interpretation
  - Invasive ductal carcinoma
    - Shape of enhancement: Variable, may reflect the mammographic or ultrasonic appearance
    - Enhancement pattern: Marginal, may cause ring enhancement depending on tumour morphology
    - Often has a "washout" or type III enhancement curve
  - Invasive lobular carcinoma
    - Usually more difficult to detect due to less contrast agent accumulation than in invasive ductal carcinoma, may have any enhancement curve type
    - Unsuitable for excluding a lobular carcinoma in situ
  - Mucinous carcinoma
    - Frequent absence of the characteristic contrast medium accumulation. Areas of high T2 signal may be visible
▶ Lesion Kinetics: Enhancement/time curves, sometimes termed the Kuhl enhancement curves
  - Type I curve: Progressive or persistent enhancement pattern, consistent over time, may reflect benign histology. <10% of malignancies have a type 1 curve
  - Type II curve: Plateau pattern—more suspicious for malignancy, cannot exclude malignancy
  - Type III curve: Washout pattern, rapid uptake which reduces during the image acquisition—highly suggestive of malignancy

► Improving the sensitivity and specificity of MR
- Fast dynamic imaging: Initial enhancement
- Diffusion weighted imaging: Diffusion restriction has some application in published research

► Diagnosis
- Focal findings identified on MRI can be initially evaluated with targeted second look ultrasound: Core biopsy under ultrasound guidance is advised of any focally suspicious MR finding
- Every suspicious finding that can be reliably delineated should be biopsied
- Findings clearly definable with mammography but not identified ultrasonically may be sampled using stereo/vacuum biopsy
- Findings clearly delineated with MR but not seen on other modalities may be referred for MR assisted biopsy where available. (if detailed second look US is unhelpful)
- Exceptional cases: Open excision biopsy
- Lymph nodes: Core biopsy

TNM Classification Breast Carcinoma

► Tx primary tumour cannot be assessed
► T0 No evidence of primary tumour
► Tis carcinoma in situ
► T1 tumour less or equal to 2 cm
► T1a: >0.1 cm to ≤0.5 cm
► T1b: >0.5 cm to ≤1 cm
► T1c: >1 cm to ≤2 cm
► T2: >2 cm to ≤5 cm
► T3: >5 cm
► T4a: Chest wall
► T4b: Skin oedema, ulceration, satellite nodules (including peau d'orange) not meeting criteria for inflammatory carcinoma
► T4c: Both T4a and T4b
► T4d: Inflammatory carcinoma

► N1: Clinically mobile nodes (ipsilateral level I, II axillary nodes)
► N1mi: Micrometastases (0.2–2 mm)
► N2: Metastasis to level I and II axillary nodes that are fixed or matted or ipsilateral internal mammary nodes in the absence of axillary nodes
► N2a: Fixed or matted axillary level I or II nodes
► N2b: Internal mammary ipsilateral metastases without axillary node metastases
► N3: Infraclavicular (level III) nodes with or without lower level I and II involvement or ipsilateral internal mammary nodes with level I and II axillary node involvement or ipsilateral supraclavicular fossa lymph node involvement with or without axillary or internal mammary nodal involvement
► N3a: Ipsilateral infraclavicular lymph node metastasis
► N3b: Axillary and internal mammary nodes
► N3c: Ipsilateral supraclavicular metastasis
► M0: No distant metastases
► M1: Distant metastases in distant organs or non-regional nodes clinically or radiologically

Inflammatory Breast Carcinoma

► Inflammatory breast cancer presents when invasive tumour spreads within subepidermal lymphatic vessels
► Breasts appear reddened and inflamed, which may progress rapidly and is unresponsive to antibiotic therapy
► **Mammo**
  • Thickening of the skin
    – Blurred tissue interfaces indicative of oedema
  • Thickening of the Cooper ligaments
  • Reticular indrawing of the fat tissue
  • Increased density of the glandular tissue
  • Rapidly progressive
► **MR**: Similar to acute mastitis, which may delay diagnosis
► **Diagnosis**: Core biopsy

Paget's Disease of the Nipple

▶ Intraepidermal carcinoma in situ
▶ Histologically Paget cells in the epidermis of the nipple and areola
▶ Clinical inflammatory reaction in the area of the nipple and areola
▶ May be associated with ductal carcinoma in situ or invasive ductal carcinoma elsewhere in the same breast. Staging MRI is indicated if clinically appropriate
▶ **Mammography**:
▶ New changes should be regarded with suspicion
  • Thickened nipple
  • Flattened nipple
  • Possibly retroareolar trabecular thickening
  • Microcalcifications—these may relate to the nipple/subareolar structures or be present elsewhere within the breast. Stereotactic biopsy should be performed of suspicious calcification
▶ **MR**: Asymmetric rapid and vigorous enhancement of the affected nipple. MRI may detect mammographically occult disease elsewhere within the breast

Other Malignancies of the Breast

▶ Angiosarcoma (primary and secondary to breast conservation/radiotherapy)
▶ Lymphoma
  • Nodular
  • Diffuse
  • Nodal
▶ Metastases

Recurrence

▶ **Mammography**: New mammographic findings should be regarded with suspicion
  • Increase in the size and density of the scar
  • New focal mammographic findings in proximity to the surgical site—lesional or microcalcification

- Change in appearance of any focal mammographic structure when compared to prior studies

Breast Prosthesis Complications

▶ Implant rupture
▶ After breast prosthesis implant a fibrous capsule forms around the implant
▶ Implant ruptures can be intracapsular (~85%) or extracapsular (~15%)
  - Intracapsular rupture: Shell around the implant defective, silicone leakage from the implant but still within the connective tissue capsule
  - US: Stepladder sign
  - MR: Linguini sign (linear structures parallel to the implant edge), irregular implant contour, implant bulges.
  - Tear drop sign: Small focal invagination of implant shell caused by minimal concealed leak of droplets of silicone
  - Differential Diagnosis: Wrinkles in the implant
    – Extracapsular rupture: Shell around the implant defective, silicone leakage from the implant, and also outside the connective tissue capsule
  - US: Silicone evident outside the connective tissue capsule with snowstorm appearance
  - MR: Silicone detection outside the connective tissue capsule
▶ Seroma
▶ Silicone deposition within the lymph nodes (axillary, thoracic)
▶ Foreign body granulomas
▶ Capsular contracture
▶ Breast implant associated anaplastic large cell lymphoma (BIA-ALCL) is a rare complication which may present many years post-surgery. Most frequently presents with a new peri-implant effusion but may form a peri-implant mass or capsular thickening. Histological evaluation of the symptomatic tissue is essential

► Free silicone injections are used as a form of breast augmentation. Radiological findings are variable, but can present mammographically as very dense, extensive cystic changes which show snowstorm appearances when assessed ultrasonically. Silicone can be found in lymph nodes and amongst the soft tissues of the thorax

Pathological Changes in the Male Breast

► Adipomastia—pseudo-gynaecomastia due to accumulation of adipose tissue
► Gynaecomastia
  • Aetiology: Hormonal imbalance due to oestrogen excess or insufficient testosterone, adolescence, testicular tumour, adrenocortical tumour, pituitary tumour, chronic illness, for example liver cirrhosis, medication
  • Types
    – Nodular type
    – Dendritic type
    – Diffuse type
► Breast carcinoma

Bones, Joints

Anatomy

Skull

► Skull sutures
  • Coronal suture: Between frontal bone and parietal bones
  • Sagittal suture: Between the two parietal bones
  • Lambdoid suture: Between the parietal bones and the occipital bone
  • Frontal suture: In the middle of the frontal scale between the two paired frontal bones
  • Squamosal suture: Between parietal bone and temporal bone
► Skull base bone
  • Frontal bone
    – Squamous part
    – Temporal fossa
    – Facies interna
    – Orbital part
    – Frontal sinus
  • Ethmoid bone
    – Crista galli
    – Perpendicular plate
    – Ethmoidal labyrinth

© The Author(s), under exclusive license to Springer Nature Switzerland AG 2026
D. Pickuth, J. T. Murchison, *Pocket Guide to Radiology*,
https://doi.org/10.1007/978-3-031-76520-9_9

- Sphenoid bone
  - Body
  - Greater wing
  - Lesser wing
  - Pterygoid process
- Occipital bone
  - Foramen magnum
  - Occipital condyle
  - Sulcus sinus sigmoidei
  - Sulcus sinus transversi
  - External occipital protuberance
  - Squamous part
- Temporal bone
  - Squamous part
  - Tympanic part
  - Petrous part
▶ Facial bones
- Maxilla
- Mandible
- Os palatinum
- Zygomatic bone
- Nasal bone
- Lacrimal bone
- Inferior nasal concha
- Vomer
▶ Pterygopalatine fossa
- Topography
  - Ventral: Maxilla
  - Dorsal: Pterygoid process
  - Medial: Palatine bone
- Connections: Nasal cavity, infratemporal fossa, orbits, middle cranial fossa, skull base, oral cavity, dental compartments

Spine

▶ Vertebrae: Vertebral body, vertebral arch, spinous processes, transverse processes, superior and inferior articular facets, laminae, vertebral foramen, vertebral canal
▶ Intervertebral components
  • Intervertebral disc
    – Nucleus pulposum
    – Anulus fibrosus
  • Neural foramina
  • Facet joints
▶ Ligaments
  • Anterior longitudinal ligament: Anterior to the vertebral body
  • Posterior longitudinal ligament: Posterior to the vertebral body
  • Ligamentum flavum: Between vertebral arches
  • Costotransverse ligament: Between transverse processes and rib
  • Interspinous ligament: Between spinous processes
  • Supraspinous ligament (on the neck nuchal ligament): Posteriorly at tip spinous processes
▶ Normal posture: Cervical lordosis, thoracic kyphosis, lumbar lordosis, sacral kyphosis

Back Muscles

▶ Autochthonous back muscles: Erector spinae muscle
  • Iliocostalis muscle
  • Longissimus muscle
  • Spinal Muscle
▶ Autochthonous back muscles: Transversospinales muscles
  • Semispinalis muscle
  • Multifidus muscles
  • Rotatores muscles

▶ Autochthonous back muscles: Spinotransversales muscles
  • Splenius cervicis muscle
  • Splenius capitis muscle
▶ Muscles between adjacent spinous and transverse processes
  • Interspinales muscles
  • Intertransversarii muscles

Shoulder Girdle

▶ Bones
  • Clavicle
  • Scapula
    – Sides: Ventral and Dorsal (Fossa supraspinata, Fossa infraspinata)
    – Margins: Medial, Lateral and Superior
    – Angle: Angulus inferior, angulus superior, cavitas glenoidalis
    – Processes: Coracoid, acromion
▶ Joints
  • Sternoclavicular joint
  • Acromioclavicular joint
  • Glenohumeral joint
▶ Anterior trunk-shoulder girdle muscles
  • Subclavius muscle
  • Pectoralis minor muscle
  • Serratus anterior muscle
▶ Posterior trunk-shoulder girdle muscles
  • Trapezius muscle
  • Levator scapulae muscle
  • Rhomboid major muscle

Shoulder Joint

▶ Bones
  • Scapula
  • Humerus
    – Humeral head, anatomical neck, greater and lesser tuberosities, humeral neck, humeral shaft, trochlea, capitel-

lum, medial and lateral epicondyles, olecranon fossa, radial fossa

▶ Ligaments
- Glenohumeral ligament
- Coracohumeral ligament
- Coracoacromial ligament

▶ Bursae
- Subacromial bursa
- Subdeltoid bursa

▶ Axilla borders
- Anterior: Pectoralis major muscle, pectoralis minor muscle
- Posterior: Subscapularis muscle, scapula, teres major muscle, latissimus dorsi muscle
- Medial: Serratus anterior muscle, thorax
- Lateral: Axillary skin
- Axilla contents
  - Axillary artery
  - Axillary vein
  - Brachial plexus
  - Axillary lymph nodes

▶ Shoulder spaces
- Triangular space: Circumflex scapular artery
- Quadrangular space: Axillary nerve, posterior circumflex humeral artery
- Triangular interval: Profunda brachii artery, radial nerve

▶ Shoulder girdle-upper arm muscles
- Deltoid muscle
- Teres minor muscle
- Teres major muscle
- Subscapularis muscle
- Coracobrachialis muscle
- Supraspinatus muscle
- Infraspinatus muscle

▶ Trunk-upper arm muscles
- Pectoralis major muscle
- Latissimus dorsi muscle

Rotator Cuff

▶ Insertion at the greater tubercle
  • Supraspinatus muscle: Abduction
  • Infraspinatus muscle: External rotation
  • Teres minor muscle: Adduction, external rotation
▶ Insertion at the lesser tubercle
  • Subscapularis muscle: Internal rotation

Elbow Joint

▶ Bones
  • Humerus
  • Radius
    – Radial head, radial neck, radial shaft, radial styloid process
  • Ulna
    – Olecranon, coronoid process, trochlear notch, radial notch
▶ Joints
  • Ulnotrochlear
  • Radiocapitellar
  • Proximal radioulnar
▶ Ligaments
  • Radial collateral
  • Lateral ulnar collateral
  • Annular
▶ Upper arm muscles
  • Extensors
    – Triceps brachii muscle
  • Flexors
    – Biceps brachii muscle
    – Brachialis muscle
    – Coracobrachialis muscle
    – Brachioradialis muscle
▶ Forearm muscles
  • Extensors: Radial and dorsal
  • Flexors: Ulnar and palmar

Carpal Tunnel

▶ Median nerve
▶ Flexor tendons
▶ Flexor retinaculum

Bones of the Hand

▶ Carpal bones (wrist)
  • Proximal row
    – Scaphoid bone
    – Lunate (lunar or moon shaped, bone)
    – Triquetrum (triangular bone)
    – Pisiform (pea shaped bone)
  • Distal row
  • Trapezium (large polygonal bone)
  • Trapezoideum (small polygonal bone)
  • Capitate
  • Hamate
▶ Metacarpal
  • Base
  • Body
  • Head
▶ Finger
  • Proximal, middle and distal phalanges

Order of Layers on the Palm of the Hand

▶ Palmar aponeurosis
▶ Superficial palmar arch, finger nerves
▶ Flexor tendons of the fingers, Lumbricals muscles
▶ Deep palmar arch, motor branches of the ulnar nerve
▶ Metacarpal bones, Palmar interossei muscles

Order of Layers on the Back (Dorsum) of the Hand

▶ Venous network, cutaneous nerves
▶ Dorsal palm fascia
▶ Extensor tendons
▶ Arterial network
▶ Metacarpal bone
▶ Dorsal interosseous muscles

Triangular Fibrocartilaginous Complex

▶ Triangular fibrocartilaginous complex
  • Insertion at the ulnar portion of the distal radius and with two portions proximally and distally at the ulnar styloid process
▶ Dorsal and volar radioulnar ligaments
▶ Ulnolunate and ulnotriquetral ligaments
▶ Ulnar collateral ligament
▶ Ulnocarpal ligament

Hip Joint

▶ Bones
  • Acetabulum
    – Ilium, Ischium, Pubis
  • Femur
    – Femoral head, fovea capitis, femoral neck, greater trochanter, lesser trochanter, femoral shaft, medial condyle, lateral condyle, intercondylar notch, Facies patellaris, medial epicondyle, lateral epicondyle
▶ Femoral neck angle
  • CCD angle (Centrum Collum Diaphyseal angle)
  • In adults about 128°
▶ Ligaments
  • Iliofemoral ligament
  • Ischiofemoral ligament
  • Pubofemoral ligament
  • Femoral head ligament

▶ Sciatic Foramen
  - Greater Sciatic Foramen
    - Cranial limit: Sacroiliac joint
    - Caudal boundary: Sacrospinous ligament
    - Structures passing through: Piriformis muscle, superior gluteal artery, superior gluteal nerve, inferior gluteal artery, inferior gluteal nerve, sciatic nerve, posterior cutaneous femoral nerve
  - Lesser Sciatic Foramen
    - Cranial boundary: Sacrospinous ligament
    - Caudal border: Sacrotuberous ligament
    - Penetrating structures: Internal pudendal artery and vein, Pudendal nerve
▶ Inguinal ligament
▶ Formed from the aponeurosis of the lower border of the external oblique muscle
▶ Extends from anterior superior iliac spine laterally to pubic tubercle medially
  - Muscular Lacuna,
    - Lateral compartment inferior to the inguinal ligament
    - Contains iliopsoas muscle, femoral nerve, lateral femoral cutaneous nerve
  - Vascular lacuna
    - Medial compartment inferior to the inguinal ligament
    - Contains femoral artery, femoral vein, deep inguinal lymph nodes
▶ Hip muscles: Gluteal muscles
  - Gluteus maximus muscles
  - Gluteus medius muscle
  - Gluteus minimus muscle
  - Tensor fasciae latae muscle
▶ Hip muscles: Small external rotators
  - Piriformis muscle
  - Gemellus superior muscle
  - Obturator internus muscle
  - Inferior gemellus muscle
  - Obturator externus muscle
  - Quadratus femoris muscle

► Hip muscles: Iliopsoas muscle
  • Psoas major muscle
  • Iliacus muscle
  • Psoas minor muscle
► Hip muscles: Adductors
  • Pectineus muscle
  • Adductor longus muscle
  • Gracilis muscle
  • Adductor brevis muscle
  • Adductor magnus muscle
► Hip muscles: Ischiocrural muscles
  • Semitendinosus muscle
  • Semimembranosus muscle
  • Biceps femoris muscle

Thigh

► Thigh muscles
  • Extensors
    – Quadriceps femoris muscle
    – Vastus medialis muscle
    – Vastus intermedius muscle
    – Vastus lateralis muscle
    – Rectus femoris muscle
    – Sartorius muscle
    – Tensor fasciae latae muscle
  • Adductors
    – Pectineus muscle
    – Adductor longus muscle
    – Adductor brevis muscle
    – Adductor magnus muscle
    – Adductor minimus muscle
    – Gracilis muscle
    – Obturator externus muscle

- Flexors
  - Semitendinosus muscle
  - Semimembranosus muscle
  - Biceps femoris muscle

Knee Joint

▶ Bones
- Femur
- Tibia
  - Medial condyle, lateral condyle, intercondylar eminence, medial and lateral intercondylar tubercles, tibial tuberosity, tibial shaft, medial malleolus
- Patella
  - Base, Apex
▶ Joints
- Medial femorotibial articulation
- Lateral femorotibial articulation
- Patellofemoral articulation
▶ Menisci
▶ Cruciate ligaments
▶ Lateral collateral ligaments
▶ Bursa
- Suprapatellar bursa
- Prepatellar bursa
▶ Adductor canal contains
- Femoral artery
- Femoral vein
- Saphenous nerve
▶ Knee joint muscles
- Quadriceps femoris muscle
  - Rectus femoris muscle
  - Vastus lateralis muscle
  - Vastus intermedius muscle
  - Vastus medialis muscle

- Sartorius muscle
- Popliteus muscle
▶ Pes anserinus
  - Sartorius muscle
  - Gracilis muscle
  - Semitendinosus muscle

Cruciate Ligaments

▶ Anterior cruciate ligament
  - Originates postero-medial aspect of lateral femoral condyle: Inserts—intercondylar area on the tibial plateau
  - With the knee extended—tense
▶ Posterior cruciate ligament
  - Originates anterolateral aspect of medial femoral condyle—inserts—posterior aspect of tibial plateau
  - Relaxed with the knee extended

Lower Leg

▶ Neuro-vascular-bundles
  - Extensor bundle
    - Anterior tibial artery and vein
    - Deep peroneal nerve
  - Fibular bundle
    - Superficial fibular nerve
  - Popliteal fossa to posterior compartment of the leg
    - Posterior tibial artery and vein
    - Tibial nerve
▶ Lower leg muscles
  - Extensor muscles
    - Tibialis anterior muscle
    - Extensor digitorum longus muscle
    - Extensor hallucis longus muscle
    - Peroneus muscle
  - Peroneal muscles
    - Peroneus longus muscle
    - Peroneus brevis muscle

- Flexor muscles
  - Superficial: Soleus, gastrocnemius, plantaris muscles
  - Deep: Posterior tibialis, flexor hallucis longus, flexor digitorum longus muscles

Ankle Joint

▶ Joints
- Upper ankle joint
  - Ankle joint
- Lower ankle joint
  - Subtalar articulation
  - Talocalcaneonavicular articulation
▶ Ligaments
- Lateral collateral ligament
  - Anterior talofibular ligament, posterior talofibular ligament, calcaneofibular ligament
- Deep deltoid ligament
- Spring Ligament (superomedial calcaneo-navicular, medioplantar oblique calcaneo-navicular and inferoplantar longitudinal calcaneo-navicular ligaments)
- Syndesmotic ligaments: Anterior and posterior inferior tibiofibular ligaments

Bones of Feet

▶ Tarsal bones
- Proximal
  - Talus: Head, neck, body
  - Calcaneus (heel bone): Peroneal tubercle, Sustentaculum tali
  - Navicular
- Distal
  - Medial cuneiform
  - Intermediate cuneiform
  - Lateral cuneiform
  - Cuboid

- ▶ Metatarsals (midfoot)
  - Base
  - Body
  - Head
- ▶ Digiti (toes)
  - Proximal phalanges
  - Middle phalanges
  - Distal phalanges

Paediatric Radiology: Anatomy

Normal Variants

- ▶ Skull
  - Accessory cranial sutures
    - Sutura intraparietalis
    - Sutura longitudinalis
  - Wormian bones
    - Inca bone
  - Focal calvarial lucency
    - Giant parietal foramina
    - Giant arachnoid granulations
- ▶ Skeleton
  - Thorax
    - Cervical rib
    - Bifid rib
  - Spine
    - Spina bifida occulta
    - Anterior arch of C1 defects
    - Segmentation defects
    - Numerical variations
    - Intervertebral disc calcification
  - Pelvis
    - Bone islands
  - Extremities
    - Benign cortical defect: Tendency to spontaneous regression

- Non-specific metaphyseal compaction bands: Growth arrest lines, lead intoxication
- Ulnar/radial spicules: Normal variant, phenylketonuria
- Physiological periosteal reaction: Accelerated growth

Bone Abnormalities

Bone Abnormalities

▶ Osteopenia
  - Due to reduced calcium content, resulting in increased radiolucency
  - Generalised: Osteoporosis, anaemia, hyperthyroidism, hyperparathyroidism, diabetes mellitus, gravidity, malnutrition, plasmacytoma, steroids
  - Localised: Immobilisation, Sudeck's atrophy, transient osteoporosis, Paget's disease
▶ Osteolysis
  - Destruction of bone tissue
  - Cancellous bone rather than compact bone
  - Morphology determined by degree of aggressiveness
  - Lodwick Classification
    - Lodwick IA: Geographical with marginal sclerosis (e.g. solitary bone cyst)
    - Lodwick IB: Geographically without marginal sclerosis and/or with cortical protrusion (e.g. epidermoid cyst)
    - Lodwick IC: Geographical with cortical penetration and/or blurred boundary (e.g. giant cell tumour)
    - Lodwick II: Moth-eaten (e.g. plasmacytoma, metastases)
    - Lodwick III: Permeative (e.g. Ewing sarcoma, osteosarcoma)
▶ Osteosclerosis
  - Increased calcium content, increased radiodensity
  - Congenital: Osteopetrosis, melorheostosis, osteopoikilosis, osteopathia striata, diaphyseal dysplasia, endostal hyperostostosis

- Neoplastic: Metastases, lymphoma, leukaemia, plasmacytoma, osteomyelosclerosis, bone tumours
- Metabolic: Heavy metal intoxication, hyperparathyroidism, renal osteopathy, Paget's disease
- Traumatic: Fracture, callus
- Vascular: Osteonecrosis, bone infarction
- Inflammatory: Osteomyelitis

▶ Periosteal reaction
- Solid: Slow growing (osteoid osteoma)
- Onion-skinned: Intermittently growing (osteomyelitis, Ewing sarcoma)
- Interrupted: Fast growing (Codman triangle, spicules) (osteosarcoma)

▶ Acroosteolysis
- Hyperparathyroidism
- Systemic sclerosis
- Raynaud syndrome
- Angiomatosis of the bones (Gorham-Stout disease)
- Thromboangiitis obliterans
- Leprosy
- Polyvinyl chloride disease

Trauma

Fracture—Clinical Signs

▶ Clinical
- Pain
- Limited function
- Massive soft tissue swelling
- Abnormal mobility
- Crepitation

▶ Radiological
- Lucent line
- Angulation
- Continuity break

Types of Fracture

▶ In children and adolescents mainly chondral fractures, in adults mainly osteochondral fractures
▶ Localisation
  • Apophyseal, epiphyseal, metaphyseal, diaphyseal
▶ Configuration
  • Compound or open (breaks skin)
  • Closed or simple (skin intact)
  • Buckle or torus (one side of bone bends—more common in children)
  • Transverse, longitudinal, oblique, spiral fracture
  • T-, Y-, V-shaped fracture
  • Comminuted, more than two pieces, splinter fracture
  • Compression fracture
  • Avulsion fracture
▶ Dislocation
  • Longitudinal dislocation with shortening
  • Longitudinal displacement with extension
  • Lateral displacement
  • Axial buckling
    – Varus malalignment
    – Valgus malposition
    – Antecurvation
  • Twisting

Special Types of Fracture

▶ Infraction
▶ Stress fracture
  • Stress fracture: Healthy bone is pathologically loaded
    – Jogging: Fibula, tibia, pelvis
    – Football: Tibia, metatarsals, navicular
    – Tennis: Ulna, metacarpals, elbow
    – Throwing sports: Ulna, humerus, spine
    – Cycling: Pelvis

- • Insufficiency fracture: Pathological bone is loaded normally
- ▶ Open or compound fracture (breaks skin)
- ▶ Pathological fracture
- ▶ Looser zones
  - • Pseudofractures of osteomalacia
  - • Pubic bone, ischium, femoral neck, femoral shaft, ribs, scapula
  - • **X-ray**: Band-like sclerosis in the cancellous bone, discrete lucency in the cortical bone
  - • Multiple as Milkman syndrome

Basics of the AO Classification of Fractures

- ▶ Step 1: Coding of the bone and the segment
  - • 1 = humerus, 2 = forearm, 3 = femur, 4 = lower leg
  - • 1 = proximal, 2 = shaft, 3 = distal
- ▶ Step 2: Typing the fracture
  - • Shaft fracture: A = simple, B = wedge, C = complex
  - • Joint fracture: A = extra-articular, B = partial joint fracture, C = complete joint fracture
- ▶ Step 3: Allocation according to complexity and prognosis
  - • 1 = easy, 2 = more difficult, 3 = difficult

Fracture Fixation Principles

- ▶ Compression
  - • Static
  - • Dynamic
- ▶ Splinting
  - • Inner
  - • Outer
- ▶ Support

Implant Types

- ▶ Screws
- ▶ External fixator

▶ Intramedullary nail
▶ Endoprostheses

Fracture Fixation Assessment

▶ Criteria
  • Prosthesis fracture
  • Prosthesis bending
  • Prosthesis dislocation
  • Lucent margin around implant
  • New fracture
  • Secondary fragment dislocation
  • Interarticular loose body
▶ Complications
  • Prosthesis failure
  • Instability
  • Laxity
  • Osteomyelitis
  • Refracture
  • Osteonecrosis

Prosthesis Infection

▶ Aetiology: Patient-dependent (obesity, diabetes, nicotine abuse, alcohol abuse), surgery-dependent, implant-dependent
▶ Stages
  • Early infection
    – Perioperative infection route
    – Classic signs of inflammation
  • Late infection
    – Haematogenous route of infection (lungs, skin, urinary tract, teeth)
    – Acute or subacute pain and looseness
▶ X-ray
  • Often inconspicuous, otherwise loosening fringe, osteolysis, periosteal reaction
  • Differential Diagnosis: Aseptic prosthesis loosening (prosthesis fracture, prosthesis mobility, prosthesis migration)

▶ **Nuclear medicine**: Positive
▶ **Diagnosis**: US aspiration of the joint cavity and culture of
pathogens, a fistula in contact with the joint or pus in the joint
cavity

Inflammation Scintigraphy

▶ **18F-FDG-PET**
▶ Indications
  • Endoprosthesis loosening
  • Prosthesis infection
  • Acute or chronic osteomyelitis
  • Fever of unknown origin
  • Leukocytosis of unclear genesis
▶ Normal findings
  • Physiological representation of liver, spleen, bone marrow
    and intestine

Fracture Healing

▶ Criteria for fracture healing
  • Age of the patient
  • Type of fracture
  • Localisation of the fracture
  • Blood supply to the fragments
  • Apposition of the fragment ends
  • Stability of the fracture
▶ Fracture morphology
▶ Initially fracture line sharp
  • With indirect fracture healing after 3–14 days fracture line
    more clearly visible
  • In the case of direct fracture healing, this is an indication of
    disturbed fracture union
  • After callus formation fracture line blurred
▶ Types of fracture healing
  • Primary (direct) fracture healing
    – Limited callus formation

- Secondary (indirect) fracture healing
  - Callus formation
  - Transformation of immature fibrous bone into mature lamellar bone
  - Callus resorbed
▶ X-ray signs of fracture healing
  - Continuous bridging of the fracture
  - Homogeneous density of the fracture callus
  - Density of fracture callus comparable with density of cortical bone
▶ Assessment of fracture healing
  - Primary fracture healing harder to assess than secondary fracture healing
  - Fracture healing of intracapsular, periosteum-free bone sections close to the joint without external callus formation
  - In case of doubtful fracture union—CT
  - Think of pathological fracture in case of unusual fracture locations
▶ Mobilisation of the patient
  - Immobilisation for lower limb fractures longer than for upper limb fractures
  - Sharp, strong callus formation necessary for mobilisation of the lower limb, fuzzy, cloudy callus formation sufficient for mobilisation of the upper limb

Fracture Healing Time

Fracture localisation	Fracture healing time (weeks)
Clavicle	4
Proximal humerus	4–5
Humeral shaft	6–8
Supracondylar humerus	4–6
Olecranon	3–4
Radius head	3–4
Forearm shaft	12
Distal radius	3–4
Scaphoid	6–16

Fracture localisation	Fracture healing time (weeks)
Metacarpal	4
Finger	3–4
Pelvis	4–10
Femoral neck	12–20
Femoral shaft	12–16
Patella	4
Lower leg shaft	12–16
Tibia shaft	8–14
Fibula shaft	4–6
Ankle joint	6–12
Midfoot	4–6
Toes	2–3
Spine	12–16

Fracture Healing Delay

▶ Aetiology: Fracture-related (unfavourable fracture alignment, soft tissue interposition, bone defects, bone sequestrum, infection, insufficient blood supply), therapy-related (instability, insufficient immobilisation, unfavourable fragment position, faulty osteosynthesis, infection), general (nicotine abuse, steroids, anticoagulants, innervation disorders)
▶ Delayed fracture healing
  • No fracture healing after 3–6 months
  • Rounding off of the fragment ends
  • Enlargement of the fracture gap
  • Marked callus
  • Material loosening
  • Lysis zones
▶ Pseudarthrosis
  • Types
    – Atrophic (areactive, avital) pseudarthrosis: No callus formation, poor vascularisation, especially in fragment necrosis
    – Hypertrophic (reactive, vital) pseudarthrosis: Good callus formation, good vascularisation, especially in fracture instability

- – Defect pseudoarthrosis
- – Infectious pseudoarthrosis
- **X-ray**
  - – Stage I: Resorption zones at the fracture edge
  - – Stage II: Marginal sclerosis and cysts
  - – Stage III: Sclerosis of the fracture margins
  - – Stage IV: Arthrosis
- **MR**
  - – Stage I: Cleft formation with fibrous content or fluid
  - – Stage II: Marginal sclerosis with cartilage coating
  - – Stage III: Subchondral necrosis, cysts, fibrosis and oedema
  - – Stage IV: Effusion and synovitis
- **US:** More precise delineation of the cause of pseudarthrosis with contrast-enhanced sonography
- Final state with pseudoarticulation at the joint

Early Fracture Complications

▶ Thrombosis
▶ Nerve damage
▶ Compartment syndrome
  - Localisation
    - – Dorsal humeral compartment
    - – Ventral humeral compartment
    - – Forearm flexor compartment
    - – Forearm extensor compartment
    - – Interossei muscles
    - – Thenar muscles
    - – Gluteal muscles
    - – Dorsal femoral
    - – Lateral femoral
    - – Tibialis anterior
    - – Superficial lower leg
    - – Deep lower leg
    - – Peroneal

- **US**
  - Acute compartment syndrome: Increased muscle diameter, diffusely increased echogenicity, facultative haematoma
  - Chronic compartment syndrome: Normal volume increase under stress, but delayed recovery

Late Fracture Complications

▶ Disuse osteopenia
▶ Complex regional pain syndrome
  - Sudeck's atrophy
  - Aetiology: Inflammation, dystrophy and atrophy of soft tissues and bones due to trauma, infection and nerve damage
  - Diffuse pain, different skin colour, diffuse soft tissue oedema, different skin temperature, limited mobility
  - **X-ray**
    - Initial phase: No skeletal changes, soft tissue swelling
    - Dystrophic phase: Patchy osteopenia (resorption first near the joint, then endosteal, intracortical, subperiosteal and subchondral)
    - Atrophy phase: Diffuse osteopenia (rarefaction of the spongy trabeculae, frame structure of the thinned cortical bone), soft tissue atrophy
    - Clinical symptoms before radiographic changes
  - **MR**
    - Bone marrow T1 hypointense, T2 hyperintense
    - Thickening of subcutis, musculature and joint capsules
    - Enhancement of the bone marrow and soft tissues
  - **Nuclear medicine**
    - Initial phase: Increased arterial blood flow
    - Dystrophy phase: No significant increase in venous blood volume
    - Atrophy phase: Avascular necrosis—photopenic region
  - **Differential Diagnosis**: Inactivity osteopenia, collagenoses, osteomyelitis, arthritis
  - **Complications**: Insufficiency fracture

▶ Osteonecrosis
▶ Osteomyelitis
▶ Myositis ossificans
▶ Osteoarthritis

Soft Tissue Injuries

▶ Fractures are often accompanied by injuries to the musculature and tendons
▶ Myotendinous injuries
- Grade I: Strain, muscle function preserved
  - US: Increase echogenicity of muscle
  - MR: Interstitial oedema and haemorrhage at the muscle-tendon junction with extension into the adjacent muscle fascicles
- Grade II: Partial rupture, limited muscle function
  - US: Echo-poor intramuscular space, regular dorsal acoustic enhancement, loss of tone, bulging
  - MR: No retraction, haematoma at the muscle-tendon junction, perifascial fluid collection
- Grade III: Complete rupture, muscle function absent
  - US: Continuity interruption, retraction, haematoma
  - MR: Retraction, haematoma, periosteal stripping at the tendon attachment site, wavy deformation of the tendon stump
▶ Muscular haematoma
  - US: Hypoechoic focus, dorsal acoustic amplification, later hyperechoic coagulation, sometimes septa, sometimes muscle swelling

Soft Tissue Injuries Associated with Fracture Types

▶ Sternal fracture
- Aortic rupture, tracheal and bronchial rupture, cardiac injury
▶ Upper rib fracture
- Aortic rupture, injury to brachiocephalic vessels, tracheal tear

▶ Left lower rib fracture
  • Splenic rupture, diaphragmatic rupture, kidney injury, duodenal haematoma
▶ Right lower rib fracture
  • Liver rupture, kidney injury
▶ Fracture of the transverse process of the lumbar spine
  • Kidney injury, pancreas injury, duodenal haematoma
▶ Pubic bone fracture
  • Urinary bladder injury, urethra injury

Soft Tissue Injuries as a Fracture Sign

▶ Spinal fracture: Paravertebral haematoma
▶ Paranasal sinus fracture: Post-traumatic air-fluid level
▶ Orbital fracture: Orbital emphysema
▶ Skull base fracture: Intracranial air
▶ Elbow fracture: Fat pad sign
▶ Knee fracture: Fat-fluid level (Holmgren sign)

Joint Effusion

▶ Clear: Joint irritation, eg OA
▶ Bloody: Internal injury
▶ Fibrinous: Inflammation
▶ Purulent: Infection
▶ Lipomatous: Bone injury

Clarification of Skull Fractures

▶ CT
▶ MR
  • In the case of craniocerebral trauma also assess craniocervical junction

Calvarial Fractures

▶ Linear fracture
▶ Splinter fracture

- ▶ Depressed fracture
- ▶ Suture diastasis
- ▶ Complicated fracture
  - • Intracranial trauma sequelae, especially in calvarial fractures over the temporal bones, near the large venous blood conduits, over the motor cortex or in depressed fractures >1 cm deep

Skull Base Fractures

- ▶ Frontobasal fractures
  - • Escher I: High frontobasal fracture
  - • Escher II: Middle frontobasal fracture
  - • Escher III: Deep frontobasal fracture
  - • Escher IV: Lateral frontobasal fracture
- ▶ Fractures of the middle skull base
- ▶ Laterobasal fractures
- ▶ Fractures of the posterior skull base

Cranial Pseudofractures

- ▶ Vascular grooves
- ▶ Sutures
- ▶ Suture variations

Orbital Fractures

- ▶ Orbital wall fracture
  - • Often component of a more complex fracture
  - • **X-ray**: Fracture line, bony displacement, suture dislocation
  - • **Diagnosis**: CT
- ▶ Orbital floor fracture
  - • Often component of a more complex fracture
  - • **X-ray**: 'Tear drop' soft tissue density below maxillary sinus roof, orbital roof air crescent, maxillary sinus fluid level
  - • **Diagnosis**: CT

▶ Blow out fracture
- Aetiology: Punch, high velocity ball sport, eg squash
- Fracture and displacement of the thin osseous walls into the maxillary or ethmoid sinuses
- Swelling, haemorrhage, diplopia, enophthalmos
- Numbness of cheek and upper lip in lesion of the infraorbital nerve in the orbital floor
- **X-ray**: Orbital floor fracture, "teardrop sign"
- **Diagnosis**: CT
- **Complications**: Trapping of ocular muscle, haemorrhage, foreign body, globe rupture, lens dislocation, orbital emphysema

▶ Blow in fracture
- Displacement of bone fragments or soft tissue into the orbit
- **X-ray**: Fracture line, fragment displacement
- **Diagnosis**: CT

Fractures of the Temporal Bone

▶ Longitudinal fracture of the petrous bone (75%)
- Direct trauma of the temporoparietal bone
- Auditory canal haemorrhage, conductive hearing loss, facial nerve palsy
- Course through external auditory canal and middle ear

▶ Temporal bone transverse fracture (25%)
- Indirect trauma to the petrous bone (occipital)
- Haematotympanum, sensorineural hearing loss, facial nerve palsy
- Course through internal auditory canal and labyrinth

▶ Evidence of a cerebrospinal fluid fistula
- Beta-2-transferrin in secretion
- Thin section CT/CT cisternography
- Thin-section MR/MR cisternography
- CSF scintigraphy with 111In-DTPA

▶ **Complications**: Cerebral haemorrhage, meningitis, brain abscess

Diagnosis of Facial Bone Fractures

▶ CT
▶ Digital volume tomography

Midface Fractures

▶ Central midface fracture
  • Le Fort I Fracture
    – Basal horizontal fracture of the maxilla,(floating palate)
    – Bones involved: Lateral nasal wall, maxilla with maxillary sinus, pterygoid process, nasal septum
  • Le Fort II Fracture
    – Pyramid-shaped break-off of the entire maxilla including the bony root of the nose (floating maxilla)
    – Skeletal parts involved: Walls of maxillary sinus, pterygoid plates, infraorbital rim, orbital floor, nasal bones
▶ Lateral midface fracture
  • Zygomatic arch fracture
  • Zygomatic fracture
▶ Combined midface fracture
  • Le Fort III fracture
    – Transverse fracture (floating face). Separation of the facial bones from the cranium including the nasofrontal junction
    – Skeletal parts involved: Nasal septum, lacrimal bone, orbital floor, frontal process of the maxilla, lateral orbital rim, zygomatic arch, nasofrontal junction

Mandibular Fractures

▶ Fractures of the mandibular body
▶ Fractures of the mandibular angle
▶ Fractures of the mandibular ramus
▶ Fractures of the temporomandibular joint

Diagnosis of Spinal Fractures

▶ AP and lateral spinal x-rays
▶ Odontoid view
▶ Swimmers view (assess cervicothoracic junction if poorly visualised on lateral radiograph)
▶ CT
▶ MR (to assess spinal cord and pre/paravertebral soft tissues)

Cervical Spine Fractures

▶ Upper cervical spine
  • Atlantooccipital dislocation
  • Atlantoaxial dislocation
  • Atlantoaxial rotational dislocation
  • Atlas fractures (C1)
    – Fracture of the anterior arch of the atlas
    – Fracture of the posterior arch of the atlas
    – Combined atlas arch fracture
    – Fracture of the lateral mass
    – Fracture of the transverse process
  • Dens fracture (C2)
    – Anderson I: Fracture of the tip of dens
    – Anderson II: Fracture of the base of the dens
    – Anderson III: Involvement of the axial body
  • Axis fractures, (C2)
    – Levine and Edwards Classification—a modification of the Effendi classification
    – Type 1: Mechanism—axial loading and hyperextension. Non-angulated C2 vertebral body. C2 body non-displaced or minimally displaced (<3 mm) C2–3 disc normal. Stable injury
    – Type 2: Anterior displacement or angulation of C2 vertebral body with >3 mm antero-posterior translation. C2–3 disc disrupted. Vertical fracture line. Unstable injury

- Type 3: Mechanism—primary flexion and rebound extension. Anterior displacement and hyperflexion of C2 vertebral body. Facet joint dislocation, either unilateral or bilateral. Horizontal/oblique fracture line. Unstable injury

▶ Middle and lower cervical spine
  • Flexion trauma
    - Flexion distortion
    - Flexion fracture
    - Joint dislocation
    - Flexion luxation fracture
    - Spinous process fracture
  • Extension trauma
    - Extension distortion
    - Lateral mass fracture
    - Extension tear drop fracture
    - Extension luxation fracture
    - Vertebral arch fracture
  • Compression trauma
    - Burst fracture

Special Forms of Cervical Spine Fractures

▶ Jefferson fracture: Fracture of the anterior and posterior arch of C1
▶ Hangman fracture: Fracture of both pars interarticularis roots of C2
▶ Tear drop fracture: Bone avulsion of the lower edge of a vertebral body

Spine and Lumbar Spine Fractures

▶ Types
  • Type A: Compression injuries of the anterior spine
  • Type B: Distraction injuries of the anterior or posterior spine
  • Type C: Unstable translational injuries of both the anterior and posterior spine

▶ Stability
- • 3 Pillars Model of Denis
- • Complete disruption of at least 2 columns is classed as unstable
  - – 1st column: Anterior two thirds of the vertebral body, annulus fibrosus, anterior longitudinal ligament
  - – 2nd column: Posterior third of the vertebral body, pars interarticularis, posterior longitudinal ligament
  - – 3rd column: Vertebral arches, vertebral joints, joint capsules

Rib Fractures

▶ Types
- • Singular rib fracture
- • Multiple rib fractures
- • Flail segment (2 or more contiguous rib fractures with 2 or more breaks per rib)

▶ Most often 4th–9th ribs

▶ Often combined with clavicle, scapula, sternum and thoracic spine fracture

▶ Accompanying injuries
- • Fractures of the three upper ribs: Trachea, bronchi, aorta
- • Of the three lowest ribs: Liver, spleen, kidneys

▶ Possible associated findings
- • Thoracic wall haematoma
- • Surgical emphysema
- • Haemothorax
- • Pneumothorax
- • Lung contusion
- • Diaphragmatic rupture
  - – Almost always left diaphragm
  - – Combination with rib fractures, splenic rupture and liver rupture

Diagnosis of Shoulder and Elbow Fractures

▶ AP Shoulder
▶ Shoulder Outlet view
▶ Shoulder Y-view
▶ Shoulder axial
▶ Clavicle AP
▶ Clavicle tangential
▶ Acromioclavicular joint AP
▶ Panorama shot with and without load
▶ SC joint weight bearing for subluxation
▶ Shoulder tangential image
▶ Elbow AP
▶ Elbow lateral
▶ Oblique view for radial head
▶ CT
▶ MR

Shoulder Fractures

▶ Clavicle fractures
  • 80% middle segment, 15% lateral segment, 5% medial segment
  • **Complication**: Excessive callus with compression of the neurovascular bundle (brachial plexus and subclavian artery)
▶ Acromioclavicular joint injuries
  • Joint stabilisers
    – Acromioclavicular ligaments
    – Coracoclavicular ligaments
    – Trapezoidodeltoid fascia
  • Joint instability
    – Tossy I: Distortion, acromion and clavicle in one plane
    – Tossy II: Subluxation with partial ligament rupture, clavicle elevation by half shaft width

- Tossy III: Luxation with complete ligament rupture, clavicle elevation by whole shaft width
- Classification of acromioclavicular dislocation also according to Rockwood

▶ Scapular fractures
  - Body fractures
  - Edge fractures
  - Coracoid fractures
  - Acromion fractures
  - Spine fractures
  - Glenoid fractures

Shoulder Dislocation

▶ Anterior
  - 95%
  - Subcoracoid (majority), subglenoid, subclavicular, intrathoracic
  - Compression fracture of the posterolateral humeral head (Hill-Sachs lesion)
  - Tear of the anteroinferior labrum (Bankart lesion)
  - Tear of the anterior joint capsule (Broca-Hartmann lesion)
▶ Posterior
  - 4%
  - Subacromial, subglenoid, subspinous
  - Compression fracture of the anteromedial humeral head (reverse Hill-Sachs lesion)
▶ Superior
  - Very rare
  - Luxatio supracoracoid
▶ Inferior
  - Very rare
  - Luxatio erecta

Rotator Cuff Disorders

▶ Impingement syndrome
  • Types
    – Primary extrinsic impingement (mechanical causes→ constricted subacromial space)
    – Secondary extrinsic impingement (glenohumeral instability → de-centered humeral head → constricted subacromial space)
    – Intrinsic impingement (lesions of the rotator cuff)
    – Internal impingement (posterosuperior in overhead sports, anterosuperior in swimming)
  • Mechanical causes of a narrowed subacromial space
    – Acromioclavicular joint arthrosis, acromial spur, hooked acromion, laterally sloping acromion, unstable os acromiale, hypertrophied coracoacromial ligament, subacromial osteophytes, caudal clavicular osteophytes, calcareous deposits, bursitis
  • In extrinsic impingement, narrowing of the subacromial space and reduced fat layers
  • Painful restriction of movement, severe abduction pain, severe external rotation pain, pressure pain, muscle atrophy, humeral head elevation
  • Painful arc
  • Stages
    – Neer I: Reversible stage; <25 years; oedema, haemorrhages
    – Neer II: Chronic inflammatory stage; 25–40 years; tendinitis, fibrosis
    – Neer III: Degenerative stage; >40 years; tendon rupture, osteophytes
  • Often simultaneous enthesopathy with degenerative changes of the tendino-osseous transition, acute tendinitis of the long biceps tendon

▶ Acute tendinitis
- **MR**: T2 tendon swollen and hyperintense (oedema), bursa hyperintense (effusions)

▶ Chronic tendinitis
- **MR**: T1 tendon hyperintense (mucoid tissue transformation), calcifications signal-free

▶ Partial rupture
- Aetiology: Impingement, trauma, overuse
- Primarily tendon of the supraspinatus muscle, less frequently of the infraspinatus or subscapularis muscles
- **MR**
  - T1 variable, T2 very hyperintense, fluid retention
  - Lower accuracy than with complete rupture
  - Therapeutic injections of local anaesthetics or steroids can lead to atypical signal changes

▶ Complete rupture
- In the event of rupture of the supraspinatus tendon, pseudo paralysis of the arm with complete loss of active abduction ability
- **X-ray**: Horizontal and/or vertical decentration of the humeral head
- **US**
  - Rotator cuff defect
  - Hypoechoic zone (oedema)
  - Hyperechoic focus (scar, calcification)
- **MR**
  - Complete interruption of continuity of the tendon
  - Occasional retraction of the tendon
  - Acute rupture: Defect T1 hypointense, T2 hyperintense, fluid retention, bursal effusion, joint effusion
  - Older rupture: Defect T1 hypointense, T2 iso- or hypointense, fat atrophy of the musculature
- Size of the tendon tear according to Bateman
  - I: <1 cm
  - II: 1–3 cm
  - III: 3–5 cm
  - IV: >5 cm

- Degrees of fat atrophy according to Goutallier
  - I: Scattered fatty streaks in the musculature
  - II: Fat mass < Muscle mass
  - III: Fat mass = Muscle mass
  - IV: Fat mass > Muscle mass
- ► Classification of arthropathy
  - Hamada Classification
    - I: Acromiohumeral distance ≥6 mm
    - II: Acromiohumeral distance <6 mm
    - III: Acromio-humeral distance <6 mm, acetabularisation of the acromion
    - IV: Acromio-humeral distance <6 mm, acetabularisation of the acromion, omarthrosis
    - V: Defect arthropathy with humeral head necrosis

Biceps Tendon Disorders

- ► Tendinitis
  - Radiating pain along the ventral upper arm
  - **MR**
    - Hyperintense tendon with marked thickening
    - Effusion in the extra-articular tendon sheath of the long biceps tendon
    - Strong enhancement of fibrovascular granulation tissue
- ► Rupture
  - Flexion weakness of the elbow, supination weakness of the forearm
  - Distal rupture usually close to the insertion at the radial tuberosity
  - Occasional co-injury of the brachialis tendon
  - Often osteophytes on the radial tuberosity, inflammation of the bicipitoradial bursa
  - **US/MR**
    - Empty intertubercular sulcus
    - Minor bleeding
    - Continuity of tendon interrupted

- Retracted tendon part
- Medialised biceps tendon
- Empty bicipital sulcus

Labral Lesions

▶ Anteroinferior segment
- Bankart lesion
  - Tearing of the labrum and capsular ligamentous apparatus from the bone and periosteum of the glenoid cavity
  - About 65% of the labrum lesions
- Perthes lesion
  - Avulsion of the labrum with detachment of the periosteum
- ALPSA lesion
  - Anterior labroligamentous periosteal sleeve avulsion
  - Avulsion and displacement of the labrum ventrally and medially between bone and periosteum
- GLAD lesion
  - Glenolabral articular cartilage disruption
  - Detachment of a cartilage fragment with the torn labrum
- HAGL lesion
  - Humeral avulsion of the glenohumeral ligament
  - Torn capsular ligament of the humerus
▶ Posterior segment
- Reverse Bankart Lesion
  - Tearing of the labrum and capsular ligamentous apparatus from the bone and periosteum of the glenoid cavity
- POLPSA lesion
  - Posterior labroligamentous periosteal sleeve avulsion
- Bennett lesion
  - Impingement or enthesopathy at the posteroinferior labrum in the form of calcifications
  - About 15% of the labrum lesions
▶ Superior section
- SLAP lesion
  - Aetiology: Fall on arm, trauma during throwing movement

- Superior labrum from anterior to posterior relative to the biceps tendon insertion on the supraglenoid tubercle
- About 15% of the labrum lesions
- Traumatisation of the long biceps tendon in the region of the attachment to the superior labrum
- Injury of the superior labrum in the anterior and posterior parts
- Often concomitant injuries of the rotator cuff and the biceps tendon
- Instability with pseudoluxation, snapping of the shoulder
- MR: Detection and classification of the SLAP lesion
- Type I: Punctate hyperintense area in the labrum
- Type II: Punctate hyperintense area in the labrum and signal enhancement between the labrum and the glenoid cavity
- Type III: Punctate hyperintense area in the labrum and evidence of a dislocated part of the labrum
- Type IV: Punctate hyperintense area in the labrum, evidence of a dislocated portion of the labrum and diffuse signal enhancement in the proximal long biceps tendon

▶ Anterosuperior segment
  • Sublabral foramen
    - Normal variant
  • Buford Complex
    - Normal variant

Clarification of Wrist and Hand Fractures

▶ Wrist dorsovolar and lateral
▶ Hand dorsovolar and oblique
▶ CT
▶ MR

Forearm and Wrist Fractures

▶ Monteggia fracture
   • Proximal ulna fracture and luxated radial head
▶ Galeazzi fracture
   • Distal radius fracture and luxated ulnar head
   • Rarer than Monteggia fracture
▶ Essex-Lopresti fracture
   • Comminuted radial head fracture with collapsed radial neck and consecutive dislocation of the distal radioulnar joint
▶ Pulled elbow injury
   • Subluxation of the radial head in children
▶ Distal radius fracture
   • Colles fracture: Distal radius fragment tilted dorsally
   • Smith fracture: Distal radius fragment tilted to palmar side
   • Barton fracture: Dorsal edge fragment broken off at the radius
   • Reverse Barton fracture: Palmar edge fragment broken off at the radius
   • Chauffeur fracture: Radial styloid fractured
   • Radial pilon fracture: Shattering of the distal radius joint surface due to axial load with radiolunate dislocation
   • **Complications**: Median paralysis, carpal tunnel syndrome
▶ Scaphoid fracture
   • Types
     – Cortical fracture
     – Trabecular fracture
   • 80% Localisation in the waist
   • In the case of uncertain X-ray findings (scaphoid series x-rays) thin-slice CT or MR
   • **MR**
     – Primary diagnosis: Bone marrow oedema, fracture line, soft tissue oedema
     – Follow-up: Differentiation of healing and non-union
   • **Complications**
     – Early complications: Ischaemic bone marrow oedema, diastasis, dislocation
     – Late complications: Delayed fracture healing, pseudarthrosis, osteonecrosis

Hand Fractures

▶ Bennett fracture
  • Intraarticular fracture of the base of the first metacarpal
▶ Rolando fracture
  • Comminuted fracture of the base of the first metacarpal
▶ Boxer fracture
  • Subcapital fracture of the fifth metacarpal
▶ Bush fracture
  • Bone avulsion from the base of the distal phalanx

Lunate Subluxation

▶ Aetiology: Trauma
▶ Results from rupture of the lunotriquetral ligament, subluxation of the lunate and carpal instability of the VISI type (volar intercalated segment instability type)
▶ **X-ray**
  • On AP image triangular shape (tip towards distal) instead of the normal rhomboid shape
  • On a lateral film, differentiation between lunate subluxation (lunate displaced to volar) or perilunate subluxation (lunate in normal position, remaining carpal bones displaced dorsally)

Scapholunate Dissociation

▶ Aetiology: Rupture or insufficiency of the scapholunate ligament due to trauma or rheumatoid arthritis
▶ Stages
  • I (predynamic): Partial rupture of the scapholunate ligament, secondary stabilisers intact, normal structural arrangement at rest and under load
  • II (dynamic): Complete rupture of the scapholunate ligament, secondary stabilisers intact, dissociation only under load (movement disorders of scaphoid and lunate)
  • III (static): Complete rupture of the scapholunate ligament, secondary stabilisers disrupted, malaligned at rest (malalignment of scaphoid and lunate)

- IV (arthritic): Complete rupture of the scapholunate ligament, secondary stabilisers dehiscent, deforming arthrosis
    - IV a: Arthrosis radioscaphoid
    - IV b: Arthrosis mediocarpal
    - IV c: Carpal collapse
▶ Carpal instabilities
- RSS type (rotational subluxation of the scaphoid)
- PISI type (Palmar intercalated segment instability)
- DISI type (Dorsal intercalated segment instability)
▶ **X-ray**
- Distance between scaphoid and lunate greater than 2 mm suspicious, greater than 3 mm definite (Terry-Thomas sign)
- Ring structure in scaphoid (signet ring sign)
▶ **MR**
- I: Tear of the scapholunate ligament
- II: Scapholunate diastasis
- III: Palmar flexion of the scaphoid
- IV: Dorsal extension of the lunate
- Reliable assessment of the individual ligament segments in MR arthrography

Lunate Pathologies

▶ Necrosis
- **MR:** Hypointense formation, enhancement initially strong, then reduced, finally absent
▶ Ulnar impaction syndrome
- **MR:** First bone marrow oedema, then chondropathy, finally cystosclerosis
▶ Intraosseous ganglion
- **MR:** Extraintraosseous ganglion components, marginal enhancement
▶ Traumatic contusion
- **MR:** Bone marrow oedema without fracture line
▶ Deforming arthrosis
- **MR:** Reduced height cartilage, subchondral oedema, subchondral sclerosis

▶ Rheumatoid arthritis
  • **MR:** Focal bone marrow oedema, contrast midline lax pannus tissue, erosive defects
▶ Osteopenia
  • **MR:** Patchy signal inclusions, focal enhancement
▶ Enostoma
  • **MR:** Hypointense formation, no enhancement
▶ Fracture
  • **MR:** Hypointense fracture line, oedematous fragments
▶ Pseudarthrosis
  • **MR:** Fluid-filled pseudarthrosis fissure, patchy fragments
▶ Chondrocalcinosis
  • **MR:** Focal bone marrow oedema, intraosseous enhancement, synovial enhancement

Triangular Fibrocartilaginous Complex

Criteria	Trauma	Degeneration
Signal intensity	Hyperintense on T2	Hyperintense on T1
Appearance	Sharply defined, band-shaped	Blurred, disc-shaped
Localisation	Eccentric	Central
Classification according to Palmer	1A: central 1B: ulnar 1C: distal 1D: radial	2A: Degeneration 2B: A + chondromalacia 2C: B + perforation 2D: C + lig. lunotriquetrum 2E: D + Arthrosis

Clarification of Pelvic and Femoral Fractures

▶ AP pelvis
▶ Pelvis obturator view (hip joint oblique)
▶ Pelvis ala view (hip joint oblique)
▶ Hip AP
▶ Hip axial (Lauenstein)
▶ Hip axial (Johansson)
▶ CT

Pelvic Fractures

▶ Types
- Type A injury (50%, stable): Pelvic rim fractures, isolated injury of the anterior pelvic ring, sacral fractures
- Type B injury (30%, rotationally unstable): Complete anterior pelvic ring rupture plus incomplete posterior pelvic ring rupture
- Type C injury (20%, rotationally and vertically unstable): Complete anterior pelvic ring rupture plus complete posterior pelvic ring rupture

▶ Stable fracture types
- Avulsion fracture
- Fracture of the sacrum
  - Sacral stress fractures
- Fracture of the iliac crest
- Fracture of the pubic rami

▶ Unstable fracture types
- Saddle fracture
- Fracture of the four pubic rami
- Fractures of the anterior and posterior pelvic rings
- Malgaigne fracture
  - Unilateral, fracture of the two ipsilateral pubic rami and sacroiliac fracture or dislocation
- Bucket handle fracture
  - Fracture of the two ipsilateral pubic rami and contralateral sacroiliac fracture or dislocation
- Open book pelvic fracture
  - Disruption of the symphysis (symphysis gap wider than 8 mm, and/or pubic rami fractures with step formation at the lower edge of the arcus symphysis) plus sacro-iliac joint disruption or iliac/sacral fractures
- Comminuted fracture

Acetabular Fractures

▶ Fracture of the posterior (ilio-ischial) pillar
- Dashboard fracture
- Often additional posterior hip dislocation

▶ Central acetabular fracture
  • Almost always additional central hip luxation
▶ Fracture of the anterior (ilio-pubic) pillar

Femoral Neck Fractures

▶ Types
  • Subcapital
  • Cervical
  • Basicervical
  • Intratrochanteric
  • Subtrochanteric
▶ **X-ray**: Difficult to recognise fracture line in osteopenia, repeat image after a few days if necessary
▶ **Complications**: Aseptic femoral head necrosis, pseudarthrosis, post-traumatic arthrosis

Femoral Head Dislocations

▶ Types
  • Posterior: Femoral head in internal rotation, adduction, flexion
  • Central: Combination with central acetabular fracture
  • Anterior: Femoral head in external rotation, abduction, flexion
▶ **X-ray**: On the post-reduction radiograph, widening of the joint space by more than 2 mm compared to the opposite side indicates an interposed fragment
▶ **Complications**: Aseptic femoral head necrosis, in case of posterior dislocation- sciatic nerve palsy

Femoro-Acetabular Impingement

▶ Pain at the onset of the disease, especially in the front of the hip, in the groin area or in the buttocks
▶ Difficulty climbing stairs or going uphill, but also discomfort after prolonged sitting

▶ **X-ray/CT/MR**
- Contour abnormalities on the femur
  - Femur sphericity
  - Femoral torsion
- Contour abnormalities on the acetabulum
- Cartilage injuries
- Labrum injuries
  - Deformity of the proximal femur (cam impingement)
  - Deformity of the acetabulum (Pincer deformity)

▶ **Complications**: Coxarthrosis

Herniation Pit

▶ Small benign oval lesions
▶ Superolateral femoral neck
▶ Transcortical synovial herniation
▶ Mechanically induced osteolysis in the area of a tightly fitting joint capsule at the femoral neck
▶ Mostly asymptomatic
▶ **MR**
- Bone marrow oedema first
- T1 hypointense, T2 hyperintense (predominantly fluid) or hypointense (predominantly connective tissue)
- Later sclerotic rim

Clarification of Knee Fractures

▶ Knee joint AP
▶ Lateral knee joint
▶ Patella axial
▶ CT
▶ MR

Knee Fractures

▶ Fracture of the femoral condyles
▶ Fracture of the proximal tibial condyles

- Tibial plateau fracture
- Lipohaemarthrosis
- **Complications**: Varus malposition, valgus malposition, arthrosis
▶ Fracture of the intercondylar eminence (tibial spine)
  - Always involves anterior cruciate ligament
  - Frequent cause of loose bodies in the knee joint
▶ Avulsion fracture of the tibial tuberosity
▶ Patella fracture
  - **Differential Diagnosis**: Patella bi- or tripartite (well-defined cortex, always located at the upper lateral edge of the patella)
▶ Knee joint dislocation
▶ Meniscus tear
  - MR for the visualisation of concomitant injuries to the cruciate and collateral ligaments
  - Unhappy or terrible triad: Medial meniscus, anterior cruciate ligament, medial collateral ligament

Meniscal Lesions

▶ Clinical meniscus signs (Steinmann I, Steinmann II, Böhler, Payr, Apley, McMurray)
▶ **MR**
  - 0: Signal-free triangular structure (normal finding)
  - I: Punctiform signal increase without connection to the surface (mucinous degeneration, magic angle artefact)
  - II: Linear signal increase without connection to the surface (extensive mucinous degeneration, tear in body of meniscus)
  - III: Linear signal increase with connection to the surface (crack)
    – III a: One surface
    – III b: Both surfaces
  - IV: Multiple signal elevations, deformation, fragmentation (complex injury)
▶ Bucket handle tear
  - Defect of the pars intermedia

- Amputation of the anterior and/or posterior horn of the meniscus
- Bucket handle fragment detection in the central joint space
- Signs of the "double anterior/posterior cruciate ligament"
  - On sagittal images, the meniscus fragment is mapped in front of the anterior/posterior cruciate ligament, so that the anterior/posterior cruciate ligament looks doubled
- Signs of the "Flipped meniscus"
  - The meniscus fragment is imaged immediately dorsal to the anterior horn, so that the anterior horn appears enlarged

▶ **Differential Diagnosis**
- Imitation of meniscus degeneration
  - Vacuum phenomenon
  - Magic angle artefact: T2 extension when fibres are oriented at a certain angle relative to the static magnetic field
  - Chondrocalcinosis
- Imitation of a meniscus tear
  - Anterior horn external meniscus: anterior meniscomeniscal ligament, lateral genicular artery
  - Posterior horn outer meniscus: anterior and posterior meniscofemoral ligaments, tendon of the Popliteus muscle

Cruciate Ligament Lesions

▶ Haemarthrosis, instability, drawer phenomenon,
▶ **MR**
- Anterior cruciate ligament
  - Continuity break
  - Global uplift and diffuse signal increase
  - Wavy course and focal signal increase
  - Bone bruise (bone marrow contusion)
  - Increased angulation of the posterior cruciate ligament

 – Lack of visualisation in anatomical position
 – Accompanying fractures
- Posterior cruciate ligament
  – Much rarer
- Accompanying injuries
  – Bone contusion
  – Fractures
  – Lesions of the posterolateral joint corner
  – Meniscus lesions
  – Cartilage damage

Lateral Ligament Lesions

▶ Lateral unfolding of the knee in a slight flexion position
▶ **MR**
- 0 (normal finding): Signal-free band-shaped structure
- I (distortion): Focal signal increase, continuity preserved; function preserved
- II (partial rupture): Ligament thinning, fibres interrupted; function limited
- III (rupture): Wavy course, contour interrupted, possibly meniscocapsular separation, femoral contusion, haemorrhage; function suspended

Articular Cartilage Lesions

▶ Pain, swelling, feeling of tension, restricted movement, knee joint effusion
▶ **MR**
- Classification according to Outerbridge
  – I: Cartilage softening, oedema
  – II: Partial thickness defect, fissure less than 1.5 cm diameter
  – III a: Surface defects <50%
  – III b: Surface defects >50%
  – IV: Subchondral bone exposed

Patellofemoral Syndrome

▶ Aetiology: Trauma, overload, malalignment, inflammation
▶ Anterior knee pain
▶ **MR**
  • Subchondral patella oedema as a sign of instability, over-loading of the bone structures or cartilage defect
  • Cartilage lesions, patellar luxation, tendon lesions
▶ **Complication**: Arthritis

Patellar Tendinitis

▶ Aetiology: Overuse-related smallest tendon ruptures due to excessive running or jumping
▶ Insertional tendinosis of the patellar tendon
▶ **US**
  • Stage I: Tendon thickening at the patellar tip <2 mm
  • Stage II: Tendon thickening at the patellar tip >2 mm
  • Stage III: Thickened patellar tendon, normal echogenicity, smooth surface
  • Stage IV: Thickened patellar tendon, increased echo-genicity, Irregular surface
  • Stage V: Partial rupture of the tendon
  • Stage VI: Total rupture of the tendon
▶ **MR**
  • Distension and signal elevation of the tendon at the inferior patellar pole (proximal fibro-osseous attachment)
  • Circumscribed oedema of the immediate vicinity

Lower Leg Fractures

▶ Fibula fracture
▶ **Complications**: Paralysis of the peroneal nerve (high step-ping, hypaesthesia), injury to the anterior tibial artery (haemor-rhage, ischaemia)
▶ Maisonneuve fracture
  • High fibula shaft fracture, complete syndesmosis rupture and medial malleolus fracture

▶ Pilon tibial fracture
  • Axial compression and flexion fracture of the distal tibial metaphysis with inclusion of the articular surface

Clarification of Ankle and Foot Fractures

▶ AP Ankle joint
▶ Lateral ankle joint
▶ Mortise view
▶ Foot dorsoplantar
▶ Foot oblique
▶ Foot lateral
▶ Lateral calcaneus
▶ Calcaneus axial
▶ CT
▶ MR

Ankle Fractures

▶ Morphology according to Lauge-Hansen
  • Direction of force: Lateral
    – Position of the foot in supination at the time of the accident: Supination-adduction injury
    – Position of the foot in pronation at the time of the accident: Pronation-abduction injury
  • Direction of force: External rotation of the talus
    – Position of the foot in supination at the time of the accident: Supination-eversion injury
    – Position of the foot in pronation at the time of the accident: Pronation-eversion injury
▶ Classification according to Weber
  • Weber A: Fracture infrasyndesmotic syndesmosis intact
  • Weber B: Fracture transsyndesmotic, syndesmosis questionably intact
  • Weber C: Fracture suprasyndesmotic, syndesmosis not intact
    – In type B and C often avulsion of a fragment at the distal posterior edge of the tibia (Volkmann triangle)

▶ **Complications**: Arthritis, pseudarthrosis, malposition, Sudeck's atrophy, infection, chondromatosis, peroneal tendon rupture

Concomitant Injuries in External Ankle Fractures

Weber	A	B	C
Injury to the syndesmosis ligaments	Never	Possible	Always
Injury to the interosseous membrane	Never	Never	Frequently
Inner ankle fracture or rupture of the inner ligament	Possible	Possible	Always

Achilles Tendon Rupture

▶ Aetiology: Athletic overload, prolonged cortisone use, rheumatoid arthritis, diabetes, gout, hyperparathyroidism
▶ Commonly 2–6 cm above the calcaneal base
▶ Interposition of fat and fluid (oedema, blood) in the rupture area
▶ Pain, palpable dent, no toe stance, limping
▶ US
  • Acute: Interrupted contour, hypoechoic defect zone, echoic edges
  • After 2 weeks: Restoration of the contour
  • After 4 weeks: Thickening of the tendon, start of remodelling
  • After 5 weeks: Completion of regeneration
  • Permanent: Thickened tendon, irregular boundary, irregular internal structure
▶ MR: Continuity interruption, fluid in the rupture site, haemorrhage

Foot Fractures

▶ Talus fracture
  • Types
    – Osteo-cartilaginous fractures (flake fractures) of the talar articular surface of the upper ankle joint after pronation and supination trauma

- – Peripheral fracture
- – Non-displaced corpus and column fracture
- – Central fracture
- • **Complications**: Due to poor vascularisation of the talus often avascular necrosis of the talus, arthritis, pseudarthrosis, osteitis
▶ Calcaneus fracture
  - • Aetiology: Fall from a height and landing on feet
  - • Types
    - – Extra-articular: Calcaneal tubercle, anterior process calcaneum, sustentaculum tali
    - – Intra-articular: Tongue type fracture, joint depression fracture
  - • 20% bilateral calcaneus fracture, 30% associated spinal fractures
  - • **Complications**: Post-traumatic dystrophy, post-traumatic tendosynovitis, buckling flatfoot, tarsal tunnel syndrome, chronic osteomyelitis, subtalar arthrosis
▶ Fracture-dislocation in the Chopart joint (transverse tarsal articulation)
  - • Dislocation usually combined with large osseous ligament tears
▶ Fracture-dislocation in the Lisfranc joint (tarsometatarsal articulation)
  - • Fracture-dislocation of the first or first and second metatarsal mediodorsally
  - • Homolateral dislocation of the first to fifth metatarsals laterodorsally
  - • Divergent dislocation with dislocation of the first metatarsal in a tibial direction and of the second to fifth metatarsals in a fibular direction
▶ Jones fracture
  - • Fracture of the base of the fifth metatarsal at the attachment site of the peroneus brevis muscle
▶ March fracture
  - • Diaphysis of the second or third metatarsal

Plantar Fasciitis

▶ Aetiology: May be triggered by increased activity
▶ Low grade inflammation of the plantar aponeurosis
▶ Pain in the heel on weight bearing
▶ X-ray: Calcaneal spur
▶ MR
  • Thickened plantar fascia
  • Intratendinous signal increase
  • Peritendinous soft tissue oedema
  • Adjacent bone marrow oedema

Os Trigonum Syndrome

▶ Aetiology: Overload
▶ Most important form of posterior ankle impingement
▶ Severe pain with forced plantar flexion
▶ Ballet dancer, dancer heel
▶ MR
  • Accessory ossicle
  • Bone marrow oedema
  • Small cysts
  • Effusion
▶ Complication: Tendosynovitis of the tendon sheath of the flexor hallucis longus muscle

Sinus Tarsi Syndrome

▶ Aetiology: Injury to the ligaments of the sinus due to supination trauma; hindfoot deformities, rheumatoid arthritis, ankylosing spondyloarthritis, gout
▶ Sinus tarsi between plantar neck of talus and cranial part of distal calcaneus
▶ Chronic pain in the lower ankle joint, unsteadiness when walking
▶ MR
  • Diffuse soft tissue in the sinus tarsi
  • Bone marrow oedema in the adjacent talus and calcaneus

- Small ganglion cysts in the tarsal sinus
- Enhancement in the entire sinus and in the lower ankle joint

Metabolic Osteopathies

Hyperparathyroidism

▶ Primary hyperparathyroidism
- Aetiology: Adenoma, hyperplasia, carcinoma
- 30% skeletal changes
- Kidney stones, skeletal changes, gastric ulcers
- Hypercalcaemia, hypophosphataemia, increased PTH
- **X-ray**
  - Brown tumours (osteodystrophia fibrosa cystica) due to localised bone resorption and intraosseous haemorrhages
  - Looser zones
  - Chondrocalcinosis
  - Pepper pot skull
▶ Secondary hyperparathyroidism
- Aetiology: Renal insufficiency, dialysis, malabsorption
- Renal osteopathy
- Frequent skeletal changes
- Bone pain, fractures
- **X-ray**
  - Osteomalacia
  - Soft tissue and vascular calcifications
  - Rugger jersey spine
▶ Shared findings
- **X-ray**
  - Osteopenia
  - Compression fractures
  - Subperiosteal bone resorption at radial mid-phalanges
  - Joint erosions
  - Acro-osteolysis

- **Nuclear medicine**
  - Diffuse increased uptake in generalised osteopathy
  - Correlation to the increase of alkaline phosphatase in serum

Osteopathies with Reduced Bone Density

Osteoporosis

▶ Aetiology
- Primary: Juvenile, premenopausal, postmenopausal, senile, idiopathic
- Secondary: Sex hormone deficiency, hyperthyroidism, steroids, malassimilation, bone dysplasias, plasmacytoma, immobilisation

▶ Types
- Low turnover osteoporosis: Low bone turnover
- High turnover osteoporosis: High bone turnover

▶ Predominance of bone resorption over bone formation

▶ Uniform reduction of ground substance and minerals with negative skeletal balance

▶ Typical osteoporosis patient
- Slender woman
- pale complexion
- Sedentary work
- Low sun exposure
- Low-calcium diet

▶ Fractures occurring with minimal trauma

▶ Fracture classification
- Grade I: Slight, <25% height reduction
- Grade II: Moderate, 25–40% height reduction
- Grade III: Severe, >40% height reduction

▶ Pain
- Fracture pain
- Rib margin pain
- Myotendopathies

▶ Pain especially in the lower thoracic and upper lumbar spine

▶ Kyphosis in the thoracic region with compensatory lordosis in the lumbar region
▶ Fractures especially of the spine and the neck of the femur
▶ **X-ray**
- Cancellous bone rarefaction
  - Radiographically—requires calcium loss of at least 30% to be detected
- Spinal end plate compression fractures
- Fish-shaped vertebrae
- Wedge compression fractures
- Vertebra plana
▶ **MR**: long T2* relaxation time in osteoporotic bone
▶ **Diagnosis**
- Dual energy X-ray absorptiometry (DXA, measurement at the neck of the femur), quantitative computed tomography (QCT, measurement at the lumbar spine), quantitative sonography (QUS, measurement at the heel)
- Categories of bone density based on DXA at the femoral neck
  - Normal bone density: No more than 1 SD (T-score >−1)
  - Osteopenia: 1–2.5 SD (T-score −1 to −2.5)
  - Osteoporosis: More than 2.5 SD (T-score <−2.5)
  - Severe osteoporosis: More than 2.5 SD (T-score <−2.5) with at least one fragility fracture
▶ Special types
- Aggressive regional osteoporosis
  - **X-ray**: Metastasis-like demineralisation
▶ Transient osteoporosis
- 40–50 years
- Successive episodes affecting the hip, knee, ankle and feet
- Complete regression in a few months
- Pain precedes decalcification by weeks
  - **MR**: T1 hypointense, T2/STIR hyperintense
▶ **Differential Diagnosis**: In the spine in osteoporotic fractures—mid-vertebral spine, symmetrical superior and inferior endplate collapses, intravertebral vacuum phenomenon; in

metastatic fractures—inhomogeneous vertebral body density, asymmetrical involvement of posterior elements, accompanying soft tissue mass

Osteomalacia

▶ Aetiology: Vitamin D deficiency (malnutrition, sunlight deficiency, malabsorption), phosphate metabolism disorder (drugs, Fanconi syndrome, tumours)
▶ Disturbance of the mineralisation of the osteoid, hindering the formation of mature cancellous and cortical bone
▶ Adult rickets
▶ Generalised bone pain, muscle weakness, multifocal pseudofractures
▶ Fractures of different ages, especially of the pelvis, sacrum, forefeet, tibial plateau and ribs
▶ **X-ray**
  • Osteopenia
  • Typical looser zones
    – Pseudofractures from osteoid callus
  • Washed-out spongiosa pattern
    – Eraser or frosted glass sign
  • Bone deformities
    – Bell shaped thorax
    – Kyphoscoliosis of the spine
    – Coxa vara
    – Heart shaped pelvis
    – Acetabular protusion
▶ Association with bone and soft tissue tumours
  • Bone and soft tissue haemangiomas
  • Giant cell tumours
  • Haemangiopericytomas
  • Malignant peripheral nerve sheath tumours
▶ **Diagnosis**: Iliac crest biopsy

Osteopathies with Increased Bone Density

Paget's Disease (Osteodystrophia Deformans)

▶ Aetiology: Excessive abnormal bone remodelling. coexistence of increased bone resorption and increased bone formation
▶ Men, middle and older age
▶ Asymptomatic or painful (spinal discomfort)
▶ Increased alkaline phosphatase, increased hydroxyproline excretion in the urine
▶ Monostotic or polyostotic (generalisation)
▶ Most frequently skull, spine, pelvis, humerus, femur
▶ X-ray/CT
  • Stage I (osteolytic): Peripherally bordered by flames on long bones
  • Stage II (osteolytic-osteosclerotic): Mixed lysis and sclerosis
  • Stage III (osteosclerotic): Increase in volume, white bone, bowing
  • All stages possible simultaneously in one bone, with osteolysis marking the area of disease progression
  • Leontiasis ossea, ivory vertebra, saber sheath tibia, basilar impression
▶ Nuclear Medicine: Increased uptake especially in phase II and III
▶ Differential Diagnosis: Metastasis, osteodystrophia fibrosa cystica generalisata Recklinghausen (affects entire skeleton), haemangioma vertebrae
▶ Complications: Pathological fracture, degenerative changes, neurological symptoms, sarcomatous degeneration, often metastatic settlement due to strong vascularisation of the diseased skeletal sections

Osteopoikilosis

▶ Aetiology: Incorporation of bone islands into the cancellous bone
▶ Transition to osteopathia striata

► **X-ray**: Symmetrical, small, roundish, sclerotic lesions close to the joint
► **Nuclear medicine**: Negative

Osteopathia Striata

► Association with Goltz-Gorlin syndrome
  • Skin atrophy
  • Telangiectasia
  • Fat tissue hernias
  • Eye anomalies
► **X-ray**: Striated condensations in the epiphyses of the long tubular bones

Melorheostosis

► In childhood, progressive hyperostosis of a limb of unclear aetiology
► Restricted mobility, soft tissue swelling, chronic pain
► Usually symptom-free in adulthood
► **X-ray**: Classic waxy candle-like hyperostosis flowing down the bone

Hyperostosis Condensans Ilii

► Women
► **X-ray**: Unilateral or bilateral sclerosis on the iliac side of the sacroiliac joint

Hypertrophic Osteoarthropathy

► Aetiology: Pulmonary (bronchial carcinoma, lung metastases, bronchiectasis) and intestinal (Crohn's disease, ulcerative colitis, Whipple's disease) diseases
► **X-ray**
  • Solid, onion-skin-like periosteal new bone formation on the diaphyses of the long tubular bones
  • Usually bilateral-symmetrical

Fluorosis

▶ Toxic osteopathy
▶ Skeletal pain, pathological fractures, muscle pain
▶ **X-ray**: Characteristic band-like compression of the base and cover plates on the spinal column

Circulatory Osteopathies

Osteonecrosis

▶ Aetiology: Local interruption of blood supply to bone in trauma, diabetes, steroids, alcohol abuse, storage diseases, decompression sickness, sickle cell anaemia, connective tissue diseases, radiotherapy
▶ Risk factors → Vascular obstruction, circulatory disturbance → Ischaemia, apoptosis→ Osteonecrosis
▶ Types
  • Perthes' disease: Femoral head
  • Ahlbäck's disease: Medial femoral condyle
  • Osgood-Schlatter disease: Tibial tuberosity
  • Blount's disease: Medial tibial plateau
  • Köhler's disease I: Navicular
  • Köhler's disease II: Metatarsal heads
  • Scheuermann's disease: Vertebral body base and cover plates
  • Friedrich's disease: Medial lower clavicle end
  • Panner's disease: Capitellum of humerus
  • Preiser's disease: Scaphoid
  • Kienböck's disease: Lunate
  • Thiemann's disease: Phalangeal bases
▶ Pathomorphologically, the osteonecroses of childhood and adulthood are similar
▶ Load-dependent pain
▶ **X-ray**
  • Stage I: Osteopenia
  • Stage II: Osteosclerosis

- Stage III: Fragmentation
- Stage IV: Joint surface collapse
- Stage V: Secondary arthrosis

▶ **MR**
- Stage I: Bone marrow oedema
- Stage II: T1 subchondral hypointensity, T2 necrosis-side hyperintensity (granulation tissue) and necrosis-distant hypointensity (sclerosis zone) (double line sign)
- Stage III: Fragmentation
- Stage IV: Joint surface collapse
- Stage V: Secondary arthrosis

▶ **CT**
- Stage I: Osteopenia
- Stage II: Increasing structural loss, changes in the asterisk sign in femoral head necrosis, sclerotic rim
- Stage III: Subchondral fracture, flattening of the condyle, fragmentation
- Stage IV: Joint surface collapse
- Stage V: Secondary arthrosis

▶ **Differential Diagnosis**: Transient osteoporosis, insufficiency fracture

Osteochondrosis Dissecans

▶ Most frequent occurrence in children, adolescents and young adults

▶ Often asymptomatic

▶ Ischaemic necrosis of an articular cartilage-bearing bone section

▶ Medial femoral condyle, Trochlea of talus, Humeral capitulum

▶ **X-ray**: Rounded or oval contour abnormality of affected articular surface osteochondral fragment may be visible within the defect or free within the joint

▶ **MR**
- I: Subchondral signal reduction
- II: Demarcation
- III: Cartilage defect, partial separation, cysts

- IV: Cartilage defect, complete separation, cysts
- V: Loose body
- Increasing loss of signal from the fragment

Bone Infarction

▶ Aetiology: Diabetes, polycythaemia, steroids, Gaucher's disease, alcohol abuse, sickle cell anaemia, diving
▶ Femur, tibia, humerus, metadiaphyseal
▶ **X-ray/CT**
- Stippled calcifications
- Sheet like central lucency with peripheral sclerosis
▶ **MR**
- Early stage (oedema) T1 low signal, T2 high signal
- Late stage (calcifications, marginal sclerosis) T1/T2 low-signal with signal-free marginal rim
- Fat detection and garland shape as differential diagnostic criteria compared to enchondroma
▶ **Differential Diagnosis:** Enchondroma
▶ **Complications:** Osteomyelitis, cyst formation, degeneration

Joint Diseases

Osteoarthritis

▶ Aetiology
- Primary: Mismatch between load and resilience
- Secondary: Post-traumatic, post-inflammatory, metabolic, endocrine
- Symmetrical involvement pattern typical for primary arthrosis
▶ Type
- Arthritis mutilans: Pain on waking or after inactivity, swelling, muscle tension, grinding, restriction of movement, deformities
- Reactive arthritis: Pain at rest, signs of inflammation

▶ Most frequently MCP, PIP, DIP, shoulder joint, hip joint, knee joint
  - Rhizarthrosis: Carpometacarpal joint I
  - Bouchard's arthrosis: PIP
  - Heberden's arthrosis: DIP
▶ **X-ray**
  - Joint space narrowing
  - Subchondral sclerosis
  - Subchondral cysts
  - Cartilage breakdown
  - Osteophytes
  - Subluxations
    - Classification of osteoarthritis according to the Kellgren-Lawrence score in grade I to grade IV (criteria: osteophytes, joint space, sclerosis, deformity)
▶ **MR**
  - Inhomogeneous cartilage signal
  - Decreasing cartilage thickness
  - Irregular cartilage surface
  - Finally uncovered cartilage
▶ **Complications**: Axial malalignments, joint instability, muscle atrophy

Neurogenic Osteoarthropathy

▶ Aetiology: Diabetes mellitus, trauma, alcohol abuse, syringomyelia, syphilis, haemorrhagic arthropathy
▶ Loss of depth sensitivity and proprioception → Relaxation and hypotonia of joint stabilising structures → Repetitive injuries → Poor alignment → Cartilage surface erosions, subchondral sclerosis → Fractures, fragmentations → Joint disorganisation
▶ Mostly arthrosis picture in excessive form
▶ Marked joint destruction excessive compared to the clinical presentation
▶ **X-ray**
  - Joint disorganisation
  - Coexistence of bone resorption, production and fragmentation

- Signs of infection
  - In the diabetic foot, indistinct bone cortex, air pockets in the adjacent soft tissues and lamellar periosteal reactions

Septic Arthritis

▶ Aetiology
- Endogenous: Osteomyelitis
- Exogenous: Joint injury, injection, puncture, surgery
▶ Especially knee and hip joint
▶ Classical signs of inflammation (calor, dolor, tumor, rubor, functio laesa)
▶ Course
- Joint empyema
- Capsular phlegmon
- Panarthritis
- Ankylosis
▶ X-ray
- Soft tissue swelling
- Osteopenia
- Joint space narrowing
- Articular surface erosion
- Geodes
- Deformation
- Mutilation
- Ankylosis
▶ MR: Early diagnosis of joint effusion, soft tissue swelling, hypervascularised pannus tissue, cartilage erosions and tendo synovitis
▶ Differential Diagnosis: Infectious arthritides have rapid progression, tuberculous arthritides have slow progression
▶ Diagnosis: Bacteriological examination of the joint aspirate

Rheumatoid Arthritis

▶ Systemic disease with a predilection for the small joints (carpal joint, metacarpophalangeal joint, proximal interphalangeal joint), relapsing course and progression in a centripetal direction

► Aggressive synovitis, which drives cartilage destruction and joint destruction through enzyme processes and pannus tissue
► 75% elevated Rheumatoid factor
► Classification criteria according to ACR/EULAR
  • Joint involvement
  • Serology
  • Symptom duration
  • Inflammation parameters
► Onset as monoarthritis in the area of the large joints possible
► Symmetrical joint swelling, morning stiffness, tendovaginitis, carpal tunnel syndrome, multiple organ involvement
► Course
  • Proliferative phase
  • Destructive phase
  • Degenerative phase
  • Burnout phase
► Syndromes
  • Felty syndrome: Rheumatoid arthritis, splenomegaly, neutropenia, lymphadenopathy, susceptibility to infection, increased incidence of malignancy
  • Caplan syndrome: Rheumatoid arthritis, silicosis, pulmonary cavitations
  • Sjögren's syndrome: Arthritis, xerostomia, keratoconjunctivitis sicca, rhinopharyngitis sicca
  • Still's syndrome: Arthritis, fevers, rash, pale red exanthema, lymphadenopathy, hepatosplenomegaly, serositis
► US
  • Stages
    – 0: Normal findings
    – I: Ligamentous synovitis
    – II: Pannus tissue
    – Accompanying findings: Tendon sheath effusion
  • Evidence of changes especially in the metacarpophalangeal joints, the tendon of the extensor carpi ulnaris muscle and the finger flexor tendons
  • Qualitative measurement of hypervascularisation using colour Doppler sonography as an indirect sign of inflammatory activity

▶ **X-ray**
- Articular signs
  - Soft tissue swelling
  - Osteopenia
  - Joint space narrowing
  - Synovial cysts
  - Ankylosis
  - Mutilation
  - Subluxations
  - Hand: Swan neck deformity, buttonhole deformity, spindle finger, ulnar deviation
- Extra-articular signs
  - Subcutaneous nodes
  - Obstructive bronchopneumonia
  - Fibrosing alveolitis
  - Pleural effusion
  - Pleural thickening
  - Pericardial effusion

▶ **MR**
- Synovitic proliferation tissue (pannus) T1 hypointense, T2 hyperintense, enhancement
- Strength of enhancement as an expression of activity
- Articular cartilage erosions
- Oedematous changes in the periarticular soft tissue
- Joint effusion
  - Significance of MR in early diagnosis (occurrence of inflammatory changes before structural changes) and in follow-up (strength of enhancement as a correlate for inflammatory activity)

Spondyloarthritides

▶ Axial spondyloarthritis
- Ankylosing spondylitis
▶ Peripheral spondyloarthritis
- Psoriatic arthritis
- Reactive arthritis (Reiter's syndrome)
- Enteropathic arthritis

Ankylosing Spondylitis

▶ Ankylosing spondylitis
▶ Most important form of axial spondyloarthritis
▶ More common in men
▶ Inflammatory back pain
  • Start <40 years
  • Slow insidious onset
  • Morning stiffness >30 min
  • Improvement with exercise
  • No improvement with rest
  • Early morning awakening due to pain
  • Occasionally also alternating buttock pain
▶ Nocturnal low back pain, loss of axial skelton mobility painful Achilles tendon insertion, restricted depth of breathing
▶ 95% HLA-B27
▶ **X-ray**
  • Sacroiliac joint
    – Usually bilateral and symmetrical involvement (sacroili-itis type picture)
    – Early signs: Joint surface erosions, reactive subchondral sclerosis, joint space narrowing
    – Late signs: Bridging, ankylosis
  • Spine
    – Vertebral body squaring
    – Spinal ligament ossification
    – Erosions at the corners of vertebral bodies with reactive sclerosis ("shiny corner sign")
    – Syndesmophytes
    – Bamboo spine
  • Ischium
    – Whiskering of ischial tuberosities due to ossification of ligamentous origins
▶ Compared to osteophytes, syndesmophytes show growth in the direction of the longitudinal axis of the vertebral body; para-syndesmophytes expand laterally and only then ventrally

▶ **MR**
  - Sacroiliitis (structural correlate: subchondral sclerosis, erosions, fat deposition, osseous bridging)
    – STIR acute inflammatory changes in the form of the typical subchondral bone marrow oedema
  - Synovitis (structural correlate: ossification, ankylosis)
  - Capsulitis (structural correlate: ossification, ankylosis)
  - Enthesitis (structural correlate: ligament degeneration)
    – Significance of MR in early diagnosis (occurrence of inflammatory changes before structural changes) and in follow-up (strength of enhancement as a correlate for inflammatory activity)
▶ **Differential Diagnosis**: Septic sacroiliitis, hyperostosis triangularis ilii, arthrosis deformans

Psoriatic Arthritis

▶ Types of psoriasis
  - Psoriasis vulgaris
  - Psoriasis arthropathica (up to one third of psoriasis patients)
  - Pustular psoriasis
▶ Well-defined inflammatory papule with parakeratotic scaling on the extensor sides of the extremities and on the scalp
▶ Köbner phenomenon (isomorphic stimulus effect, disease-specific skin reaction to non-specific stimuli)
▶ Spotted nails, oil stain nails, crumb nails
▶ Types of psoriatic arthritis
  - Asymmetric oligoarthritis
  - Symmetric polyarthritis
  - Distal interphalangeal arthritis
  - Mutilating arthritis
  - Ankylosing spondyloarthritis
▶ Oligoarthritis, fibroostitis, dactylitis
▶ **X-ray**
  - Sacroiliitis type picture
  - Parasyndesmophytes

- Joints
  - Bone proliferations
  - Joint erosions
  - Metadiaphyseal compact erosions
  - Diaphyseal periostitis
- Enthesitis often on the calcaneus

▶ **MR**: Significance of MR in early diagnosis (occurrence of inflammatory changes before structural changes) and in follow-up (strength of enhancement as a correlate for inflammatory activity)

▶ **US**: Qualitative measurement of hypervascularisation by means of colour Doppler US as an indirect sign of inflammatory activity

▶ **Nuclear medicine**:
- Radiographic involvement of the small joints
- Tracer accumulation in soft tissue

▶ **Differential Diagnosis**: Rheumatoid arthritis

▶ **Complications**: Destruction, mutilation, ankylosis

Reactive Arthritis

▶ Reiter's syndrome
▶ Aetiology: Post-infectious disease (intestinal infection, urethritis, conjunctivitis)
▶ Predominantly men
▶ Mostly asymmetric and oligoarticular joint involvement
▶ Fever, urethritis, prostatitis, conjunctivitis, iridocyclitis, polyarthritis, fasciitis, exanthema, hyperkeratosis, balanitis
▶ **X-ray**
- Sacroiliitis type picture
- Parasyndesmophytes
- Erosive destructive arthropathy in joints of the lower extremity with tender accompanying periosteal ossifications
- Enthesitis of ischium/trochanters
- Achilles bursitis

Enteropathic Arthritis

▶ Aetiology: Ulcerative colitis, Crohn's disease, Whipple's disease, coeliac disease, pseudomembranous colitis
▶ **X-ray**
  • Oligo- and polyarthritides of the knee and ankle joints
  • More rarely sacroiliitis type picture

Pustular Arthroosteitis

▶ Pustulosis palmoplantaris or pustular psoriasis
▶ SAPHO syndrome
  • Synovitis
  • Acne
  • Pustulosis
  • Hyperostosis
  • Osteitis
▶ **X-ray**: Sclerosing changes in vertebral bodies and large tubular bones with or without sternocostoclavicular hyperostosis
▶ **Nuclear medicine**: Bull's Head Sign

Metabolic Arthropathies

▶ Gout
  • Aetiology
    – Primary: Metabolic
    – Secondary: Haematological, endocrine, vascular, renal
  • Sodium urate crystals
  • Especially men
  • Podagra, tophi
  • **US**
    – Intra-articular hyperechoic structures
    – Partial dorsal acoustic shadowing
    – Hyperechoic band at the transition area between cartilage and synovia (double contour sign)
    – Intra-articular hyper-perfusion in active synovitis
    – Erosive changes in chronic synovitis

- **X-ray**
  - Mostly metatarsophalangeal joint, rarely knee and small wrist joints
  - Acute stage: No changes
  - Late stage: Joint space narrowing, joint surface ulcerations, spiky periosteal calcifications, destruction, tophi
- **CT**: Specific and quantitative imaging of urate deposits with dual energy CT
- **MR**: Tophus T2 hyperintense or hypointense
- **Differential Diagnosis**
  - When in doubt, think of gout
  - DD of acute polyarticular gout: Acute rheumatic fever
  - DD of chronic recurrent gout: Rheumatoid arthritis, ankylosing spondylitis, psoriatic arthritis

► Chondrocalcinosis
  - Pyrophosphate crystals
  - Especially men
  - **Ultrasound**: Hyperechoic structures in the cartilage itself
  - **X-ray**
    - Arthrosis signs
    - Cartilage calcification of the knee, hand and elbow joints
    - Calcification of tendons, ligaments and symphysis
    - Scapholunate necrosis and collapse

► Hydroxyapatite disease
  - Hydroxyapatite crystals
  - **X-ray**
    - Arthrosis signs
    - Calcifying tendinitis of the shoulder joint
    - Extra-articular calcifications
    - Milwaukee shoulder with high-grade destruction of the joint

► Haemochromatosis
  - Iron deposits
  - **X-ray**
    - Arthrosis signs
    - Hooked osteophytes at the metacarpophalangeal joints
    - Cartilage calcification of the knee and wrist joint

- ▶ Wilson's arthropathy
  - Copper deposits
  - **X-ray**
    - – Evidence of arthropathy
    - – Osteoporosis with secondary spontaneous fractures
- ▶ Ochronosis (Alkaptonuria)
  - Homogentisic acid deposits
  - **X-ray**
    - – Evidence of arthropathy
    - – Multiple calcifications in all intervertebral discs

Synovial Chondromatosis

- ▶ Aetiology: Transformation of synovial tissue into cartilage, resulting in loose cartilaginous bodies in the joint space
- ▶ Pain, stiffness and jarring due to numerous free intra-articular bodies
- ▶ **X-ray**: Multiple round loose bodies in the joint which may calcify

Tendon Diseases

Tendinosis

- ▶ **US**
  - Acute tendinosis: Hypoechoic thickening, loss of fibrillary pattern, normal tendon sheath
  - Chronic tendinosis: Increasing echogenicity, increasing inhomogeneity, contour irregularities, calcifications
  - General: Diffuse or nodular thickening

Tenosynovitis

- ▶ **US**: Halo phenomenon, obstructed gliding, hyperechoic tendon thickening, thickened tendon sheath, secondary tendon changes, calcifications

Insertion Tendinopathies

▶ Lateral Epicondylitis (tennis elbow)
  • Aetiology: Chronic overload reaction of the common extensor tendon at the lateral epicondyle
  • US
    – Hypoechoic attachment thickening of the tendon
    – Widening of the hypoechoic cartilaginous insertion
    – Hyperechoic intertendinous calcification and bony irregularity at tendon insertion
  • MR
    – Swollen tendon
    – Diffuse oedema
    – Significant enhancement
    – Fluid accumulation around the tendon in peritendinitis
  • Differential Diagnosis: Focal synovitis, bursitis, radial tunnel syndrome
▶ Medial Epicondylitis (golfer's elbow)
  • Aetiology: Chronic overload reaction of the common flexor tendon at the medial epicondyle

Compression Syndromes

▶ Carpal tunnel syndrome
  • Aetiology
    – Acute: Fracture
    – Chronic: Idiopathic
  • 30–60 years, women, often bilateral
  • Brachialgia paraesthetica nocturna
  • Eliciting distal symptoms by tapping over the carpal tunnel (Tinel-Hoffmann sign)
  • MR
    – Protrusion of the flexor retinaculum
    – Proximal swelling, distal flattening of the median nerve
    – T2 hyperintensity, enhancement
    – Effusion around the tendon sheath
  • Differential Diagnosis: In secondary carpal tunnel syndrome, exclusion of space-occupying processes (tumours, ganglia, synovitis, haemorrhages)

► Ulnar tunnel syndrome
  • Aetiology
    – Acute: Blow, cut, hamate fracture
    – Chronic: Walking aids, cycling, tools
  • Guyon's box between pisiform and hamate hook volar ulnar side
  • Ulnar nerve, ulnar artery

Muscle Diseases

Fibromyalgia

► Chronic musculoskeletal pain in various parts of the body with generally increased pain sensitivity
► Increased pressure pain at defined test points
► Joint pain, muscle pain, spinal pain, morning stiffness, sleep disorders, exhaustion, concentration problems, depression
► Women more often than men
► Prevalence of the disease increased in rheumatism patients
► MR: Possible STIR oedema zones in affected regions

Disuse Atrophy

► US: Reduced muscle cross-sectional area, reduced muscle diameter, isoechoic musculature, normal septum appearance, normal fascial appearance

Myositis

► US: Hypoechoic areas, anechoic surrounding reaction, septa, foci of gas possible muscle swelling, possible adipose tissue involvement

Muscle Abscess

► US: Hypoechoic or hyperechoic foci, hyperechoic inclusions, cyst formation, hyperechoic rim

Muscle Cyst

▶ **US**: Anechoic space, round-oval shape, smooth wall, dorsal acoustic amplification, lateral acoustic shadow
▶ **Differential diagnosis**: Haematoma, synovial cyst, tumour, myositis, muscle abscess, vascular aneurysm, echinococcus cyst

Benign Muscle Tumours

▶ Rhabdomyoma
▶ Leiomyoma
▶ Haemangioma
▶ Lymphangioma
▶ Elastofibroma
▶ Lipoma
▶ Neurofibroma
▶ Peripheral nerve sheath tumours
▶ Desmoid

Malignant Muscle Tumours

▶ Rhabdomyosarcoma
▶ Leiomyosarcoma
▶ Liposarcoma
▶ Lymphoma
▶ Metastasis

Bone Tumours

Clarification of Bone Tumours

▶ **X-ray**: Basic diagnostics, initial assessment
▶ **CT**: Cortical destruction, periosteal reaction
▶ **MR**: Soft tissue infiltration, bone marrow infiltration
▶ Contrast agent: Viability, biopsy site
▶ **Scintigraphy**: Multiplicity, activity

- ▶ Biopsy
  - Open surgery: Primary bone tumours, indeterminate diagnosis
  - Percutaneous radiological: Metastases, plasmacytoma, malignant lymphoma, inflammatory processes
- ▶ Bone lesion assessment
  - Acronym: LAMA
    - Localisation
    - Age
    - Morphology
    - Aggressiveness

Localisation of Bone Tumours

- ▶ Epiphyseal
  - Giant cell tumour
  - Chondroblastoma
- ▶ Metaphyseal
  - Enchondroma
  - Chondromyxoid fibroma
  - Aneurysmal bone cyst
  - Osteochondroma
  - Osteosarcoma
- ▶ Diaphyseal
  - Ewing sarcoma
  - Reticulum cell sarcoma

Multi-focal Skeletal Locations

- ▶ Benign
  - Fibrous dysplasia
  - Ollier's disease
  - Maffucci syndrome
  - Paget's disease
  - Eosinophilic granuloma
- ▶ Malignant
  - Metastases
  - Malignant lymphoma
  - Plasmacytoma

Epiphyseal Bone Processes

▶ Giant cell tumour
▶ Chondroblastoma
▶ Degenerative cyst
▶ Intraosseous ganglion
▶ Pigmented villonodular synovitis

Eccentric Bone Processes

▶ Giant cell tumour
▶ Chondroblastoma
▶ Osteochondroma
▶ Adamantinoma
▶ Aneurysmal bone cyst
▶ Non-osseous bone fibroma

TNM Classification Bone Tumours

▶ T1: ≤8 cm
▶ T2: >8 cm
▶ T3: Discontinuous in primary affected bone
▶ N1: Regional
▶ M1a: Lung metastases
▶ M1b: Other distant metastases
  • Separate classifications for different localisations

Skeletal Scintigraphy

▶ 99mTc-MDP, 99mTc-DPD or 18F-sodium fluoride PET
▶ Recording the metabolic activity of the bone
▶ Phases
  • Phase 1
    – After injection, perfusion phase
    – Represents arterial flooding
  • Phase 2
    – 1–5 min p. i., blood pool phase
    – Represents venous pooling

- Phase 3
  - >2 h post injection, skeletal phase
  - Represents osseous metabolism
► Normal findings
- Uptake in young people stronger than in older people
- Accumulation in regions with a lot of bone mass greater than in regions with little bone mass
- Physiological representation of the kidneys, ureters and urinary bladder
► Bone processes
- Acute inflammatory or traumatic processes positive in all three phases
- Soft tissue processes positive only in perfusion and blood pool phase
- Osteoblastic metastases positive only in skeletal phase
- Osteolytic metastases often negative in all phases

Chondrogenic Skeletal Neoplasms

► Osteochondroma
- Cartilaginous exostosis
- 5–30 years, most common benign bone tumour
- Femur, humerus, metaphyseal, metadiaphyseal
- **X-ray/CT**: Cartilage cap bone exostosis
- **MR**
  - Exostosis with fat marrow
  - No cortical bone between exostosis and bone
  - T2 Cartilage cap hyperintense, perichondrium hypointense
- **Nuclear medicine**: Variable
- **Complication**: Growth disturbance
  - Multiple cartilaginous exostoses, especially in men and with a tendency to degeneration
  - Cartilage cap thickness >2 cm after growth completion suspicious for chondrosarcoma
► Enchondroma
- Arises within bone
- 20–80 years

- Phalanges, femur, diaphyseal, metaphyseal
- Lodwick IA-IB
- In short bones almost always benign, in long tubular bones degenerative tendency
- **X-ray/CT**
  - Sharply demarcated osteolysis with thinned and bulging cortical bone (scalloping), marginal sclerosis, calcifications
  - Pathological fractures
- **MR**: T1 isointense, T2 very hyperintense, lobulated contour, septations, matrix mineralisations, enhancement peripherally or of septations
- **Nuclear medicine**: Strongly positive
- **Differential Diagnosis:** Bone infarct
- Ollier's disease (enchondromatosis): Multiple enchondromas, confined to one side of the body, risk of malignant transformation
- Maffucci syndrome (enchondromatosis): Multiple enchondromas, cutaneous haemangiomas, risk of malignant transformation
- Signs of degeneration: Pain, increase in size, cortical destruction, soft tissue process
  - **CT**: Cortical erosions, cortical penetration

▶ Chondroblastoma
- 10–30 years, rare
- Femur, humerus, epiphyseal, eccentric
- Lodwick IB-IC
- **X-ray/CT**
  - Osteolysis, marginal sclerosis
  - Spotty calcifications in the centre
- **MR**: Inhomogeneous image of matrix calcifications, cyst formations, rim and perifocal oedema
- **Nuclear medicine**: Strongly positive

▶ Chondromyxoid fibroma
- 15–25 years
- Tibia, femur, metaphyseal
- Lodwick IB-IC
- **X-ray/CT**: Osteolysis, marginal sclerosis, septation
- High risk of recurrence
- **Differential Diagnosis**: Aneurysmal bone cyst

▶ Chondrosarcoma
- 50–70 years, after plasmacytoma, osteosarcoma and Ewing sarcoma most frequent malignant bone tumour
- Pelvis, shoulder girdle, femur, metadiaphyseal
- Primary or secondary at the base of an enchondroma or osteochondroma
- The closer to the trunk a cartilage-producing tumour is, the more likely it is a chondrosarcoma
- **X-ray/CT**
  - Osteolysis, lobulation, matrix calcifications, soft tissue expansion
  - Slow growth, indistinct, osteolytic margins as growth progresses
- **MR**
  - Severe bone expansion
  - Cortical erosions
  - Destroyed compact bone
  - Inhomogeneous enhancement
  - Heterogeneous soft tissues
- **Nuclear medicine**: Positive

Osteogenic Skeletal Neoplasms

▶ Osteoid osteoma
- 5–25 years, 10% of all benign bone tumours
- Femur, tibia, diaphyseal
- Nocturnal pain with significant relief after ASA or NSAIDs
- Lodwick IA
- **X-ray/CT**
  - Long bones: Spindle-shaped osteosclerosis (surrounding sclerosis) with central osteolysis (nidus) in the diaphysis
  - Spine: Small osteolysis with central mineralisation in the vertebral arch, scoliosis
  - Detection of the nidus on CT

- **MR**
  - Nidus T1 isointense, T2 hyperintense, strong arterial enhancement
  - Surrounding sclerosis signal-free
  - Regional bone marrow and soft tissue oedema (prostaglandin secretion)
  - Accompanying oedema can mimic aggressive tumour
  - Reactive synovitis and joint effusions in intra-articular osteoid osteomas
- **Nuclear medicine**: Double density sign (strong uptake nidus, weak uptake sclerosis)
- **Differential Diagnosis**: Osteoblastoma, Brodie abscess
- **IR**: Radiofrequency ablation (removal of the nidus crucial for therapy)
- **Complications**: Growth acceleration in lesions near the epiphyseal fossa, recurrence

▶ Osteoblastoma
- 10–30 years, men, rare
- Spine, tarsal bones
- Lodwick IB-IC
- **X-ray/CT**
  - Sharply defined osteolysis with an expansive character and weak sclerosis
  - Cystic portions in secondary aneurysmal bone cyst
- **MR**: T1 isointense, T2 hyperintense, strong enhancement, perifocal oedema
- **Nuclear Medicine**: Strongly positive
- **Differential Diagnosis**: Aneurysmal bone cyst, Brodie abscess

▶ Osteoma
- 20–50 years
- Skull, paranasal sinuses, mandible
- **X-ray/CT**: Sharply defined sclerosis
- **Nuclear medicine**: Negative
- Gardner syndrome: Multiple osteomas, dental anomalies, epidermoid cysts, intestinal polyposis

▶ Osteosarcoma
- 10–20 years or >50 years, most frequent malignant bone tumour after plasmacytoma
- Femur, tibia, humerus, metaphyseal
- Lodwick III
- 50% mixed, 30% osteosclerotic, 20% osteolytic
- **X-ray/CT**
    - Wide zone of transition cortical interruption, periosteal reaction (Codman triangle, spicules)
    - Soft tissue component
    - Pathological fractures
    - Metastases as skip lesions proximal to the primary tumour, in other bones, lungs and lymph nodes
- **MR**: Inhomogeneous signal behaviour, focal haemorrhages, cystic components, clear enhancement
- **Nuclear medicine**: Strongly positive
- Parosteal osteosarcoma
    - 20–40 years
    - Metaphysis of the distal femur
    - Lobulated exophytic, cauliflower mass with dense ossification
    - Thin radiolucent line between tumour and cortex (String sign)
- Telangiectatic osteosarcoma
    - Imaging similar to aneurysmal bone cyst

Fibrohistiocytic Skeletal Neoplasms

▶ Malignant fibrous histiocytoma
- 50–70 years
- Pelvis, femur, tibia, metaphyseal, eccentric
- Lodwick IC-II
- **X-ray/CT**: Aggressive osteolysis
- **Nuclear medicine**: Strongly positive
- Also develops at the edge of bone infarcts

Round Cell Tumour Skeletal Neoplasms

▶ Eosinophilic granuloma
- 5–15 years
- Skull, mandible, spine, ribs
- Lodwick I-II
- **X-ray**
  - Geographic osteolysis
  - Button sequestrum and multiple lesions on the skull (geographic skull)
  - Vertebra plana
- **MR**: T1 isointense, T2 hyperintense, marked periosteal reactions, circular soft tissue oedema, strong enhancement
- **Nuclear medicine**: Variable
- **Differential Diagnosis**: Osteomyelitis, Ewing sarcoma

▶ Ewing sarcoma
- 10–20 years, men
- Pelvis, femur, tibia, diaphyseal
- Under 20 mainly long bones, over 20 flat bones
- Lodwick II-III
- **X-ray/CT**
  - Patchy, permeative bone destruction
  - Lamellar, onion-skin-like periosteal thickening
  - Moth-eaten picture with osteolyses and osteoscleroses
  - Extra-osseous soft tissue component
  - Pathological fractures
- **MR**
  - Non-specific picture, extraosseous soft tissue component, peritumoral oedema
  - Full-body examination to exclude multifocal skeletal involvement (skip lesions)
- **Nuclear medicine**: Positive
- **Differential Diagnosis**: Acute osteomyelitis (blurred boundary)

Giant Cell Tumour

▶ Giant cell tumour
- Osteoclastoma
- 20–40 years
- Femur, tibia, radius, epiphyseal, eccentric
- Lodwick IB-IC
- **X-ray/CT**
  - Osteolytic, radiolucent, well-defined non sclerotic margins,
  - Excentric location, frequent trabeculation
  - Spontaneous fractures
  - Extends to the joint
- **MR**
  - T1 isointense, T2 hyperintense, with haemosiderin deposits signal reductions
  - Cystic areas with blood degradation products and fluid-fluid levels
  - Homogeneous enhancement
- **Nuclear medicine:** Strongly positive or peripherally positive with central defect
  - High recurrence tendency
  - Degeneration frequency 15%

Vascular Skeletal Neoplasms

▶ Haemangioma
- 30–60 years
- Spine, skull, ribs, femur, tibia, humerus
- Frequent asymptomatic incidental finding
- Symptomatic in case of intrusion into the spinal canal or neural foramina
- Rare haemangiomatosis with multiple skeletal involvement and involvement of visceral organs
- **X-ray/CT**
  - Coarse, thickened vertical trabeculae
  - Honeycomb or accordion appearance
  - Pathological fractures

- **MR**
  - Picture depends on predominant component (lipoma-tous, vascular; the more aggressive the lesion, the less lipomatous and the more vascular components)
  - Lipomatous: T1 hyperintense, T2 hyperintense, loss of signal in case of fat suppression (STIR)
  - Vascular: T1 isointense, T2 very hyperintense, very hyperintense with fatty suppression (STIR)
  - Variable enhancement
- **Nuclear medicine**: Strongly positive

Lipoma

▶ Lipoma
- Any age, rare
- Long tubular bones, calcaneus
- **X-ray/CT**
  - Well-defined osteolysis, thin sclerotic shell
  - Centrally often small calcification (fat necrosis)
- **MR**: T1 very hyperintense, T2 hyperintense, loss of signal with fat suppression

Other Skeletal Neoplasms

▶ Chordoma
- 50–80 years
- Sacrum, clivus, vertebral body
- **X-ray/CT**
  - Osteolysis, local destruction, local recurrence
  - May extend across intervertebral disc space
- **MR**: Lobular structure, fibrous septations, amorphous cal-cifications, high T2 signal
▶ Adamantinoma
- 20–30 years, men, rare
- Tibia, diaphyseal, eccentric
- Lodwick IA-IC
- **X-ray/CT**: Lucent distension with surrounding sclerosis

Tumour-Like Skeletal Neoplasms

▶ Bone island (enostoma)
- 20–50 years
- Vertebral body, pelvis, hand, foot
- **X-ray/CT**
  - Round, oval or elongated sclerosis
  - Cancellous bone structure can be traced into sclerotic foci (not in osteosclerotic bone metastases)

▶ Glomus tumour
- Usually distal phalanx of hand
- **X-ray/CT**: Erosion of the outermost cortex without periosteal reaction

▶ Aneurysmal bone cyst
- 10–20 years
- Tibia, femur, fibula, vertebral arches, metaphyseal, eccentric
- Primary or, less frequently, secondary to other bone lesions such as osteoblastoma, chondroblastoma or giant cell tumour
- Lodwick IB-IC
- **X-ray/CT**: expansile lucent lesion with thinned cortical bone and eggshell-like periosteal ossification
- **MR**
  - Cystic portion, septation, fluid level due to blood degradation products (fluid-fluid level), rim, solid portion
  - Enhancement of the septa
- **Nuclear medicine**: Strongly positive
- **Differential Diagnosis**: Telangiectatic osteosarcoma, chondromyxoid fibroma

▶ Non-osseous bone fibroma
- Fibrous cortical defect
- 10–20 years
- Tibia, femur, metaphyseal, eccentric
- Lodwick IA
- **X-ray/CT**
  - Grape-like lesion
  - Sharply defined osteolysis
  - Typical marginal sclerosis

- **Nuclear medicine**: Negative
- After growth completion- spontaneous healing with sclero-therapy
- **Differential Diagnosis**: Adamantinoma (adult)
- Jaffé-Campanacci syndrome: Non-osseous bone fibromas, café au lait macules

▶ Juvenile bone cyst
▶ Solitary bone cyst
- 0–20 years, men
- Humerus, femur, metadiaphyseal
- Lodwick IA-IB
- **X-ray/CT**
  - Concentric distention of the bone
  - Significant thinning of the cortical bone
  - No periosteal reaction
  - Pathological fractures
- **MR**
  - T1 hypointense, T2 hyperintense
  - Often periosteal shell
- **Nuclear medicine**: Peripherally positive with central defect

▶ Epidermoid cyst
- 20–40 years
- Skull, distal phalanx
- Lodwick IA
- **X-ray/CT**: Sharply defined osteolysis

▶ Intraosseous ganglion
- Lodwick IA
- **X-ray/CT**
  - Subchondral osteolysis
  - Sometimes connection with the joint space
  - No ossification
  - No signs of arthrosis

▶ Fibrous dysplasia
- 5–25 years
- Femur, tibia, ribs, skull
- 80% monostotic, 20% polyostotic
- Lodwick IA-IC

- **X-ray/CT**
  - Expansile, intramedullary
  - Ground-glass opacity (frosted glass phenomenon)
  - Shepherd's crook deformity of femur
  - Detection of a ground glass matrix on CT
▶ McCune Albright Syndrome: Café au lait spots, precocious puberty, polyostotic fibrous dysplasia

Bone Metastases

▶ Clinical: 75% of all bone metastases from breast, prostate, bronchial, thyroid and renal cell carcinoma
▶ Especially spine, pelvis, humerus, femur, skull, ribs
▶ Rarely distal to the elbow or knee joint
▶ **MR**
  - Full-body MR
  - T1 hypointense, T2 hyperintense, STIR hyperintense, enhancement
  - Diffuse signal change, depleted fat signal, convex vertebral body contour, posterior elements of vertebrae affected, destroyed end plates, accompanying soft tissue process
  - Osteoplastic metastases in all sequences hypointense
  - Advantage compared to scintigraphy
    - Greater sensitivity
    - Exact anatomical assignment
    - Also detection of osteolytic metastases and metastases without cortical involvement
    - Precise morphological mapping
    - Higher specificity
▶ **Differential Diagnosis**: Haematopoiesis (localisation), haemangioma (T1 hyperintense), osteoporosis (band-shaped signal alteration, preserved fat signal, concave vertebral body contour, normal posterior elements, intact endplates, no soft tissue process), bone island (pronounced signal reduction in all sequences), plasmacytoma (variable signal alterations due to differing disease patterns)

▶ **Nuclear medicine**: Solitary or multiple lesions
▶ **X-ray**
  • Osteolytic, osteosclerotic, mixed
  • Asymmetric manifestation
  • Blurred margins
  • Frequently pathological fractures
  • Rarely periosteal reaction
▶ **CT**
  • Stability assessment
  • Limitations in assessment of bone marrow infiltration
▶ **IR:** Vertebroplasty, Kyphoplasty

Bone Marrow Diseases

▶ Reconversion (mature yellow marrow replaced by haemopoi-
  etic red marrow)
  • Chronic anaemia, chronic infections, chronic heart failure,
    hyperparathyroidism, competitive sports, nicotine abuse
▶ Infiltration
  • Metastases, plasmacytoma, lymphoma, leukaemia, polycy-
    thaemia
▶ Suppression
  • Aplastic anaemia, radiotherapy, chemotherapy
▶ Fibrosis
  • Osteomyelosclerosis

Bone Marrow Oedema

▶ Oedema equivalent
▶ Pathologically-anatomically diverse entities as cause
▶ Types
  • Vascular-ischaemic
    – Bone marrow oedema syndrome
    – Osteochondrosis dissecans
    – Osteonecrosis
  • Mechanical-traumatic
    – Bone contusion
    – Stress response

- Reactive
  - Osteoarthritis
  - Operation
  - Bone tumour

Plasmacytoma

▶ Mostly IgG, IgA or light chain plasmacytomas
▶ Older people
▶ Skeletal pain, hypercalcaemia syndrome (nausea, vomiting, tiredness, polydipsia, polyuria), general symptoms
▶ Paraproteins in the serum, plasma cell infiltration of the bone marrow, end organ damage by plasma cells
▶ CRAB criteria
  - Hypercalcaemia
  - Renal insufficiency
  - Anemia
  - Bone lesions
▶ Extramedullary myeloma in nasopharynx and lymph nodes
▶ Types
  - Solitary myeloma (brown tumours)
    - Long bones
    - **X-ray/CT**: Cystic expanding lesion (soap bubble image), sharp demarcation
  - Multiple myeloma
    - Spine, pelvis, skull, ribs
    - **X-ray/CT**: Varying sizes, sharply defined lytic bone lesions, smooth curved central cortical defects (endosteal scalloping)
  - Myelomatosis
    - Spine
    - **X-ray/CT**: Stringy rarefied spongiosa (osteoporosis-like), diffuse manifestation
▶ **MR**
  - Type I: Normal-appearing bone marrow with little interstitial infiltration
  - Type II: Focal affection
  - Type III: Diffuse infestation
  - Type IV: Combined focal and diffuse involvement

- • Type V: Salt and pepper pattern
  - – Classification according to MYRADS
▶ In multiple myeloma, initial diagnosis with whole-body low-dose CT and whole-body MR
▶ **Nuclear medicine**: Often negative
▶ **Differential diagnosis**: Metastases (indistinct margins, destruction of the cortical bone, asymmetric manifestation), osteoporosis
▶ **Complications**: Antibody deficiency syndrome, anaemia, renal insufficiency, haemorrhage, second neoplasia, amyloidosis, polyneuropathy

POEMS Syndrome

▶ Symptom complex
  - • Polyradiculitis
  - • Organomegaly
  - • Endocrinopathy
  - • Monoclonal M protein
  - • Skin lesions
▶ **X-ray**: Multiple osteosclerotic foci

Langerhans Cell Histiocytosis

▶ Aetiology: Clonal proliferation of Langerhans cell type histiocytes and organ infiltration together with lymphocytes, eosinophils and histiocytes
▶ Types
  - • Monosystemic: Unifocal (monostotic bone involvement, solitary lymph node involvement, solitary skin, lung or CNS involvement), multifocal (polyostotic bone involvement, multiple lymph node involvement)
  - • Multisystemic: Two or more organs, with or without organ dysfunction
▶ Manifestations
  - • Eosinophilic granuloma
  - • 5–15 years

- Monosystemic
- Skull, mandible, spine, ribs
- Lodwick I-II
- **X-ray**: Geographic osteolysis, on the skull often radiopaque sequestrum (button sequestrum) and multiple lesions (geographic skull), vertebra plana
- **MR**: T1 isointense, T2 hyperintense, marked periosteal reactions, circular soft tissue oedema, strong enhancement
- **Nuclear Medicine**: Negative
- **Differential Diagnosis**: Osteomyelitis, Ewing sarcoma

▶ Hand-Schüller-Christian syndrome
- 1–5 years
- Multisystemic
- Diabetes insipidus, exophthalmos, multiple osteolyses, pulmonary fibrosis

▶ Letterer-Siwe Disease
- 0–3 years
- Multisystemic
- Generalised organ infiltration
- **Complications**: Fractures, bone deformities, growth disorders
- **Nuclear medicine**: Positive

Mastocytosis

▶ Aetiology: Clonal proliferation of mast cells
▶ Urticaria pigmentosa, gastrointestinal complaints, flush symptomatology
▶ **X-ray**: Lytic, sclerotic or mixed. Most common diffuse sclerosis, involving axial skeleton and ends of long bones
▶ **Nuclear medicine**: Positive
▶ **Diagnosis**: Clinical, serum tryptase, mast cell infiltrates in organ biopsies

Leukaemia

▶ Types
- Acute leukaemias: Acute myeloid leukaemia, acute lymphatic leukaemia
- Chronic leukaemias: Chronic myeloid leukaemia, chronic lymphocytic leukaemia, hairy cell leukaemia

▶ **X-ray**
- Osteopenia
- Metaphyseal anomalies
- Osteolytic lesions
- Periosteal reaction
- Osteosclerosis

▶ **MR**
- Diffuse infiltration of the spine
- Absence of fatty marrow in the epiphyses

Myelofibrosis

▶ Aetiology: Independent disease or end-state of myeloproliferative disorders
▶ Blood-forming bone marrow replaced by fibre-rich connective tissue
▶ Middle aged to elderly
▶ Anaemia symptoms, upper abdominal discomfort, hepatosplenomegaly
▶ **X-ray**
- Generalised homogeneous osteosclerosis, of the spine, ribs and proximal long bones
- Ground glass appearance of the bone structure
▶ **MR**: T1/T2/STIR homogeneous massively hypointense bone marrow

Soft Tissue Tumours

- ▶ Lipoma
  - • **MR**
    - – Signal behaviour like subcutaneous fat tissue
    - – Often capsule, fibrous septa, no enhancement
- ▶ Haemangioma
  - • **MR**
    - – T1 hypointense, T2 very hyperintense
    - – Significant signal reduction due to recurrent haemorrhages
    - – Round areas of signal drop-out due to flow void or phleboliths
    - – Clear enhancement, tortuous vessels
- ▶ Peripheral nerve sheath tumour
  - • **MR**
    - – T1 isointense, T2 very hyperintense
    - – Inhomogeneous signal in cysts, haemorrhages, necroses
    - – Target-like enhancement (strong enhancement in the myxomatous periphery, weak enhancement in the fibrosed centre)
- ▶ Liposarcoma
  - • The lower the degree of differentiation, the lower the fat content
- ▶ Rhabdomyosarcoma
- ▶ Synovial sarcoma

TNM Classification Soft Tissues Tumours

- ▶ T1: ≤5 cm
- ▶ T2: >5 cm to ≤10 cm
- ▶ T3: >10 cm to ≤15 cm
- ▶ T4: >15 cm
- ▶ N1: Regional
- ▶ M1: Distant metastases
  - • Separate classifications for different localisations

Pigmented Villonodular Synovitis

▶ Aetiology: Proliferative synovial disease with involvement of joints, bursae and tendon sheaths
▶ Types
  • Diffuse
  • Nodular
▶ 30–40 years
▶ Mostly knee joint or hip joint
▶ Pain, swelling, recurrent serosanguinous joint effusions
▶ **X-ray**
  • Joint space narrowing
  • Multilobulated osteolysis in the region near the joint
▶ **MR**
  • Synovial proliferations
  • Low signal due to susceptibility effects of haemosiderin in all sequences
  • Diffuse enhancement
  • Osseous erosions
  • Subchondral cysts
▶ **Differential Diagnosis**
  • Haemophilic arthropathy
  • Amyloid arthropathy
  • Rheumatoid arthritis in the stage of cicatricial pannus
▶ All also hypointense synovium, but typical history and polyarticular occurrence

Ganglion

▶ Aetiology: Gelatinous masses originating from ligamentous, tendinous or osseous structures and spreading in the vicinity of joints
▶ Often around the wrist

Baker's Cyst

▶ Aetiology: Protrusion of the dorsal joint capsule of the knee joint between the gastrocnemius muscle and the semimembranosus muscle as a result of internal knee damage
▶ Mass in the popliteal fossa with fluctuation and possibly pain
▶ **Differential Diagnosis**: Vascular aneurysm
▶ **Complications**: Compression effect, rupture, leakage

Bone Infections

Osteomyelitis

▶ Acute osteomyelitis
  • Aetiology: Endogenous form (sepsis), exogenous form (trauma); Staphylococcus aureus, Pseudomonas aeruginosa
  • Long tubular bones, spine
  • Pain, functional impairment, general symptoms
  • Early stage
    – **X-ray**: Loss of fat plains, soft tissue swelling, no bone changes
    – **US**: Soft tissue swelling and displacement of the fat lines
    – **Nuclear medicine**: Perfusion phase strongly positive
  • Late stage
    – **X-ray**: Regional osteopenia, loss of trabecular bone, cortical loss, periosteal reaction/thickening
  • **MR**: T1 hypointense compared to fat marrow, T2 hyperintense, Enhancement
  • **Differential Diagnosis**: Ewing sarcoma
  • **Complications**: Bone necrosis, sequestration, periostitis, subperiosteal abscess, soft tissue phlegmon, recurrence, multifocality, epiphyseolysis, growth disturbance

▶ Brodie abscess
  • Subacute osteomyelitis with good immune status
  • Near the knee joint
  • Few symptoms
  • **X-ray:** Sharply demarcated osteolysis with sclerotic margin
  • **Nuclear Medicine**: Positive
  • **MR**
    – T2 Abscess hyperintense, sclerosis hypointense
    – Often channel-like configuration
  • **Differential Diagnosis**: Osteoid osteoma (circular configuration)
▶ Plasma cell osteomyelitis
  • Few symptoms
  • **X-ray**
    – Pronounced sclerosis around polygonal lucencies
    – Rarely sequestrum
▶ Sclerosing osteomyelitis
  • Often mandible
  • **X-ray**: Sclerosis and distension of the affected bone section without destruction and sequestration
▶ Chronic osteomyelitis
  • Aetiology: Post-traumatic, after acute haematogenous osteomyelitis, postoperative
  • **X-ray**
    – Florid picture of cortical thickening, sclerosis and osteolysis
    – Sequestrum
    – Fistulas
  • **Nuclear medicine**: Perfusion phase mostly negative
▶ Tuberculous osteomyelitis
  • Aetiology: Tuberculosis
  • Especially lower thoracic and upper lumbar spine
  • Gibbus formation, paraplegia, drop abscesses
  • On the phalanges of children—spina ventosa with spindle-shaped distension

Spondylitis

▶ Loss of the boundary between vertebral body and interverte-
bral disc
▶ Paraspinal extension possible
▶ **MR**: T1 hypointense, T2 hyperintense, inhomogeneous
enhancement
▶ **Complication**: Abscess

Spondylodiscitis

▶ Aetiology: Infectious, tuberculous
▶ Course of infectious spondylodiscitis compared to tuberculous
spondylodiscitis
  • Faster
  • Monosegmental
  • High inflammation parameters
  • Early disc involvement
▶ Lumbar spine as the most frequent localisation
▶ Back pain, fever, chills, feeling ill
▶ Early signs
  • **X-ray/CT**
    – Reduced height intervertebral space
    – First erosion, then destruction of the adjacent endplate
    – Paravertebral abscesses
  • **MR**
    – T1 Intervertebral disc, superior and inferior endplate
      hypointense
    – T2 Intervertebral disc, superior and inferior endplate
      hyperintense
    – Enhancement
  • **Differential Diagnosis**: Erosive osteochondrosis, acute
    osteoporotic fracture, neoplastic bone marrow infiltration
▶ Late signs
  • **X-ray/CT**
    – Sclerosis
    – Osteophytes

  – Block vertebrae
  – Cysts
  – Gibbus
- **MR**: T1 hyperintense medullary cavity due to fatty regeneration

Connective Tissue Disorders

▶ Lupus erythematosus
- Aetiology: Autoimmune disease
- Benign discoid form (DLE), aggressive systemic form (SLE)
- Predominantly younger women
- Butterfly facial rash, thick scaly patches on skin, hair loss, Raynaud symptoms
- Arthralgias, myalgias, lymphadenopathy
- Pleurisy, pericarditis, serositis
- Lupus nephritis determines prognosis
- **X-ray**
  – Hand and feet, periarticular osteoporosis, symmetrical polyarthritis, deforming non-erosive arthropathy due to ligamentous laxity
▶ Systemic sclerosis
- Scleroderma
- Types
  – Localised scleroderma: Often affects only the skin or organs just deep to the skin including muscle and bone. Raynaud symptoms, finger swelling, tightness of skin of fingers, microstomia
  – Diffuse scleroderma: Trunk-localised oedema, subsequent sclerosis, early organ involvement (oesophagus, lungs)
  – Cutaneous scleroderma: Calcinosis, Raynaud phenomenon, oesophageal dysmotility, sclerodactyly, telangiectasia, arthritis (CRESTA syndrome)
- Predominantly middle-aged women

- **X-ray**
  - Hand—periarticular osteopenia
  - Erosions
  - Phalangeal osteolysis (acro-osteolysis)-resorption of distal phalanx
  - Soft tissue calcinosis
▶ Dermatomyositis
  - Predominantly women of all ages
  - Lilac erythema, poikiloderma, myositis, glomerulonephritis
  - **X-ray**
    - Periarticular hand skeletal osteoporosis
    - Soft tissue calcinosis
▶ Mixed connective tissue disease
  - Sharp's syndrome
  - Overlapping symptoms of the different collagenases
  - **X-ray**: Mixed picture of the connective tissue diseases

Sarcoidosis

▶ Hand as the most frequent localisation of skeletal sarcoidosis
▶ **X-ray**
  - Patchy sclerosis, osteolysis
  - Polycystic changes in the hand
  - Often periosteal ossification, soft tissue swelling
▶ **Nuclear medicine**: Multilocular signal uptake

Diabetes Mellitus

▶ **X-ray**
  - Neurogenic osteoarthropathy
  - Progressive demineralisation
  - Skeletal deformities
  - Stress fractures

Varicose Veins

▶ Aetiology: Venous outflow obstruction, also of the veins of the periosteum, leads to periosteal bone formation
▶ X-ray: Solid or onion-skinned periosteal ossifications on the tibia or fibula

Haemoglobinopathies

▶ Sickle cell disease
  • X-ray: Bone infarcts, osteonecrosis, H-shaped vertebrae
▶ Thalassaemia
  • X-ray: Diffuse osteopenia, hair-on-end appearance of skull

Diffuse Idiopathic Skeletal Hyperostosis

▶ DISH
▶ Forestier's disease
▶ Increasing prevalence among older people
▶ Neck pain, back pain, restricted movement
▶ X-ray/CT
  • Calcifications or ossifications at the ventral or lateral edge of at least four adjacent vertebral bodies
  • Normal intervertebral spaces, no signs of osteochondrosis
  • No ankylosis of the intervertebral joints, no ankylosis of the sacroiliac joints
▶ MR: Bone marrow in the neo-ossifications

Paediatric Radiology: Bones, Joints

Birth Trauma

▶ Soft tissues
  • Cephalhaematoma
  • Subgaleal haematoma
  • Caput succedaneum
  • Sternocleidomastoid haematoma

▶ Nervous system
- Erb-Duchenne upper plexus palsy
- Inferior plexus paresis (Klumpke)
- Peripheral facial nerve palsy
- Hypoxic-ischaemic encephalopathy
- Subdural haematoma
- Skull fracture
- Brain contusion

▶ Skeleton
- Clavicle fracture
- Epiphyseolysis

▶ Organs
- Liver rupture
- Rupture of the spleen
- Adrenal cortical haemorrhages

Bone Maturity

▶ Assessment criteria
- Degree of closure of the epiphyseal joints of the long bones
- Number, shape and size of the bone nuclei
- Determination of bone age by comparison with the normal controls

▶ Ossification times
- Capitate 3 months
- Hamate 3 months
- Triquetrum 3 years
- Lunate 4 years
- Trapezium 5 years
- Scaphoid 6 years
- Trapezoid 6 years
- Pisiform 10 years

Achondroplasia

▶ Aetiology: Autosomal dominant inheritance
▶ Disruption of enchondral ossification
▶ Most common skeletal dysplasia

► Disproportionate short stature due to short femur length
► Frontal bossing, depressed nasal bridge, short extremities, trident hands, increased lumbar lordosis, normal intelligence
► **X-ray**
  • Narrow spinal canal
  • Small rectangular vertebral bodies
  • Broadened tubular bones

Cleidocranial Dysostosis

► Aetiology: Autosomal dominant inheritance
► Missing or hypoplastic clavicles, enlarged fontanelles with delayed closure
► Bulging forehead, delayed eruption of teeth, open symphysis, narrow pelvis
► **X-ray**: Ossification disorders of clavicles, fontanelles, spine and pelvis

Marfan Syndrome

► Aetiology: Autosomal dominant inheritance
► Tall stature, arachnodactyly, funnel chest, kyphoscoliosis, ectopia lentis, aortic valve insufficiency, aortic aneurysms

Ehlers-Danlos syndrome

► Aetiology: Collagen maturation disorder with varying heredity
► Hyperlaxity, skin lesions, joint hypermobility, joint instability, dislocations, scoliosis

Osteogenesis Imperfecta

► Aetiology: Various disorders of collagen synthesis and periosteal bone formation
► Main types
  • Type I: Autosomal dominant inheritance, mild
  • Type II: Autosomal recessive inheritance, lethal
  • Type III: Autosomal recessive inheritance, deforming
  • Type IV: Autosomal dominant inheritance, moderate

▶ Other types mostly with recessive inheritance
▶ Blue sclerae, short stature, bone fragility, ligament laxity, dental changes, otosclerotic hearing loss
▶ **X-ray**
- Deformed long bones
- Biconcave vertebral bodies
- Pectus excavatum
- Osteoporosis
- Thinning of the cortex
- Multiple fractures

Vitamin D-Resistant Hypophosphataemic Rickets

▶ Aetiology: X-linked dominant inheritance
▶ Girls are usually much less affected than boys
▶ Hypophosphataemia, no hyperaminoaciduria, normocalcaemia
▶ Short stature, bow legs, spontaneous fractures

Chondrodystrophia Calcificans

▶ Aetiology: X-linked dominant inheritance
▶ Asymmetric shortening of the long tubular bones
▶ Moderate short stature, asymmetric cataracts, alopecia circumscripta, asymmetric ichthyosis

Meckel's Syndrome

▶ Aetiology: Autosomal recessive inheritance
▶ Occipital encephalocele, microcephaly, cleft lip and palate, polydactyly, polycystic kidneys

Mucopolysaccharidoses

▶ Aetiology: Mostly autosomal recessive inheritance, disorders in the degradation of glycosaminoglycans due to enzyme defects
▶ Facial dysmorphia, growth disorders, joint contractures, hernias, hepatosplenomegaly, corneal opacity, retardation

▶ Most importantly dysostosis multiplex (mucopolysaccharidosis type I, Hurler's disease)
▶ **X-ray**
  • Generalised osteoporosis
  • Thoracolumbar gibbus
  • Shortened and widened long bones
  • Oval or beaked vertebral bodies
  • Oar-shaped ribs
  • Abnormal pelvic shape

Haemophilia A

▶ Aetiology: X-linked recessive inheritance
▶ Factor VIII deficiency
▶ Bleeding into subcutaneous tissues, muscles, joints and mucous membranes after minor trauma
▶ **X-ray**: Chronic deforming joint disease with very pronounced bone destruction, bone density preserved, squaring of femoral condyles
▶ **MR**
  • Joint destruction with arthritis picture
  • Susceptibility artefacts due to blood degradation products

Down's Syndrome

▶ Aetiology: Additional chromosome 21; free trisomy (95%), translocation trisomy (2.5%) or mosaic trisomy (2.5%)
▶ Craniofacial dysmorphia
  • Brachycephaly
  • Epicanthal fold
  • Flat broad nasal root
  • Open mouth
  • Furrowed tongue
  • Macroglossia
  • Hypertelorism
▶ Extremities
  • Brachydactyly
  • Short wide hands
  • Sandal Gap

► Other features
- Mental disability
- Muscular hypotonia
- Delayed reflexes
- Increased susceptibility to infection
- Joint hyperflexibility
- Hip dysplasia
- Cardiac defects
- Leukaemia

Prader-Willi Syndrome

► Aetiology: Microdeletion syndrome
► Short stature, muscular hypotonia, hyperphagia, obesity, hypogonadism, underachievement

Pes Equinovarus

► Congenital clubfoot
► Foot points downwards and inwards, talocalcaneal parallelism,
► Boys twice as often as girls
► In 50% bilateral

Osteopetrosis

► Albers-Schönberg disease
► Marble bone disease
► Types
- Early-presenting type
  - High-grade anaemia, significant hepatosplenomegaly, septic infections
  - **X-ray**: Generalised compression and thickening of the entire skeleton, medullary canal no longer delineated, bone in bone appearance
- Late presenting type
- Often no signs of disease
  - **X-ray**: Less pronounced and delayed changes
► **Complications**: Fractures, coxarthrosis, scoliosis

Diaphyseal Dysplasia (Camurati-Engelmann Disease)

▶ Aetiology: Autosomal dominant inheritance, defect in TGFB1 gene
▶ Infants
▶ Osteoblastic overactivity, limb pain and muscle weakness
▶ X-ray: Symmetrical fusiform cortical widening and sclerosis of the long tubular bones
▶ Differential Diagnosis: Endosteal hyperostosis van Buchem (autosomal recessive), endosteal hyperostosis Worth (autosomal dominant)

Gaucher's Disease

▶ Initially hepatosplenomegaly, failure to thrive
▶ Then opisthotonus, dysphagia
▶ Early death
▶ X-ray: Erlenmeyer flask deformity of the long bones

Lipoatrophic Diabetes Mellitus

▶ Absence of fatty tissue
▶ Diabetes mellitus, hirsutism, skull facies, gigantism, acanthosis nigricans
▶ X-ray
  • Congenital form: Premature epiphyseal joint closure, epimetaphyseal sclerosis
  • Acquired form: Increased bone density

Madelung Deformity

▶ Deviation of the radius in the direction of the ulna and the palm (bayonet position) due to a hereditary growth disorder of the distal radius epiphysis

Radioulnar Synostosis

▶ Congenital ossification between the radius and ulna, mostly in the proximal third of the forearm

Rickets

▶ Aetiology: Deficient mineralisation of the osteoid in the growing bone
▶ Types
  • Calcipenic rickets
  • Phosphopenic rickets
  • Congenital hypophosphatasia
▶ Growth zones of the metaphyses particularly affected
▶ Hypocalcaemia symptoms, skeletal changes, myopathy
▶ Craniotabes, bell thorax with Harrison's groove and rosary, kyphosis while sitting
▶ Bowed legs,
▶ Nerve hyperexcitability
▶ X-ray
  • Rachitic rosary
  • Widened epiphysis
  • Concavity of the distal metaphyses
  • Skeletal deformation
  • Greenstick fractures
▶ Differential Diagnosis: Non-accidental injury

Special Types of Fracture

▶ Greenstick fracture
  • Fracture of the cortical bone on the tension side (convexity), bending on the compression side (concavity)
  • One third of long bone fractures
  • Importance of sonography for the detection of fractures in childhood
▶ Bending fracture
  • Only bending of the long bone
  • Most frequent occurrence on the forearm

▶ Buckle fracture
- Compression trauma in the longitudinal axis, protrusion of the periosteum and cortical bone, compression of the spongiosa
- Metaphysis of the distal radius and distal ulna

▶ Tibial spiral fracture
- Fine spiral fracture of the tibia with preserved continuity of the bone
- Fracture of the age of learning to walk

▶ Epiphyseal injuries
- Injuries of the epiphyseal joints typical for growth age
- Epiphysis involved in up to 20% of all fractures
- Classification
  - Salter-Harris I/Aitken 0: Epiphyseolysis; proliferative zone not injured, no growth disturbance
  - Salter-Harris II/Aitken I: Epiphyseolysis and metaphyseal fracture; proliferative zone not injured, no growth disturbance
  - Salter-Harris III/Aitken II: Epiphysis and epiphyseal fracture; proliferative zone injured, growth disturbance possible
  - Salter-Harris IV/Aitken III: Epiphyseolysis, metaphyseal fracture and epiphyseal fracture; proliferative zone injured, growth disturbance possible
  - Salter-Harris V/Aitken IV: Epiphyseal compression; proliferative zone injured, growth arrest

▶ Suspected Non-Accidental Injury
- Unexplained behavioural disorders, psychomotor developmental delays
- Multiple haematomas on unusual parts of the body
- Burns, bite marks, hairline fractures
- Radiographic fractures of different ages
- Implausible explanation for injury, trivialising explanations
- Skeletal screening according to the child protection guideline
- X-rays of the spine and pelvis only as a supplement to seek evidence of other fractures

- Thoracic oblique radiographs and repetition of skeletal screening in case of negative skeletal status and reasonable suspicion of physical abuse
- **X-ray**
    - Metaphyseal corner fractures
    - Skull fracture
    - Sutural diastasis
    - Subdural haemorrhage
    - Cortical hyperostosis in the region of the diaphyses of long tubular bones
    - Mandible fractures
    - Clavicle fractures
    - Scapular fractures
    - Posterior rib fractures
- **Nuclear medicine**
    - Fractures in the acute stage (after 1 day) positive in all phases
    - Fractures in the subacute stage (4–12 weeks) positive in the skeletal phase
    - Fractures in the healing stage (>6 months) negative in all phases
- Other injuries with high specificity
    - Subdural haematomas
    - Intestinal wall haematoma
    - Hollow organ perforation
    - Injured upper abdominal organs

Perthes' Disease

▶ Aetiology: Aseptic femoral head necrosis
▶ 4–8 years, boys significantly more often than girls
▶ Occasional bilateral but not simultaneous occurrence
▶ Movement restriction, pain, leg length discrepancy
▶ Restriction of abduction and internal rotation in the hip joint
▶ Stages
- Initial/necrosis stage
- Fragmentation stage

- Reossification stage
- Healed stage
▶ Classification according to the lateral epiphyseal height according to Herring
  - A: Lateral epiphyseal column not reduced in height
  - B: Lateral epiphyseal column <50% reduced in height
  - C: Lateral epiphyseal column >50% reduced in height
▶ Early diagnosis
  - **MR**: T1 hypointensity in the femoral head
  - **Nuclear medicine**: Photopenic femoral head in all phases
▶ **X-ray**
  - Early signs
    - Soft tissue swelling
    - Lateralisation, fragmentation, sclerosis and flattening of the femoral head
    - Joint effusion
  - Late signs:
    - Deformed, flattened femoral head
    - Shortening of the femoral neck
    - Coxa vara
    - Joint space narrowing
    - Subluxation
▶ **US**
  - Femoral head changes
  - Synovitis
  - Effusion
▶ Healing outcomes
  - I: Normal joint
  - II: Spherical femoral head, optional coxa magna, abnormal acetabulum, shortening of femoral neck
  - III: Non-spherical femoral head, facultative coxa magna, abnormal acetabulum, shortening of femoral neck
  - IV: Coxa plana with abnormal acetabulum
  - V: Coxa plana with normal acetabulum
▶ **Differential Diagnosis**: Coxitis fugax, epiphyseolysis capitis femoris, juvenile idiopathic arthritis, purulent coxitis

Irritable Hip (Transient Synovitis)

▶ Aetiology: Inflammation in a hip commonly occurring after a respiratory viral infection
▶ 3–10 years
▶ Radiating pain, relieving posture, limping gait, restricted mobility
▶ Mildly raised temperature or afebrile
▶ Normal laboratory values, at most slight CRP increase
▶ US: Evidence of effusion
▶ X-ray: Normal findings

Juvenile Idiopathic Arthritis

▶ Types
  • Systemic arthritis
    – Still's syndrome
    – Fevers, rash, arthritis
    – Pale red rash
    – Lymphadenopathy, hepatosplenomegaly, serositis
  • Seronegative polyarthritis
    – Infantile and more frequent form of progression
    – Possible cure
  • Seropositive polyarthritis
    – Adolescent and rarer form of progression
    – Swift progression
  • oligoarticular juvenile idiopathic arthritis
    – Fewer than five joints involved
    – Peak incidence 2–3 years
    – Limping without complaint
    – Females most commonly
    – Uveitis—but otherwise absence of systemic features
  • Psoriatic arthritis
    – Arthritis
    – Psoriasis
    – Dactylitis
    – Nail abnormalities

- • Enthesitis-associated arthritis
  - – Arthritis
  - – Enthesitis
- ▶ Manifestation of an inflammatory systemic disease at the joint
- ▶ Synovitis of large and small joints
- ▶ Swelling, pain, redness, overheating, restriction of movement
- ▶ Ankylosis
- ▶ Involvement of the cervical spine in 65% (fifth limb of the juvenile rheumatic)
- ▶ US
  - • Joint effusion
  - • Synovial hypertrophy
- ▶ X-ray
  - • Early stage
    - – Periarticular soft tissue swelling
    - – Osteopenia near the joint
    - – Osseous hypertrophy
    - – Pronounced periosteal reaction
  - • Late stage
    - – Erosions
    - – Synostoses
    - – Ankyloses
    - – Subluxations

Brain, Spinal Cord

Anatomy

Brain

▶ Medulla oblongata
▶ Pons
▶ Midbrain
- Cerebral peduncles (Crura cerebri)
- Tegmentum
- Tectum (quadrigeminal plate)
  - Superior colliculus
  - Inferior colliculus
▶ Diencephalon
- Thalamus
- Hypothalamus
  - Mammillary bodies
  - Tuber cinereum
  - Pituitary infundibulum
  - Neurohypophysis
  - Optic chiasm
  - Optic tract
- Epithalamus
  - Pineal gland
  - Habenula
  - Posterior commissure

© The Author(s), under exclusive license to Springer Nature Switzerland AG 2026
D. Pickuth, J. T. Murchison, *Pocket Guide to Radiology*,
https://doi.org/10.1007/978-3-031-76520-9_10

- • Subthalamus
  - – Globus pallidus
  - – Subthalamic nucleus
- ▶ Telencephalon
  - • Frontal lobe
  - • Parietal lobe
  - • Temporal lobe
  - • Occipital lobe
- ▶ Cerebellum
  - • Cerebellar hemispheres
  - • Vermis

Deep Nuclei

- ▶ Mesencephalon
  - • Substantia nigra
    - – Pars compacta
    - – Pars reticularis
- ▶ Diencephalon
  - • Thalamus
  - • Subthalamic nucleus
  - • Globus pallidus
- ▶ Telencephalon
  - • Striatum
    - – Caudate nucleus
    - – Putamen

Internal Capsule

- ▶ Anterior limb
  - • Medial lenticulostriate arteries and recurrent artery of Heubner (from anterior cerebral artery)
- ▶ Genu
  - • Lateral lenticulostriate arteries (from middle cerebral artery)
- ▶ Posterior limb
  - • Anterior choroidal artery

- Corticospinal fibres of the pyramidal tract in somatotopic order
  - Front: Upper limb
  - Centre: Trunk
  - Rear: Lower limb

Basal Ganglia Cross Section

▶ Topographical anatomy in axial basal ganglia section from inside to outside
- Thalamus
- Internal capsule
- Globus pallidus
  - Globus pallidus internus
  - Medial medullary lamina
  - Globus pallidus externus
  - Lateral medullary lamina
- Putamen
- External capsule
- Claustrum
- Extreme capsule
- Insula
▶ Lentiform nucleus consisting of globus pallidus and putamen

Venous Sinuses

▶ Superior sagittal sinus
- At the upper edge of the falx cerebri
▶ Inferior sagittal sinus
- At the inner edge of the falx cerebri
▶ Straight sinus
- At the junction of the falx cerebri and tentorium cerebelli
▶ Occipital sinus
- Along the inner table of the occipital bone draining to the confluence of the sinuses
▶ Transverse sinus
- At the posterior edge of the tentorium cerebelli

▶ Sigmoid sinus
  • Between the transverse sinus and jugular foramen
▶ Cavernous sinus
  • Next to the pituitary gland
▶ Superior and inferior petrosal sinuses
  • Between the cavernous sinus and the sigmoid sinus on the petrous bone

Cisterns

▶ Cisterna magna
▶ Suprasellar cistern
▶ Interpeduncular cistern
▶ Ambient cistern
▶ Prepontine/premedullary cisterns
▶ Quadrigeminal cistern

Internal Carotid Artery

▶ C1: Cervical segment
▶ C2: Petrous segment
▶ C3: Foramen lacerum segment
▶ C4: Cavernous segment
▶ C5: Clinoid segment
▶ C6: Ophthalmic segment
▶ C7: Terminal segment

Middle Cerebral Artery

▶ M1: Sphenoidal segment
▶ M2: Insular segment
▶ M3: Opercular segment
▶ M4: Terminal (cortical) segment

Vertebral Artery

▶ Segments
  • V1: Preforaminal segment
  • V2: Foraminal segment

- V3: Atlantic (extradural) segment
- V4: Intracranial (intradural) segment
▶ Branches
  - Anterior spinal artery
  - Posterior inferior cerebellar artery
  - Basilar Artery
    - Anterior inferior cerebellar artery
      - labyrinthine (auditory or internal auditory) artery- (originates AICA ~85%, basilar ~15%, vertebral ~5%)
  - Pontine artery
  - Superior cerebellar artery

Circle of Willis

Anterior cerebral artery → Anterior communicating Artery ← Anterior cerebral artery

↑   ↑

Internal carotid artery   Internal carotid artery

↓   ↓

Middle cerebral artery   Middle cerebral artery

↓   ↓

Posterior communicating artery   Posterior communicating artery

↑   ↑

Posterior cerebral artery ← Basilar Artery → Posterior cerebral artery

External Carotid Artery

▶ Superior thyroid artery
▶ Ascending pharyngeal artery
▶ Lingual artery
▶ Facial artery
▶ Occipital artery
▶ Posterior auricular artery
▶ Superficial temporal artery
▶ Maxillary Artery
  - Middle meningeal artery

Spinal Cord Cross-Section

▶ Ventral (anterior) column
  • Anterior corticospinal tract: Voluntary motor activity
  • Anterior spinothalamic tract: Sensory, coarse touch and pressure
  • Extrapyramidal motor pathways: Non-volitional motor pathways
▶ Lateral column
  • Lateral corticospinal tract: Voluntary motor activity
  • Lateral spinothalamic tract: Pain and temperature sensation
  • Spinocerebellar tracts: Cerebellar information
  • Extrapyramidal motor pathways: Non-volitional motor pathways
▶ Dorsal (posterior) column
  • Proprioception, vibration, fine touch
    – Fasciculus gracilis (column of Goll): Medial
    – Fasciculus cuneatus (column of Burdach): Lateral

Spinal Arteries

▶ Anterior spinal artery (unpaired), posterior spinal artery (paired)
▶ Supply
  • Vertebral artery
  • Posterior intercostal arteries
  • Lumbar artery

Nervous System

▶ Central
  • Brain (without cranial nerve nuclei)
  • Spinal cord (without anterior horn ganglion cells)
▶ Peripheral
  • Cranial nerve nuclei
  • Anterior horn cells
  • Nerve root

- Plexus
- Peripheral nerve
- Neuromuscular junction
- Muscle

Cranial Nerves

▶ I: Olfactory—sensory—smell
▶ II: Optic—sensory—vision
▶ III: Oculomotor—motor (somatic and parasympathetic)—muscle innervation of eyeball, pupil and upper eyelids
▶ IV: Trochlear—motor—innervation of superior oblique muscle of eye
▶ V: Trigeminal—sensory and motor—chewing and sensation of face, teeth and anterior tongue
▶ VI: Abducens—motor—abduction of eye, lateral rectus muscle
▶ VII: Facial—sensory and motor—movement of facial muscles, taste, salivary glands
▶ VIII: Vestibulocochlear—sensory—equilibrium and hearing
▶ IX: Glossopharangeal—sensory and motor—taste, swallowing, elevation of pharynx and larynx, parotid salivary gland, sensation to posterior tongue and upper pharynx
▶ X: Vagus—sensory and motor—taste, swallowing, phonation, elevation of palate, parasympathetic supply to visceral organs
▶ XI: Accessory—motor—trapezius muscle and sternocleido-mastoid muscles -turning head and shrugging shoulders
▶ XII: Hypoglossal—motor—tongue movement

Nerve Plexuses

▶ Cervical plexus
- Segments: C1-C4
- Location: In front of the origins of the medial scalene muscle and the levator scapulae muscle
- Area supplied: Head, neck, diaphragm, shoulder
▶ Brachial plexus
- Segments: C5-T1

- Location: Above the clavicle to the armpit
- Area supplied: Shoulder, arms, chest, back
► Lumbar plexus
  - Segments: L1-L4
  - Location: At the origin of the psoas major muscle
  - Area supplied: Hip, genitals, thigh, lower leg
► Sacral plexus
  - Segments: L4-S3
  - Location: Inside of the piriformis muscle
  - Area supplied: Buttocks, thigh, lower leg, foot
► Coccygeal plexus
  - Segments: S4-S5 plus usually one coccygeal segment
  - Location: Anterior to the coccyx
  - Area supplied: Skin of coccyx and anus

Reflexes

► Biceps tendon reflex: C5-C6
► Triceps tendon reflex: C7-C8
► Abdominal skin reflexes: T6-T12
► Cremasteric reflex: L1-L2
► Adductor reflex: L2-L4
► Patellar tendon reflex: L3-L4
► Tibialis posterior reflex: L5
► Achilles tendon (ankle) reflex: S1-S2
► Bulbocavernosus reflex: S3-S4
► Anal reflex: S3-S5

Paralysis

Characteristics	Central paralysis	Peripheral paralysis
Reflexes	↑	↓
Babinski reflex	+	−
Atrophy	−	+
Muscle tone	↑	↓

Radicular Syndromes

Syndrome	Weakness	Reflex loss	Dermatome
C5	Deltoid and biceps muscles	Biceps	Shoulder and upper arm lateral
C6	Biceps and brachioradialis	Biceps	Above elbow lateral, forearm radial, thumb and index finger radial
C7	Triceps, pronator teres and pectoralis major	Triceps	Forearm dorsal, middle three fingers
C8	Small hand muscles	Hoffmann, Triceps	Forearm dorsal, ring and little finger
L3	Quadriceps femoris and iliopsoas	Patellar	From the greater trochanter over the thigh medially to the knee
L4	Quadriceps femoris and tibialis anterior	Patellar	From the hip and lateral thigh towards the medial ankle
L5	Extensor hallucis longus and extensor digitorum brevis	Tibialis posterior	From the thigh to the knee joint laterally, along the edge of the tibia, over the dorsal side of the foot to the big toe and adjacent toe
S1	Peronei, triceps surae (calf muscles) and gluteus maximus	Achilles	Back of upper and lower leg to outer ankle and edge of foot, small toe area and sole of foot laterally

Skin Innervation

- ▶ Clavicle: C4
- ▶ Lateral upper arm: C5
- ▶ Lateral forearm and thumb: C6
- ▶ 2nd–4th finger: C7
- ▶ 5th finger and medial forearm: C8
- ▶ Forearm and medial upper arm: T1
- ▶ Nipple: T5
- ▶ Navel: T10
- ▶ Groin: L1

▶ Upper half of the front of the thigh: L2
▶ Lower half of the front of the thigh: L3
▶ Tibial side of the lower leg: L4
▶ Fibular side of lower leg and 1st–2nd toe: L5
▶ 3rd–5th toe and dorsolateral lower leg: S1

Brain

Vascular Syndromes

▶ Anterior choroidal artery
  • Hemiplegia, hemisensory loss, contralateral hemianopia
▶ Anterior cerebral artery
  • Unilateral leg weakness, urinary incontinence
▶ Middle cerebral artery
  • Brachiofacial hemiparesis, hemisensory deficits, gaze paresis, ataxia
▶ Posterior cerebral artery
  • Contralateral hemisensory loss, hemianopia
▶ Basilar Artery
  • Nuclear oculomotor palsy, vertical gaze palsy, ataxia, hypersomnia
▶ Superior cerebellar artery
  • Hemiataxia, dysarthria, dizziness, nausea
▶ Anterior inferior cerebellar artery
  • Tinnitus, dysarthria, vertigo
▶ Posterior inferior cerebellar artery
  • Wallenberg syndrome—affects swallowing, balance and vision

Aetiology of Ischaemic Infarcts

▶ Microangiopathic infarction
  • Lacunar infarct
    – Aetiology: Hypertension
    – Smaller lesions in the basal ganglia, thalamus, capsule and pons
    – État lacunaire (Status lacunaris) as a severe manifestation
    – Smallest penetrating cerebral arteries

- Subcortical arteriosclerotic encephalopathy
  - Binswanger's disease
  - Type of vascular dementia
  - Aetiology: perivascular myelin loss and increased gliosis of the cerebral medullary layer due to longstanding hypertension, omission of the U-fibres; vascular dementia in the later course
  - Diffuse subcortical lesions
  - Confluent periventricular lesions over a large area
  - Often brain volume reduction
- CADASIL (Cerebral autosomal dominant arteriopathy with subcortical infarcts and leukoencephalopathy)
  - Aetiology: Genetic defect on chromosome 19q12 due to mutation of the Notch 3 gene; non-arteriosclerotic and non-amyloid related angiopathy; most common familial stroke syndrome; No association with hypertension; Migraine, depression, stroke, dementia
  - Symmetrical involvement of the anterior temporal lobe, external capsule
  - Diffuse leukoencephalopathy, microhaemorrhages, lacunar infarcts
▶ Haemodynamically induced infarction
- Border zone infarction (watershed infarction)
  - Aetiology: Hypotensive state causing perfusion deficits in terminal supply areas between the vascular territories (watershed)
  - External (cortical) border zone infarcts: In the frontal cortex (between the anterior and middle cerebral arteries), in the occipital cortex (between the middle and posterior cerebral arteries), in the paramedian white matter (between the anterior and middle cerebral arteries); embolic or haemodynamic aetiology
  - Internal (deep / subcortical) border zone infarcts: Typically in the centrum semiovale, mostly between lenticulostriate and middle cerebral arteries; haemodynamic; increased risk of stroke
- Hypoxic-ischaemic encephalopathy
  - Aetiology: Anoxia e.g. cardiac arrest, drowning

- Hypodensity of the basal ganglia and cortex, relative preservation of the cerebellum
- Cerebral oedema, sulcal effacement
▶ Thromboembolic infarction
  • Territorial infarction
    - Aetiology: Arterio-arterial or cardioembolic, rarely autochthonous arteriosclerotic
    - Middle cerebral artery, posterior cerebral artery, anterior cerebral artery

Diagnosis of Ischaemic Infarction

▶ Acute phase
  • **CT**
    - Early signs: Reduced density of basal ganglia, lack of differentiation between grey and white matter, hyperdense artery (e.g. MCA, basilar artery), swollen gyri, sulcal effacement, demarcation from 6 to 12 h
    - Perfusion CT: Reduced blood flow, CBF decreased (penumbra), CBV decreased (core)
    - Haemorrhagic transformation of the infarct can occur, especially after 1–2 days
    - Infarct can become isodense at 2–3 weeks (fogging effect)
    - Determination of the ASPECTS score on the initial CT
  • **CTA**
    - Detection of vascular occlusion
    - Localisation of the vascular occlusion
    - Information on brain perfusion
    - Information on collateral supply
    - Planning of intervention
  • **MR**
    - T2 hyperintense, ill-defined, weakly space-occupying (after around 6 h of onset of the infarct)
    - DWI: High signal intensity due to low diffusion movement of the water protons in the infarct oedema

- – ADC: Low signal intensity from a few minutes to around 9 days after symptom onset
- – PWI: Immediately after gadolinium administration (first pass) significant signal reduction of the perfused brain tissue with persistently high signal intensity in the non-perfused infarct areas
- – Irreversible ischaemia (core): Areas with changes in PWI and DWI
- – Reversible ischaemia (penumbra): Areas with changes in PWI but not in DWI
- – Ischaemic tissue: MTT increased, TTP increased
- **MRA**: Vascular occlusion
- **MRS**
  - – Irreversible ischaemia: Drop in NAA
  - – Reversible ischaemia: Increase in lactate
▶ Subacute phase
- **MR**
  - – T2 sharply defined, hyperintense, space-occupying
  - – From day 3 patchy, from day 6 strong enhancement
  - – Enhancement of infarction from day 3 to week 6 due to impaired blood-brain barrier and/or reactive luxury perfusion
▶ Chronic stage
- **MR**
  - – T2 very sharply demarcated, CSF signal intensity, not space-occupying
  - – No enhancement
  - – Adjacent sulci and ventricles dilated
▶ **Differential Diagnosis**
- **CT**: Hyperdense vascular sign with high haematocrit values in all cerebral arteries, misinterpretation as early infarct sign possible
- **MR**
  - – FLAIR physiological linear signal elevations around the frontal and occipital horns of the lateral ventricles due to normal subependymal gliosis or increased interstitial fluid content, misinterpretation as microangiopathic changes possible

- – DWI signal elevations due to shine through effects in microangiopathy, misinterpretation as acute infarcts possible
- – Assessment of the ADC map for differential diagnosis
▶ **Complications**: Haemorrhagic transformation, ischaemic cerebral oedema, seizures, dysphagia, respiratory disturbance

Therapy of Ischaemic Infarction

▶ Three-compartment model
- • Infarct core
  - – Cerebral blood flow (CBF) <10 ml/100g/min
  - – Irreversibly damaged brain parenchyma
- • Infarct penumbra
  - – CBF 10–25 ml/100g/min
  - – Functionally disturbed and structurally intact brain parenchyma
  - – Transition to infarct core if ischaemia persists
- • Oligemic brain parenchyma
  - – CBF 25–80 ml/100g/min
  - – Functionally and structurally intact brain parenchyma
- • Normal brain parenchyma
  - – CBF >80 ml/100g/min
  - – Functionally and structurally intact brain parenchyma
▶ Measures to accelerate recanalisation
- • Pre-hospital
  - – Educating the population
  - – Optimisation of the rescue service
  - – Mobile stroke units
  - – Pre-hospital LAMS score
  - – Optimisation of patient handover
  - – Use of telemedicine
- • Hospital
  - – Stroke Unit
  - – CT or MR without delay
  - – Coagulation and blood count

- After exclusion of bleeding, immediate intravenous thrombolysis if indicated
- CTA or MRA for the detection of proximal intracranial vascular occlusions
- Transport to angiography
- Sedation or intubation anaesthesia without delay
- Mechanical thrombectomy/endovascular therapy
► Clarification by means of MR and MRA
  • Mismatch imaging
    - Patients with a clear mismatch between small DWI lesion and extensive PWI deficit may benefit from late recanalisation (in advanced time windows or unknown time window)
  • Collateral formation
► Possible contraindications for local/systemic thrombolysis
  • Exceeding the therapeutic window
    - Intravenous thrombolysis: Time window 4.5 h (up to 6 h)
    - Mechanical thrombectomy: Time window up to 24 h
  • Spontaneous regression of the neurological symptoms
  • Acute bleeding
  • Coagulopathy
  • Recent surgery
  • Demarcated infarct
    - Cerebral microangiopathy, major diffusion defects and multiple microhaemorrhages as confirmed risk factors for thrombolysis-associated haemorrhage
► IR
  • Mechanical thrombectomy
    - In cases of large intracranial vessel occlusion and in the absence of extensive ischaemic damage in downstream brain tissue
    - E.g. internal carotid artery, middle cerebral artery
    - Time window up to 6 h, in selected patients in advanced time windows up to 24 h
    - Additional systemic thrombolysis

- Local intra-arterial thrombolysis
  - e.g. vertebral artery, basilar artery
  - Clinical indications: Crossed symptoms with homolateral cranial nerve deficits and contralateral paralysis or sensory disturbances
  - Time window up to 24 h
▶ Procedure for mechanical thrombectomy
  - Neurovascular Intervention Centre ("Mothership")
  - Thrombus aspiration (aspiration catheter), thrombus extraction (stent retriever)
  - Minimise the risk of vascular injury by probing with inverted wire, avoiding microcatheter passage against high resistance and using size-matched thrombectomy instruments
▶ Procedure for local intra-arterial thrombolysis
  - Placement of the microcatheter tip (2 F) into the proximal part of the thrombus
  - 0.9 mg/kg bw rt-PA, of which 10% as bolus, remainder over 1 h, maximum 90 mg rt-PA
  - Bleeding as a complication
▶ When diagnosing acute proximal intracranial vessel occlusion in a hospital without the possibility of mechanical thrombectomy, a "bridging concept" should be used
  - After starting intravenous thrombolysis with rt-PA, transfer to a centre with endovascular therapy options should take place immediately ("drip and ship")
▶ Mechanical thrombectomy must not delay the initiation of intravenous thrombolysis and intravenous thrombolysis must not delay the initiation of mechanical thrombectomy
▶ Patients with acute basilar artery occlusion should be treated with mechanical thrombectomy and, if there are no contraindications, additionally with intravenous thrombolysis

Moyamoya Disease

▶ Progressive stenosis and occlusion of the distal internal carotid artery and proximal anterior and middle cerebral arteries
▶ Occurrence mainly in Asia

▶ Cause of ischaemic strokes in children

▶ Cerebral infarctions, cerebral haemorrhages, headaches, seizures

▶ **Angio**: Nebulous collateral circulation via lenticulostriate, leptomeningeal and pial vessels ("puff of smoke")

Venous Sinus Thrombosis

▶ Aetiology
  • Local
    – Extradural infection: Throat infections, osteomyelitis, mastoiditis
    – Intradural infection: Meningitis, abscess, empyema
    – Trauma
    – Neoplasm
  • Systemic
    – Dehydration
    – Hormonal e.g. pregnancy, oral contraceptive pill
    – Hypercoagulopathy
▶ Localisation
  • Superior sagittal sinus
  • Transverse sinus
  • Sigmoid sinus
  • Cavernous sinus
▶ Young women
▶ Acute headache, focal deficits, central paresis, clouding of consciousness, seizures, psychoses
▶ In the case of thrombosis of the internal cerebral veins—bilateral infarctions of the basal ganglia, thalamus, hypothalamus and cerebellum
▶ Early diagnosis crucial
▶ **CT**
  • Hyperdense sinuses
    – Cord sign—cord-like hyper-attenuation on non-enhanced CT
  • Filling defect in the venous sinus
    – + enhancement of the adjacent dura—empty delta sign

- Collaterals filled with contrast medium
  - dilated superficial veins
▶ **MR**
  - Stage I (1st–5th day): Thrombus T1 isointense, T2 hypointense
  - Stage II (5th–15th day): Thrombus T1 hyperintense, T2 hyperintense
  - Stage III (from day 15): Thrombus T1 hypointense, T2 hypointense
  - Stage IV (from several months): Signal inhomogeneities in the sinus
    - T2* Signal cancellation due to thrombus (blooming)
▶ **MRA**: Filling defect in the sinus
▶ Accompanying findings
  - Brain oedema
  - Stasis haemorrhages and infarctions in the drainage area of the sinus
  - Ventricular compression
▶ **Differential Diagnosis**: Slow venous flow, increased haematocrit, prominent arachnoid granulations, inter-sulcal subarachnoid haemorrhage, hypoplastic sinus

Intracranial Haemorrhage

▶ Aetiology
  - Basal ganglia haemorrhage: Hypertension
  - Parenchymal and subarachnoid haemorrhage: Aneurysm
  - Lobar haemorrhage: Vascular malformation, tumour, infarction, amyloid angiopathy
▶ Focal deficits, raised intracranial pressure, seizures
▶ **CT**
  - Acute: Hyperdense, space-occupying, perilesional oedema
  - Subacute: Isodense, peripheral enhancement
  - Chronic: Hypodense, not space-occupying
▶ **MR**
  - Hyperacute
    - Oxyhaemoglobin, <24 h
    - T1 isointense, T2 hyperintense, T2* hypointense, DWI hyperintense

- Acute
  - Deoxyhaemoglobin, 1–3 days
  - T1 isointense, T2 hypointense, T2* hypointense, DWI hyperintense
- Early subacute
  - Intracellular methaemoglobin, 3–7 days
  - T1 hyperintense, T2 hypointense, T2* severely hypointense, DWI hyperintense
- Late subacute
  - Extracellular methaemoglobin, 7 days—1 month
  - T1 hyperintense, T2 hyperintense, T2* hypointense, DWI invisible
- Chronic
  - Haemosiderin and ferritin, >1 month
  - T1 hypointense, T2 hypointense, T2* hypointense, DWI invisible
▶ **Differential Diagnosis**: Haemorrhagic brain tumour with peripheral enhancement (follow-up to differentiate)
▶ **Complications**: Cerebral oedema, hydrocephalus
▶ Amyloid angiopathy
- Most common cause of recurrent bleeding in elderly patients without hypertension
- Transient focal neurological episodes
- Subacute dementia
- **MR**
  - Lobar haemorrhage
  - T2* microbleeds (lobar distribution)
  - Superficial siderosis
  - White matter hyperintensities/ small vessel disease
  - Cortical infarcts
▶ Microhaemorrhages (microbleeds)
- Focal haemosiderin deposits after circumscribed haemorrhage
- More frequent occurrence in amyloid angiopathy, hypertension and old age
- **MR**: T2* round, measuring <10 mm, hypointense lesions

- Causes for multiple black dots on T2*
  - Hypertensive microbleeds
  - Cerebral amyloid angiopathy
  - Multiple small cavernomas
  - Diffuse axonal injury

Subarachnoid Haemorrhage

▶ Aetiology: Aneurysm, arteriovenous malformation, trauma
▶ Worst-ever headache, photophobia, meningism, reduced level of consciousness, cranial nerve palsies, seizures, intraocular haemorrhage
▶ Severity according to Hunt and Hess
  - I: Mild headache, mild meningism
  - II: Severe headache, severe meningism, cranial nerve palsies
  - III: Somnolence, confusion, focal symptoms
  - IV: Stupor, hemiparesis, extensor phenomena
  - V: Coma
▶ **CT**
  - Blood in basal cisterns, interpeduncular cistern, prepontine cistern, lateral fissure, interhemispheric fissure, over convexity
  - Possible extension into the ventricular system
  - Possible hydrocephalus
  - Infarcts
▶ **MR**
  - Detection of bleeding (FLAIR is most sensitive)
▶ In case of clinical suspicion and negative imaging, cerebrospinal fluid (CSF) puncture to confirm the diagnosis
▶ Aneurysm detection with CTA, MRA (first line) or DSA
▶ **Angiography**: To find the source of haemorrhage
  - If four-vessel angiography does not demonstrate pathological findings:
    - If subarachnoid haemorrhage is only present in perimesencephalic cisterns, a venous source of haemorrhage is probable

- Otherwise, re-angiography after a few days for further clarification
- In 20% of subarachnoid haemorrhages no source of haemorrhage is detectable even with re-angiography

▶ **Differential Diagnosis**: Migraine, meningitis, vertebral dissection, brain tumour

▶ **Complications**: Recurrent haemorrhage, vasospasm with the risk of infarction, hydrocephalus

Aneurysms

▶ Aetiology: Vessel wall weakness, vessel wall degeneration

▶ High-risk group: Autosomal-dominant polycystic nephropathy with aneurysms in 25%

▶ Localisation
- Anterior communicating artery
- Bifurcation of the middle cerebral artery
- Posterior communicating artery
- Carotid siphon
- Basilar artery
- Origin of the ophthalmic artery
- Anterior choroidal artery

▶ 98% saccular (berry) 2% fusiform

▶ 10–20% multiple

▶ 85% in the anterior circulation, 15% in the posterior circulation

▶ Rupture risk factors
- Size
- Symptoms
- Posterior circulation
- Female sex
- Higher age
- Smoking
- Hypertension

▶ Subarachnoid haemorrhage, cranial nerve deficits (oculomotor palsy), hemiparesis

▶ **CTA/MRA**
- Sensitivity of CTA higher than MRA
- Limitations of MRA
    - Very small aneurysms
    - Thrombosed aneurysms
    - Very slow flow

▶ **Angio**
- Objectives of the DSA
    - Identification of the vessel of origin
    - Characterisation of the aneurysm neck
    - Position of the aneurysm
    - Morphology of the aneurysm
    - Detection of a second aneurysm
- Limitations of DSA
    - Thrombosed aneurysms

▶ **Differential Diagnosis**: Vascular loop, dilated vascular infundibulum, tumour

▶ **Diagnosis**: Four-vessel angiography

▶ **IR**
- Elimination (coiling, stenting, flow modulation)
- In case of angiographically-proven, haemodynamically relevant, vasospasm, intra-arterial application of vasodilator drugs (nimodipine, papaverine)

▶ **Complications**: Recurrent haemorrhage, vasospasm with the risk of infarction, hydrocephalus

Vascular Malformations

▶ Arteriovenous malformation
- Grading according to Spetzler-Martin
    - Size: Small (<3 cm) = 1, medium (3–6 cm) = 2, large (>6 cm) = 3
    - Eloquence of adjacent brain: No = 0, yes = 1
    - Deep vascular component: No = 0, yes = 1
    - Total score: 1–5
- Local arteriovenous shunt without interposed normal capillary bed

- Dilated feeding artery, arteriovenous convolutions (nidus), dilated draining veins
- Steal phenomena in neighbouring vascular territories
- Bleeding, ischaemia, headache, seizures
- **CT**
  - Hyperdense vascular convolution/ nidus
  - Dilated internal or external cerebral veins
  - Enhancement
- **MR**
  - T2 round flow void
  - T2 adjacent hyperintense foci due to ischaemia and gliosis, hypointense foci due to haemosiderin
  - Significant enhancement
- **Angio**
  - Enlarged arterial feeder
  - Nidus
  - Early draining and markedly dilated veins
  - Possible arterial or venous aneurysmal changes
  - Risk of overlooking the malformation during active bleeding
- **IR**: Embolisation
▶ Arteriovenous fistulas
- Local arteriovenous shunt at dural level
- Localisation includes:
  - Transverse sinus
  - Cavernous sinus
- Classification according to Cognard and Merland
  - Type I: Venous drainage into the dural venous sinus with antegrade flow
  - Type II: Venous drainage into the dural venous sinus with retrograde flow/reflux into other sinuses or veins
  - Type II a: Retrograde flow in the dural venous sinus
  - Type II b: Retrograde flow into cortical veins
  - Type III: Direct drainage into cortical veins
  - Type IV: Direct drainage into cortical veins, additional venous ectasia
  - Type V: Drainage into spinal perimedullary veins

- Depending on the type of fistula: Ringing in the ears, exophthalmos, visual disturbance, chemosis, headaches, cranial nerve palsies
- Risk of bleeding varies with type
- **Angio**
  - Solitary arterial feeder, multiple arterial feeders or direct fistula from larger artery such as internal carotid artery
  - Fistula via a diffuse vascular network into the dural sinus with early filling
  - Depending on the type of fistula, may also be contrast filling of cortical veins or the superior ophthalmic vein
- **IR**: Embolisation
► Cavernous malformation
- Cavernoma
- Cerebral venous malformation from dilated sinusoidal spaces
- Seizures, headaches
- Only slightly increased risk of bleeding
- **CT**
  - Hyperdense round lesion
  - Calcification (around 50%)
  - No perilesional oedema
  - Minimal enhancement
- **MR**
  - Mostly signal inhomogeneous lesions with blood in all stages of degradation
  - Mulberry-like, honeycomb or popcorn-like structure
  - Often T2* hypointense rim
- **Complications**: Bleeding
► Developmental venous anomaly
- Wide drainage vein with venous inflow
- Preferentially found in the frontal lobe and cerebellum
- Frequent association with other vascular malformations
- Mostly incidental finding without clinical relevance
- **MR**
  - Dilated draining veins
  - Transcerebral, umbrella or star-shaped structure
  - Usually strong enhancement

▶ Capillary telangiectasia
  • Thin-walled ectatic blood vessels of the capillary type
  • Preferentially affect the pons
  • Frequent association with developmental venous anomaly (transitional malformation)
  • Mostly incidental finding without clinical relevance
  • **MR**
    – T1 hypo- to isointense, T2 iso- to hyperintense, T2* hypointense
    – Flat, brush-like or stippled structure
    – Usually weak enhancement

Vasculitis

▶ Aetiology: Heterogeneous disease group with vessel wall inflammation, leukocyte infiltration, vessel stenoses, microaneurysms, thromboses
▶ Types
  • Idiopathic primary vasculitis
  • Vasculitis in primary systemic vasculitides
  • Vasculitis in collagen vascular disease
  • Infection-related or infection-associated vasculitis
  • Drug- or substance-induced vasculitis
  • Vasculitis associated with lymphoproliferative disorders and other malignancies
▶ Headache, nausea, myalgias, focal deficits, encephalopathy, seizures
▶ Inflammatory parameters, vasculitis serology
▶ **MR**
  • Multifocal hyperintensities, some with contrast enhancement (ischaemic infarcts, inflammatory infiltrates)
  • In granulomatosis with polyangiitis, dural thickening with enhancement near the granulomatous involvement (orbital, nasal, paranasal)
  • **Differential Diagnosis:** Embolic cerebral infarcts, multiple sclerosis

► **MRA/Angio**
  • Multiple calibre changes of the intracranial arteries
  • No atherosclerosis of the extracranial arteries
  • Irregular stenoses, occlusions
  • Small aneurysms
► **Nuclear medicine**: 99mTc-HMPAO, 99mTc-ECD

Vascular Compression Syndromes

► Aetiology: Contact between artery and cranial nerve, damage to the cranial nerve due to pulsation trauma
► Types
  • Trigeminal neuralgia: Contact of trigeminal nerve with SCA or AICA
    – Sharp shooting pain in the area of innervation for a few seconds
  • Hemifacial spasm: Contact of facial nerve with PICA or AICA
    – Unilateral twitching of the facial musculature innervated by the facial nerve
  • Glossopharyngeal neuralgia: Contact of glossopharyngeal nerve with PICA or vertebral artery
    – Sharp pharyngeal pain associated with swallowing, always unilateral manifestation
► **MR**
  • No CSF signal between artery and cranial nerve
  • Cranial nerve displacement
  • Atrophy of the cranial nerve

Bacterial Infections

► Meningitis
  • Source of infection: Haematogenous, local extension of infection (sinusitis, mastoiditis, otitis media, cerebrospinal fluid fistula, osteomyelitis), traumatic
  • Causes:
    – Purulent (bacterial) meningitis

- – Lymphocytic (viral, aseptic) meningitis
- – Chronic (tuberculous) meningitis
- Headache, fever, neck stiffness, clouding of consciousness, vomiting, seizures
- Nuchal rigidity, Brudzinski sign, Kernig sign
- Elevated CSF WBC count
- **MR**
- Enhancement of the leptomeninges or pachymeninges
- Bacterial meningitis mostly frontoparietal, tuberculous meningitis mostly basal
- Parenchymal lesions with concomitant cerebritis or additional brain abscesses
- **Differential Diagnosis**: Meningeal enhancement in leptomeningeal metastasis (carcinomatous meningitis), after surgery, intracranial hypotension and after cerebrospinal fluid puncture
- **Complications**: Hygroma, abscess, empyema, cerebritis, ependymitis, ventriculitis, hydrocephalus, cerebral oedema, infarction, sinus vein thrombosis

▶ Brain abscess
- Source of infection: Local spread of infection (sinusitis, otitis, mastoiditis; localisation mostly frontotemporal), traumatic (brain injuries, brain surgery; localisation mostly superficial), haematogenous (pneumonia, endocarditis; often multiple)
- Initially purulent cerebritis, then bacterial brain abscess
- Headache, vomiting, fever, raised intracranial pressure, somnolence, seizures
- **MR**
  - – Central restricted diffusion
  - – Grey-white matter junction as the most frequent localisation
  - – Early cerebritis: Focal cerebral oedema
  - – Late cerebritis: Ill-defined margin, ring enhancement
  - – Early abscess: Well-defined margin, ring enhancement
  - – Later abscess: Capsule thickens, central cavity reduces
- **MRS**: Pathological lactate peaks

- **Differential Diagnosis**: Glioblastoma, metastases, toxoplasmosis, tuberculosis, demyelinating lesion
- **Complications**: Daughter abscesses, meningitis, ependymitis, ventriculitis

▶ Septic encephalitis
- Source of infection: Bacterial endocarditis, acute sepsis
- **MR**
  - Multiple small brain abscesses
  - Microhaemorrhages or haemorrhage
  - Multiple ischaemic infarcts

▶ Empyema
- Causes: As for brain abscess
- Epidural empyema biconvex, subdural biconcave
- Fever, headache, hemiparesis, clouding of consciousness, meningism, seizures
- **CT/MR**: Enhancement at the medial border of the empyema
  - Restricted diffusion

▶ Neuroborreliosis
- Cause: Borrelia burgdorferi
- Initially flu-like symptoms, then radicular pain, peripheral paresis and inflammatory cerebrospinal fluid syndrome, finally vasculitic complications, motor deficits and development of dementia
- **MR**
  - T2 focal hyperintensities, some may enhance
  - Cranial nerve enhancement
  - Meningeal enhancement
  - Normal findings also possible

▶ Neurotuberculosis
- Aetiology: Mycobacterium tuberculosis
- Types
  - Leptomeningeal tuberculosis
  - Pachymeningeal tuberculosis
  - Parenchymal tuberculosis
- Initially nonspecific symptoms, then basal meningitis, finally seizures

- **MR**
  - Leptomeningeal tuberculosis: Enhancement of basal meninges, hydrocephalus, cerebral infarcts in supratentorial regions, meningeal calcifications, ependymal calcifications
  - Pachymeningeal tuberculosis: Dural masses with homogeneous enhancement
  - Parenchymal tuberculosis: First granulomas with nodular or ring enhancement, finally calcifications with regional brain atrophy
- **Differential Diagnosis:** Misinterpretation of new non-enhancing lesions under effective tuberculostatic therapy as progression of the disease (increased release of tuberculoprotein by destroyed tubercle bacilli, thereby triggering an inflammatory reaction)

Viral Infections

► Herpes simplex encephalitis
  - Stages
    - Initially flu-like symptoms
    - Encephalitic stage
    - Psychotic stage
  - Fever, headache, confusion, temporal lobe seizures, aphasia, quadrantanopia
  - High mortality, severe long-term damage
  - **MR**
    - Initial findings: T2 hyperintensities medial temporal lobe, anterior temporal lobe, insula, cingulate. Involvement of the limbic system, asymmetric, no or minimal enhancement in early stages
    - Progressive findings: Involvement of other cortical regions, gyral and less commonly meningeal enhancement, petechial haemorrhages at the grey-white matter junction
    - Late findings: Cystic or gliotic residue with focal or diffuse brain atrophy
  - **Diagnosis**: CSF PCR test for HSV

▶ Cytomegalovirus encephalitis
  • Often opportunistic infection in immunocompromised patients
  • Ventriculitis due to destruction of the ependymal lining of the ventricular system
  • MR: Periventricular T2 hyperintensities and subependymal enhancement
▶ Epstein-Barr virus encephalitis
  • Encephalitis in the course of primary infection or in the case of viral reactivation, can cause transverse myelitis, trigger Guillain-Barré syndrome
  • Association with nasopharyngeal carcinoma and Burkitt's lymphoma
  • MR: Diffuse multifocal hyperintensities including basal ganglia, thalamus, cortical involvement
▶ Varicella zoster virus encephalitis
  • Often opportunistic infection in immunocompromised patients
  • MR
    – Multifocal cortical, cerebellar hyperintensities, cranial nerve involvement
    – With vasculitis (immunocompromised): Ischaemic lesions at the transition between grey and white matter, territorial cerebral infarcts
▶ Progressive multifocal leukoencephalopathy
  • Aetiology: Subacute opportunistic infection due to reactivation of the JC-Virus
  • In AIDS, leukaemia, lymphoma, sarcoidosis, immunomodulation, immunosuppression
  • Cortical blindness, aphasia, confusion, dementia, hemiparesis, ataxia
  • MR: T2 asymmetric, peripheral, confluent hyperintensities in the parieto-occipital white matter, subcortical U-fibres involved, rarely signs of mass effect, no enhancement, no brain atrophy
  • Differential Diagnosis: HIV encephalitis, acute disseminated encephalomyelitis

▶ HIV encephalitis
  • Cognitive, behavioural and motor disturbance, subcortical dementia
  • MR: T2 symmetrical, central, confluent hyperintensities in the white matter, U-fibres not involved, rarely signs of mass effect, no enhancement, later cerebral atrophy
  • Opportunistic infections in AIDS
    – Often toxoplasmosis
    – Less frequently tuberculosis, cryptococcosis, candidiasis, nocardiosis, aspergillosis, cytomegaly
▶ Measles virus encephalitis
  • Types
    – Post-infectious measles virus encephalitis: recurrent fever, seizures, neurological deficits
    – Subacute measles virus encephalitis: refractory seizures
    – Subacute sclerosing panencephalitis: mental changes, speech changes, involuntary movements
  • MR: in subacute sclerosing panencephalitis, initially T2 hyperintensities in white matter, basal ganglia and corpus callosum, later brain atrophy

Mycoses

▶ Neuroaspergillosis
  • Aetiology: Aspergillus
  • Extrapulmonary manifestation of invasive aspergillosis
  • Manifestation as brain abscesses, granulomas, meningitis, ventriculitis
  • CT: Calcifications
  • MR
    – T2 parenchymal hyperintensities, ring enhancement, restricted diffusion, haemorrhagic
    – Dural enhancement where there has been intracranial spread from fungal sinusitis
  • Complications: Haemorrhagic cerebral infarcts, fungal aneurysms

- ▶ Neurocandidiasis
  - Aetiology: Candida
  - Subacute basal meningoencephalitis
  - **MR**: Multiple microabscesses
- ▶ Neurocryptococcosis
  - Aetiology: Cryptococcus neoformans
  - Fever, headache, neck stiffness
  - **MR**: Cryptococcomas with enhancement, dilated perivascular spaces in basal ganglia, meningeal enhancement

Helminthoses

- ▶ Neurocysticercosis
  - Aetiology: Taenia solium
  - Classification according to Escobar
    - I: Simple vesicle
    - II: Colloidal vesicle
    - III: Granular nodule
    - IV: Calcified nodule
  - Clinical picture of chronic meningitis
  - **CT**: Depending on stage: Cyst with dot (scolex), hyperdense cyst with wall enhancement, enhancing nodule, calcifications
  - **MR**: Cyst with marginal nodule through the scolex as an important diagnostic criterion
  - **Differential diagnosis**: In stage I neuroepithelial cyst, in stage II glioblastoma and metastasis, in stage III tuberculoma and brain abscess, in stage IV cavernous haemangioma
- ▶ Echinococcosis
  - Aetiology: Echinococcus granulosus, Echinococcus multilocularis
  - Hydatid disease
  - Epileptic seizures, increased intracranial pressure
  - **CT**: Solitary round cysts with hypodense cyst contents and sharp isodense rim, occasional cyst wall calcification, no perilesional oedema, no enhancement

Protozoonoses

▶ Toxoplasmosis
  • Aetiology: Toxoplasma gondii
  • Structure of the toxoplasmosis lesion: Central necrosis, in the middle inflammatory tissue, peripherally pathogen cysts
  • In immunocompetent persons—flu symptoms, swelling of the lymph nodes
  • In immunocompromised patients—severe diffuse encephalitis
  • **CT/MR**: Peripherally enhancing lesions with marked perilesional oedema in basal ganglia, grey-white matter junction and thalami, haemorrhagic component, later calcification
  • **Differential Diagnosis**: Lymphoma, neurotuberculosis, mycoses
▶ Malaria
  • Aetiology: Plasmodium falciparum most common
  • Unconsciousness, seizures, headache, temporary paralysis
  • **MR**: Cerebral oedema, disseminated microhaemorrhages, infarcts

Prion Diseases

▶ Sporadic Creutzfeldt-Jakob disease (sCJD)
  • Subacute spongiform encephalopathy
  • First cognitive symptoms such as mood swings, depression, fatigability, forgetfulness, then neurological symptoms such as tone abnormalities, pyramidal signs, fasciculations, myoclonus, finally dementia
  • Shorter duration of illness, higher age at death
  • **MR**: DWI/T2/FLAIR hyperintensity in caudate nucleus and putamen, thalamus, cerebral cortex
  • **Differential Diagnosis**: Alzheimer's disease, Lewy body disease

- ▶ Variant Creutzfeldt-Jakob disease (vCJD)
  - From cattle
  - Early psychiatric symptoms, painful sensory symptoms, ataxia, myoclonus, chorea, dystonia, eventually dementia
  - Longer duration of illness, lower age at death
  - **MR**: DWI/T2/FLAIR bilateral hyperintensity in the pulvinar of the thalami

Neurosarcoidosis

- ▶ Basal granulomatous meningoencephalitis with involvement of cranial nerves and basal cerebral vessels
- ▶ Peripheral facial nerve palsy, hypothalamic disorders (diabetes insipidus, amenorrhoea), various visual disorders (optic atrophy, papilloedema), focal seizures
- ▶ **MR**
  - Diverse morphologies
  - T2 periventricular and medullary hyperintensities
  - Single or multiple supratentorial and infratentorial lesions
  - Solitary extra-axial mass
  - Leptomeningeal enhancement
  - Cranial nerve enhancement

Limbic Encephalitis

- ▶ Aetiology: Non-infectious cerebral inflammation mainly affecting mesial temporal structures
- ▶ Types
  - Paraneoplastic
  - Non-paraneoplastic
- ▶ Memory impairment, temporal lobe seizures, affective disorder
- ▶ **MR**
  - T2/FLAIR mesial temporal hyperintensity and oedema, often bilateral
  - Can have enhancement
  - Can progress to brain atrophy

Multiple Sclerosis

▶ Inflammation and neurodegeneration as main components of the disease
▶ 10–50 years, women > men
▶ Repeated relapses, different parts of the central nervous system affected, progressive disability
▶ Lhermitte's (neck flexion) sign, retrobulbar neuritis, diplopia, nystagmus, internuclear ophthalmoplegia, paraplegia, spasticity, urinary incontinence
▶ **MR**
  - T2/FLAIR focal hyperintensities
    - ≥3 mm in the longitudinal axis
  - Dissemination in space
    - Periventricular (Dawson's fingers perpendicular to lateral ventricles)
    - Juxtacortical
    - Corpus callosum
    - Infratentorial
    - Spinal
    - Optic nerve
  - Dissemination in time
    - Enhancing: Homogeneous or peripheral (often incomplete); enhancement usually transient lasting up to 1 month and at most up to 4 months; no enhancement after systemic steroid administration (sealing of the blood-brain barrier)
    - Non-enhancing
▶ McDonald criteria
  - Spatial distribution
    - ≥1 T2 lesion in at least 2 of 4 areas (periventricular, juxta/cortical, infratentorial, spinal)
  - Plus temporal distribution
    - Simultaneous detection of enhancing and non-enhancing lesions in one examination or
    - Evidence of a new T2 lesion and/or an accumulating lesion in the course, regardless of the time of the initial examination

▶ **Differential Diagnosis**
- Small vessel disease
  - Over 50 years
  - Mostly confluent lesions
  - Spared subcortical U-fibres
  - No spinal lesions
- CADASIL
- Acute disseminated encephalomyelitis
  - After infections
  - Monophasic course of disease
  - Rare linear lesions
  - Rarely optic nerve lesions
- Neuromyelitis optica
- Various vasculitic syndromes
- Neurosarcoidosis
- Progressive multifocal leukoencephalopathy
- Cerebral metastases

▶ Spinal multiple sclerosis
- 10% only spinal and no cerebral lesions
  - 75% cervical localisation, 50% multiple occurrence
  - Mostly dorsolateral, mostly ovoid

▶ **Diagnosis**: Overall picture from clinical evaluation, electrophysiology (visual evoked potentials, auditory evoked potentials, somatosensory evoked potentials), laboratory diagnostics (oligoclonal bands, elevated IgG, basic myelin protein) and MRI

▶ Procedure for incidental MRI findings typical of multiple sclerosis (radiologically isolated syndrome): Regular follow-up, alternatively watch and wait

Acute Disseminated Encephalomyelitis

▶ Aetiology: Para-infectious, post-vaccine, post-chemotherapy
▶ Monophasic disease
▶ Usually presents in children
▶ Initially fever, headache, vigilance disorders, then hemi-symptoms, cerebellar signs, optic neuritis

▶ **MR**
- T2 multifocal white matter hyperintensities with irregular asymmetric distribution
- Brainstem, thalamic involvement
- In spinal lesions—often blurred demarcation due to perilesional oedema
- Infratentorial lesions in the cerebellum or middle cerebellar peduncle
- No mixed picture of enhancing and non-enhancing lesions

▶ **Differential Diagnosis:** Multiple sclerosis

Overview of Brain Tumours

▶ Frequency
- 10% of all tumours

▶ Localisation
- 85% intracranial, 15% intraspinal
- Mostly supratentorial in adults, infratentorial in children
- Extra-axial mostly benign, intra-axial mostly malignant

▶ Rough distribution
- 40% Brain metastases
- 35% Gliomas
- 15% Meningiomas
- 5% Vestibular schwannomas
- 5% Pituitary adenomas

▶ Presenting symptoms
- Headache
- Intracranial pressure
- Seizures
- Psychological changes

Localisation of Brain Tumours

▶ Intra-axial supratentorial
- Glioblastoma, astrocytoma, oligodendroglioma, lymphoma, metastasis

► Extra-axial supratentorial
  • Meningioma
► Intra-axial infratentorial
  • Cerebellum
    – Metastasis, medulloblastoma, haemangioblastoma, astrocytoma
  • Brainstem
    – Astrocytoma, glioblastoma
► Extra-axial infratentorial
  • Cerebellopontine angle
    – Vestibular schwannoma, meningioma, epidermoid, arachnoid cyst
  • Jugular foramen
    – Glomus tumour
  • Clivus
    – Chordoma, chondroma, chondrosarcoma
  • Foramen magnum
    – Meningioma, neurofibroma
► Pituitary fossa
  • Pituitary adenoma, craniopharyngioma, meningioma, Rathke's pocket cyst
► Corpus callosum
  • Astrocytoma, glioblastoma, lymphoma
► Pineal gland
  • Pineal cyst, pineocytoma, pineoblastoma, teratoma, glioma, meningioma
► Ventricle
  • Glioma, choroid plexus papilloma, ependymoma, neurocytoma, meningioma, colloid cyst

Age Predilection of Brain Tumours

► Under 2 years
  • Astrocytoma, teratoma, medulloblastoma, embryonal tumours
► Older children, adolescents
  • Supratentorial: Astrocytoma, oligodendroglioma, craniopharyngioma, pineal tumours

- Infratentorial: Astrocytoma, medulloblastoma, ependymoma
▶ Adults
  - Supratentorial: Astrocytoma, oligodendroglioma, meningioma, pituitary adenoma
  - Infratentorial: Vestibular schwannoma, meningioma, epidermoid, haemangioblastoma

Main Findings with Brain Tumours

▶ **MRI**
  - Tumours: T1 hypointense, T2 hyperintense
  - Melanin, high protein, subacute haemorrhage, fat: T1 hyperintense
  - Iron, melanin, calcifications, chronic haemorrhage, high cell density, collagen-rich stroma: T2 hypointense
▶ Malignancy criteria
  - Indistinct tumour margin
  - Tumour necrosis
  - Tumour neovascularisation
  - Tumour heterogeneity
  - Bone invasion
▶ Tumours which may contain calcifications
  - Oligodendroglioma
  - Craniopharyngioma
  - Ependymoma
  - Choroid plexus papilloma
  - Meningioma
  - Teratoma
  - Chordoma

Astrocytoma

▶ Pilocytic astrocytoma
  - WHO Grade I
  - 10–20 years
  - Cerebellum, optic pathway, pons

- **MR**: Solid tumour component, cystic tumour component, high ADC values, hardly any perilesional oedema, strong enhancement of solid component
- **Differential Diagnosis**: Haemangioblastoma
▶ Glioblastoma
  - WHO grade IV
  - 90% primary glioblastomas, 10% secondary glioblastomas (from previously known lower grade gliomas)
  - 50–70 years
  - Multicentricity possible
  - **MR**
    - Irregular thick margins, central necrosis
    - Significant perilesional oedema
    - Peripheral irregular enhancement
    - Mass effect
    - Necrosis
    - Bleeding
  - **Differential Diagnosis**: Abscess, metastasis
  - Determination of the extent of a glioma in the context of radiotherapy planning as well as differentiation of a tumour recurrence from therapy changes also by 11C-methionine or 18F-fluoroethyltyrosine PET
  - Neuroradiological response criteria for malignant gliomas according to the RANO criteria (Response assessment in neuro-oncology)
    - Complete response: No contrast enhancing lesion, T2/FLAIR stable or smaller, no new lesion
    - Partial response: Contrast enhancing lesions ≥50% smaller, T2/FLAIR lesions stable or smaller, no new lesion
    - Stable disease: Contrast enhancing lesion <50% smaller but <25% larger, T2/FLAIR lesions stable or smaller, no new lesion
    - Progressive disease: Contrast enhancing lesions ≥25% larger, T2/FLAIR lesions larger, any new lesions
▶ Gliomatosis cerebri
  - Growth pattern of infiltrative gliomas

- Not an independent tumour entity
- Rapid progression within a few months
- Bihemispheric and also infratentorial spread
- **MR**
  - T1 homogeneously hypointense, T2 homogeneously hyperintense
  - Diffuse spread
  - Minimal mass effect
  - Minimal or no enhancement
- **Differential Diagnosis**: Low-grade astrocytoma, leukodystrophy, encephalitis

Oligodendroglioma

► 50% of oligodendrogliomas contain parts of astrocytomas (mixed gliomas)
► Calcifications characteristic, but absence does not exclude the diagnosis
► Seizures most common initial symptom
► **CT**: Hypodense, space-occupying, cortical or subcortical, skull remodelling, nodular or gyriform calcifications
► **MR**: Calcifications as susceptibility artefacts

Ependymoma

► Originate from the ependymal cells of the ventricular walls and central canal
► Meningeal seeding and spinal metastases possible
► Posterior fossa most common location—fourth ventricle
  - Floor of fourth ventricle—brainstem side
► Soft tumour, passes through foramina of Luschka and Magendie
► **MR**
  - Calcification, cystic spaces common, can contain haemorrhage
  - Heterogeneous enhancement
  - No perilesional oedema
  - Associated hydrocephalus

▶ Always also perform MR of the entire neuraxis (including spine)
▶ **Differential Diagnosis**: Medulloblastoma

Medulloblastoma

▶ Localisation in the cerebellar vermis, bulging into fourth ventricle
▶ Common brain tumour in childhood
▶ Ataxia, nausea, vomiting, headache
▶ **MR**
  • Heterogeneous signal pattern—cysts/necrosis
  • Heterogeneous enhancement
  • Round shape, infiltrating growth
  • Calcification occurs, less common than ependymoma
  • Restricted diffusion due to high cellularity (hyperattenuating on CT)
  • Hydrocephalus
  • Drop metastases
▶ Always also perform MR of the entire neuraxis
▶ **Differential Diagnosis**: Ependymoma

Meningioma

▶ Aetiology: Slow-growing, extra-axial meningothelial tumour originating from the covering cells of the arachnoid
▶ Most frequent localisations and typical initial symptoms
  • Convexity: Seizures
  • Falx cerebri: Foot weakness, epilepsy
  • Tuberculum sellae: Visual disturbances
  • Tentorium cerebelli: Cerebellar symptoms
  • Sphenoid wing: Visual disturbances
  • Olfactory groove: Anosmia
  • Cerebellopontine angle: Hearing loss, vertigo
  • Foramen magnum: Brainstem symptoms
▶ Multiple in 10%
▶ Mostly benign, rarely atypical, very rarely anaplastic

▶ **CT/MR**
- Broad-based tumour base
  - Dural tail sign
  - Especially in sphenoid wing meningiomas, often sheet-like (en plaque) or intraosseous growth (hyperostotic)
- Sharply defined
- Often perilesional oedema
- Expansive growth
- No infiltration
- Intratumoral calcifications
- Strong enhancement
- Meningeal enhancement
- Possible sinus infiltration

▶ **Differential Diagnosis:** Esthesioneuroblastoma (olfactory neuroblastoma), vestibular schwannoma (cerebellopontine angle meningioma)

▶ **IR:** Embolisation selected cases

Lymphoma

▶ Aetiology: Malignant extra-nodal lymphoma with diffuse cerebral infiltration and without extracerebral manifestation, cerebral lymphoma rare manifestation of systemic lymphoma

▶ Especially in immunocompromised patients

▶ Non-specific symptoms, focal deficits, neuropsychiatric symptoms

▶ **CT**
- Hyperdense mass
- Periventricular position
- Slight perilesional oedema
- Homogeneous enhancement

▶ **MR:** T1 hypointense, T2 isointense or slightly hypo- or hyperintense, restricted diffusion

▶ Subependymal, meningeal and intraocular spread

▶ Always also MR of the entire neuraxis

▶ **Differential Diagnosis:** Glioblastoma, metastasis, abscess, multiple sclerosis, acute disseminated encephalomyelitis

▶ **Diagnosis**: Biopsy before steroid administration
▶ Size reduction under steroid administration typical for lymphoma, but not conclusive

Pituitary Adenoma

▶ Types
  • Classification according to hormone production
    – Non-functioning (endocrine inactive) adenomas: Bitemporal hemianopia
    – Prolactin-producing adenomas: Galactorrhoea, amenorrhoea, hirsutism, headaches, loss of libido, impotence
    – Somatotropin-producing adenomas: Acromegaly, sella enlargement, headache, menstrual disorders, visual disturbances, hyperhidrosis
    – Corticotropin-producing adenomas: Cushing's disease
  • Classification according to size
    – Microadenomas: Diameter up to 10 mm
    – Macroadenomas: Diameter more than 10 mm
  • Classification according to growth
    – Expansive growth: Expansion of osseous structures
    – Invasive growth: Infiltration of the osseous structures
▶ Haemorrhage with consecutive oedema possible (pituitary apoplexy)
▶ **CT/MR**
  • Ballooning of the sella
  • Thinning of the sella floor
  • Increase in pituitary height
  • Displacement of the pituitary stalk
  • Compression of the optic chiasm
▶ **MR**: Delayed enhancement and slower washout of adenomas compared to normal pituitary tissue (contrast dynamics)
▶ Enhancement in pituitary adenomas
  • Tumour: Minimal enhancement
  • Anterior pituitary: Low enhancement

- Posterior pituitary: Moderate enhancement
- Pituitary stalk: Strong enhancement

▶ Differential Diagnosis: Craniopharyngioma, meningioma, Rathke's pocket cyst (roundish cyst between anterior and posterior pituitary, smooth border, no enhancement), dermoid, epidermoid

Craniopharyngioma

▶ Aetiology: Epithelial tumour from the former Rathke's pouch
▶ Mostly combined intra- and suprasellar localisation
▶ In children (adamantinomatous type) tumour often calcified, in adults (papillary type) rare. Adamantinomatous and papillary types are now considered distinct entities
▶ Visual disturbances, anterior pituitary insufficiency, bitemporal hemianopia, occasionally hydrocephalus
▶ CT (adamantinomatous)
  - Mixed picture with hypodense (cysts), isodense (tumour) and hyperdense (calcifications) components
  - Enhancement of the solid parts only
▶ MR: Signal intensity dependent on cyst content
▶ High recurrence rate
▶ Differential Diagnosis: Rathke's pocket cyst (roundish cyst, smooth boundary, no enhancement)

Haemangioblastoma

▶ Association with von Hippel Lindau syndrome
▶ Most often cerebellum
▶ Mostly in adults
▶ MR: Large space-occupying cyst with eccentrically contrast enhancing tumour component
▶ Always MR of the entire neuroaxis due to multifocal occurrence
▶ Differential Diagnosis: Pilocytic astrocytoma, ganglioglioma, pleomorphic xanthoastrocytoma

Colloid Cyst

▶ Ventral part of the III ventricle, fornix region
▶ Symptoms of developing hydrocephalus
▶ **CT**: Hyperdense mass
▶ **MR**
  • T1 hyperintense, T2 variable
  • Displacement or blockage of the foramina of Monro with consequent hydrocephalus
  • Peripheral enhancement of cyst wall
▶ **Differential Diagnosis**: Cyst of the septum pellucidum (medium-sized, elongated, follows CSF signal)

Esthesioneuroblastoma (Olfactory neuroblastoma)

▶ Aetiology: Tumour originating from the olfactory nerve or the olfactory epithelium
▶ Classification according to Kadish
  • Type A: Tumour in the nasal cavity
  • Type B: Spread to the paranasal sinuses
  • Type C: Further extension
▶ Growth from the superior nasal cavity through the cribriform plate into the anterior cranial fossa
▶ Obstruction of the nasal cavity, epistaxis, anosmia
▶ **MR**
  • Homogeneous mass with intermediate signal. Dumbbell-shape as it passes through cribriform plate
  • Avid enhancement
  • T2 differentiation of solid tumour and cystic parts or necrotic zones
▶ **Differential Diagnosis**: Olfactory meningioma, paranasal sinus carcinoma

Chordoma

▶ Aetiology: Locally destructive midline tumour from the cells of the notochord
▶ 50–70 years

▶ At the base of the skull—clivus
▶ Headache, diplopia, cranial nerve symptoms
▶ **CT/MR**
  • Destructive midline lesion
  • Extraosseous portion
  • Very high T2 signal
  • Strong enhancement
  • Calcifications
  • Bone fragments
  • Haemorrhage
▶ **Differential Diagnosis:** Chondrosarcoma, plasmacytoma, metastasis

Phacomatoses

▶ Neurofibromatosis I (90%)
  • Neurofibromas, gliomas including optic nerve glioma
▶ Neurofibromatosis II (10%)
  • Vestibular schwannomas, meningiomas
▶ Tuberous sclerosis
  • Subependymal hamartomas, subependymal giant cell astrocytomas, cortical and subcortical tubers, parenchymal cysts
▶ von Hippel-Lindau syndrome
  • Haemangioblastomas, endolymphatic cell tumours
▶ Sturge-Weber syndrome
  • Vascular malformations

Brain Metastases

▶ Aetiology: Bronchial carcinoma, breast carcinoma, gastrointestinal carcinoma, renal cell carcinoma, melanoma
▶ Types
  • Brain metastasis
  • Calvarial metastasis
  • Leptomeningeal metastasis
  • Pachymeningeal metastasis
▶ At time of diagnosis, a third of patients have one metastasis, a third have two metastases, and a third have multiple metastases

▶ Headache, hemiparesis, seizures, cranial nerve palsies, intracranial pressure signs
▶ **CT/MR**
  • Small masses with large volume of oedema
  • Sharp boundary, multiple lesions, known primary tumour
  • Homogeneous, inhomogeneous, nodular or circular enhancement
  • Necrosis, bleeding
▶ **MR**: T1 hyperintense with melanoma as primary tumour
▶ **Differential Diagnosis**
  • Solitary focus: Glioblastoma, resorbing haematoma, infarction, thrombosed vascular malformation
  • Multiple foci: Abscesses, tuberculosis, sarcoidosis, toxoplasmosis, cysticercosis

Carcinomatous Meningitis/Leptomeningeal Metastasis

▶ Aetiology: Solid tumours, leukaemias, lymphomas, brain tumours
▶ Polyradicular symptoms, cranial nerve symptoms, central symptoms (headache, nausea, vomiting), visual disturbances, meningitic symptoms
▶ **MR**
  • Lobular or smooth thickening and enhancement of the meninges
    – cerebral
    – spinal
  • Enhancement of the ependyma, the basal cisterns and the tentorium
  • Brain metastases
  • Hydrocephalus
▶ **Diagnosis**: CSF cytology

Differential Diagnosis of Intracranial Processes

Criteria	Brain abscess	Cystic necrotic anaplastic glioma or glioblastoma	Brain metastasis
MR T2	Signal behaviour of the cystic component dependent on protein content, hypointense capsule, pronounced perilesional oedema	Hyperintense cyst contents, no continuous rim, marked perilesional oedema	Hyperintense cyst contents, no continuous rim, round lesion at grey-white matter junction, variable perilesional oedema
MR T1	Signal behaviour of the cyst content dependent on protein content, isointense capsule, pronounced perilesional oedema	Hypointense cyst contents, no continuous rim, marked perilesional oedema	Hypointense cyst contents, no continuous rim
MR T1 + KM	Strong ring enhancement, smooth border on the outside	Irregular, thick rim of strong peripheral enhancement	Strong ring enhancement
Diffusion MR	ADC reduction in the cystic component	ADC increase in the cystic component	ADC increase in the cystic component
Perfusion MR	Hardly any increase in rCBV in the solid portion compared to normal brain tissue	Increase of rCBV in the solid portion compared to normal brain tissue by 100% or more	Increase of rCBV in the solid portion compared to normal brain tissue by 100% and more

Spectroscopy of Intracranial Processes

Spatial growth	Choline	Creatine, creatine phosphate	N-acetyl aspartate, N-acetyl aspartyl glutamate	Lactate	Lipids	Amino acids
Astrocytoma grade I	+	-	-			
Glioblastoma	+++	- - -	- - -	++	++	
Brain metastasis	++	- - -	- - -	+	+++	

(continued)

Spatial growth	Choline	Creatine, creatine phosphate	N-acetyl aspartate, N-acetyl aspartyl glutamate	Lactate	Lipids	Amino acids
Brain abscess	-	- -	- - -	+	+	++
Cerebral infarction	-	-	-	+++		

Epilepsy

▶ Aetiology: Chronic disease with repeated spontaneous episodic changes in perception or behaviour due to abnormal synchronisation of cortical neuron assemblies
▶ **MR**
  • Hippocampal sclerosis
    – T1 atrophy of the hippocampus, T2 signal increase in the hippocampus
  • Benign brain tumours
    – 40% gangliogliomas, 30% astrocytomas, 15% oligodendrogliomas; 80% temporal
  • Focal cortical dysplasia
  • Migration and gyration disorders
    – Heterotopias, lissencephaly
    – Polymicrogyria, schizencephaly
  • Vascular lesions and post-traumatic epilepsies
    – Cavernomas
    – Contusions
  • Inflammatory foci
▶ Postictal changes during magnetic resonance imaging follow-up
  • Cortical/subcortical T2/FLAIR hyperintensity
  • Signal alterations of the pulvinar
  • Focal leptomeningeal enhancement
▶ **Nuclear Medicine**
  • 99mTc ethyl cysteinate dimer (ECD)
  • Ictal increased perfusion, interictal reduced perfusion of the epileptogenic focus

▶ **Differential Diagnosis**: Syncope, hyperventilation tetany, drop attack, paroxysmal dyskinesias, psychogenic seizures

Alzheimer's Disease

▶ Aetiology: Synapse dysfunction, amyloid plaques, neurofibrillary degeneration, immunological changes, deposition of beta-amyloid (extracellular) and tau protein (intracellular)
▶ Risk factors: Age, nicotine abuse, physical inactivity, depression, hypertension, diabetes, obesity, lack of mental stimulation
▶ Most common cause of dementia in old age
▶ Memory disorders, orientation disorders, word-finding disorders
▶ Disproportionate short-term memory impairment
▶ Cortical dementia, psychiatric symptoms, progressive deterioration
▶ **MR**
  • Temporal lobe, particularly hippocampal and parahippocampal increased brain atrophy
    – Automated hippocampal volumetry
  • Atrophy of the precuneus with widening of the marginal and parieto-occipital sulci
  • Increased perivascular spaces
  • PWI hypoperfusion of the hippocampus
  • Findings with variants
    – Posterior cortical atrophy: Parieto-occipital atrophy
    – Logopenic variant of primary progressive aphasia: Left temporoparietal atrophy
    – Frontal variant: Frontal atrophy
▶ **Magnetic Resonance Spectroscopy (MRS)**: Decreased N-acetylaspartate, increase myoinositol
▶ **Nuclear Medicine**: 18F-FDG-PET, hypometabolism in temporal and parietal lobes, particularly posterior cingulate cortex and precuneus
▶ **Differential Diagnosis**: Vascular dementia, pseudodementia in depression, Pick's disease

Vascular Dementia

- ▶ Aetiology: Territorial infarcts, embolic infarcts, strategic infarcts, haemodynamic infarcts, cerebral microangiopathy, cerebral haemorrhages, cerebral vasculitis, amyloid angiopathy
- ▶ Neurological deficits due to vascular brain lesions, temporal relationship to cognitive impairment
- ▶ Small infarcts with bilateral localisation can also lead to dementia (e.g. bilateral infarcts in the hippocampus and thalamus)
- ▶ Executive deficits are more in the foreground of the clinical picture than cognitive deficits
- ▶ **MR**
  - Generalised brain atrophic changes
  - Pronounced vascular lesions—territorial and lacunar infarcts, small vessel ischaemic changes
  - Numerous strategic infarcts
    - Internal capsule
    - Thalamus
    - Caudate nucleus
- ▶ **MR spectroscopy (MRS):** First increase in lactate, then strong decrease in lactate and N-acetylaspartate (NAA)

Frontotemporal Lobar Degeneration

- ▶ Aetiology: Presenile degenerative brain disease preferentially affecting the frontal and temporal lobes
- ▶ Variants
  - Behavioural variant
  - Primary progressive aphasia
- ▶ Depending on the variant, frontal brain syndrome with changes in personality, social behaviour, emotionality or aphasia. Progressive dementia
- ▶ **MR:** Atrophy accentuated in the frontal and temporal lobes or atrophy of language-relevant areas

Friedreich Ataxia

▶ Children, young people
▶ Progressive ataxia, absent reflexes, disturbance of dorsal column sensation, development of dysarthria
▶ MR: Cervical spinal cord atrophy

Amyotrophic Lateral Sclerosis

▶ Motor neurone disease
▶ Aetiology: Degeneration of anterior horn cells, motor nerve nuclei and pyramidal tract
▶ Atrophic paresis, muscular atrophy, bulbar symptoms (dysarthria, dysphagia), fasciculations, spasticity
▶ No sensory disturbance
▶ MR
  • T2 Hyperintensities and later volume loss along the pyramidal tracts (especially in the area of the internal capsule and cerebral peduncles)
  • T2*/T2 Hypointensities along the precentral gyrus (iron deposition)
  • Cortex atrophy
▶ Complications: Frontal dementia

Parkinson's Disease

▶ Aetiology: Uncontrolled aggregation of alpha-synuclein in the substantia nigra, pathoanatomical evidence of Lewy bodies in the substantia nigra, deficiency of dopamine in the basal ganglia as a consequence
▶ Akinesia, rigidity, tremor
▶ Accompanying symptoms including anosmia, psychological symptoms
▶ MR
  • T2 Hypo-intensities in the putamen and in the pars compacta of the substantia nigra
  • In chronic cases, generalised brain atrophy

▶ **Nuclear Medicine**
- 123 I-ioflupane SPECT (DaT scan), loss of uptake in the basal ganglia
- 123I-mIBG

▶ **Differential Diagnosis**: Akinetic-rigid syndrome, atypical Parkinson's syndromes

Atypical Parkinson's Syndromes

▶ Multisystem atrophy
- Types
  - Striatonigral degeneration
  - Olivopontocerebellar degeneration
- Autonomic symptoms such as urinary bladder dysfunction and orthostatic hypotension
- Additional symptoms depending on the subtype
- **MR**
  - T2 hypo-intensity in the putamen
  - Atrophy of the putamen
  - T2 hyperintense rim of putamen (lateral margin)
  - T2 hyperintensities in the middle cerebellar peduncle, pons (hot cross bun sign), cerebellum
  - Dilatation of the fourth ventricle (atrophy of surrounding structures)
▶ Progressive supranuclear palsy
- Progressive supranuclear gaze palsy, postural instability, falls backwards (Richardson's syndrome)
- **MR**
  - Midbrain atrophy
  - Hummingbird sign (flat or concave upper border of midbrain—usually convex)
  - T2 periaqueductal midbrain hyperintensities
▶ Corticobasal degeneration
- FTLD-tau with inclusions of tau protein
- Unilateral limb apraxia with myoclonus, dystonia, bradykinesia and rigidity of the affected limb
- **MR**: Asymmetric frontoparietal atrophy (pre- and postcentral gyri, posterior frontal lobe, superior parietal lobule)

Huntington's Disease

▶ Aetiology: Autosomal dominant inheritance
▶ Arrhythmic hyperkinesias, grimacing, phonation disorders, speech disorders, swallowing disorders, rigidity, athetotic hyperkinesias
▶ Hyperhidrosis, hypersalivation
▶ Personality disorders, dementia
▶ MR
  • Atrophy of the caudate heads with widening of the frontal horns of the lateral ventricles
  • T2 Hypo-intensities in the putamen and caudate nucleus

Wilson's Disease

▶ Aetiology: Abnormal copper storage in liver, brain and cornea due to caeruloplasmin deficiency
▶ Tremor, dysarthria, dysphagia, dementia syndrome, jaundice, hepatosplenomegaly, thrombocytopenia
▶ Kayser-Fleischer corneal rings
▶ Decreased serum copper, decreased caeruloplasmin level
▶ MR
  • T2 hyperintensities in basal ganglia (particularly putamen), thalamus, midbrain tegmentum, pons and dentate nuclei
  • T2 hypointensities in the central putamen
  • Brain atrophy

Pantothenate Kinase-Associated Neurodegeneration

▶ Hallervorden-Spatz Disease
▶ Chorea, rigidity, dementia beginning between the ages of 5 and 15
▶ MR: T2 hyperintensities in the inner segments of the globus pallidus, almost complete loss of signal in the outer segments (tiger eye sign)

Hydrocephalus

▶ Disproportion of the width of internal and external CSF spaces
▶ With moderate increase in intracranial pressure: Headache, nausea, vomiting, photophobia, sensitivity to noise
▶ In acute hydrocephalus, progressive reduction in consciousness, Cushing's reflex, disorders of pupillary and bulbar motor function (anisocoria, gaze divergence), brainstem reflex failure
▶ Hydrocephalus ex vacuo
  • Aetiology: Brain atrophy, cerebral infarction
  • CT/MR: generalised or focal dilatation of the ventricles
▶ Obstructive hydrocephalus
  • Aetiology: Malformation e.g. aqueduct stenosis, haemorrhage, infection, tumour
  • Impaired CSF flow
  • CT/MR
    – Dilatation of the ventricles proximal to the site of obstruction
    – Passage of CSF into adjacent white matter- transependymal oedema. Feature of acute hydrocephalus
▶ Non-obstructive hydrocephalus
  • Increased CSF production (Choroid plexus papilloma, carcinoma) or impaired cerebrospinal fluid resorption (Subarachnoid haemorrhage, meningitis, sinus vein thrombosis, trauma)
▶ Normal pressure hydrocephalus
  • Special form of non-obstructive hydrocephalus
  • Aetiology: Idiopathic or consequence of cerebral haemorrhage, craniocerebral trauma, meningitis
  • Hakim triad: Gait disorder, urinary incontinence, dementia
  • Paraspasticity, pyramidal sign
  • Often substantial clinical improvement after multiple CSF puncture
  • Clinical findings, imaging and CSF dynamics contribute to diagnosis
  • CT/MR
    – Plump dilated ventricles
    – Ballooned frontal horns

     – Narrow high frontoparietal sulci, widened sylvian fissures
     – Acute callosal angle
     – Evans index (frontal horn width/maximum diameter cranial interior) >0.3
- **MR CSF flow measurement**: Increase in CSF flow velocity in the aqueduct, volume flow of 24.5 ml/min as threshold value

Raised Intracranial Pressure

▶ Aetiology: Intracranial mass, inflammation, trauma, CSF drainage disturbance, toxins, altitude sickness
▶ Headache, vomiting, apathy
▶ Drowsiness, respiratory disorders, bradycardia, hypertension, pupil dilation
▶ Papilloedema, oculomotor nerve palsy, abducens palsy
▶ **CT/MR**
   • Ventricular narrowing
   • Transependymal oedema
   • Late stage
     – Increased convolutional markings/ copper beaten skull (in children)
     – Empty sella turcica
     – Osteopenic dorsum sellae
▶ Brain swelling
   • Seriously ill patient, life threatening situation
   • Herniation syndromes
     – Subfalcine
     – Uncal
     – Ascending transtentorial
     – Descending transtentorial
     – Tonsillar
     – Extracranial
▶ **Complications**: Ischaemia, cerebrospinal fluid circulation disorders, death

Brain Oedema

Criteria	Vasogenic oedema	Cytotoxic oedema
Aetiology	Tumour, trauma, bleeding, abscess	Ischaemia, infection
Pathophysiology	Disrupted blood-brain barrier	Hydropic cell swelling
Location	Extracellular	Intracellular
Distribution pattern	White matter	Grey and white matter

Idiopathic Intracranial Hypertension

▶ Pseudotumour cerebri
▶ Benign intracranial hypertension, markedly elevated CSF pressure, no focal brain lesion
▶ Young women, increased BMI
▶ Often in pregnancy or in the postpartum period
▶ Headache, vomiting, dizziness, tinnitus, nystagmus, decrease in visual acuity, papilloedema
▶ MR
  • Extension of the suprasellar cistern to sella turcica (empty sella)
  • Flattening of the posterior globe at the entry point of the optic nerve
  • Dilated cerebrospinal fluid space around the optic nerve
  • Normal ventricular size
  • Stenosis of the lateral portions of the transverse sinuses

Osmotic Demyelination Syndrome (Central Pontine Demyelination)

▶ Aetiology: Over-rapid compensation of hypernatriaemia
▶ Limb weakness, dysarthria, dysphagia, gaze paralysis, tetraparesis, decerebration
▶ MR: T2 Hyperintensity of the central sections of the pons without space-occupying component. Restricted diffusion
▶ Differential Diagnosis: Pontine glioma, pontine microangiopathy

Posterior Reversible Encephalopathy Syndrome (Acute Hypertensive Encephalopathy)

▶ Aetiology: Hypertension, kidney disease, pre-eclampsia, eclampsia, malaria
▶ Headache, confusion, visual disturbances, seizures
▶ Prognosis is usually good with rapid treatment
▶ MR
  • T2 cortical and subcortical patchy hyperintensities
  • Symmetrical or asymmetrical, classically parieto-occipital predominance
  • DWI usually normal, sometimes areas of restricted diffusion
  • Patchy enhancement
▶ **Complications**: Haemorrhage, oedema with mass effect, herniation

Toxic Leucoencephalopathy

▶ Aetiology: Radiotherapy, chemotherapy, alcohol
▶ Acute encephalopathy, disorders of oculomotor function, psychoorganic changes
▶ MR: Diffuse white matter damage
▶ **Differential Diagnosis:** Hypertensive encephalopathy (changes reversible)

Wernicke's Encephalopathy

▶ Aetiology: Vitamin B1 deficiency (thiamine deficiency), often in context of alcohol excess
▶ Diplopia, ataxia, cognitive disorders
▶ Korsakoff's psychosis
  • Disorientation
  • Amnestic disorders
  • Confabulations
▶ MR
  • T2 symmetrical hyperintensities around the 3rd ventricle (thalami, hypothalamus), mammillary bodies, periaqueductal grey (periventricular regions). Can have restricted diffusion, contrast enhancement

- Atrophic mammillary bodies
- Infratentorial (vermis) and frontal (cingulate gyrus) brain volume reduction—chronic alcohol use

Subacute Combined Degeneration of the Cord

▶ Aetiology: Vitamin B12 (cobalamin) deficiency
▶ Proprioception and vibration sense loss, fatigue, weakness, tingling paraesthesia, gait instability
▶ Hunter glossitis
▶ Megalocytic anaemia
▶ MR: T2 hyperintensities in the dorsal columns of the cervical and thoracic spinal cord, mild cord enlargement

Schizophrenia

▶ Delusions, delusional perception, hallucinations, ego disorders (thought induction, thought propagation, extraneous influence, depersonalisation, derealisation), formal thought disorders, affective disorders, catatonic symptoms
▶ Radiological diagnostics to exclude organic causes
▶ MR
  - Volume reduction, especially in prefrontal and superior temporal cortex areas
  - Dilatation of the ventricles
  - Numerous fMRI findings regarding e.g. psychomotor function, acoustics, attention, working memory
▶ Nuclear medicine: 18F-FDG-PET (hypometabolism in the frontal lobe)

Generalised Brain Atrophy

▶ Degree of atrophy
  - Mild atrophy: Widening of the sulci, slight dilatation of the ventricles
  - Moderate atrophy: Volume reduction of the gyri, moderate dilatation of the ventricles

- Severe atrophy: Knife-like appearance of the gyri, significant dilatation of the ventricles

▶ **MR**
- T2 periventricular cap-shaped hyperintensities due to disruption of the ependymal cell wall with subependymal gliosis and loss of myelin
- White matter punctate hyperintensities due to perivascular myelin loss
- Large confluent hyperintensities due to ischaemic tissue damage

Focal Brain Atrophy

▶ Trauma
▶ Haemorrhage
▶ Infarct
▶ Inflammation
▶ Radiotherapy

Cerebellar Atrophy

▶ Alcohol abuse
▶ Phenytoin use
▶ Hypothyroidism
▶ Alzheimer's disease (with cerebral atrophy)
▶ Olivopontocerebellar degeneration (variant of multiple system atrophy)

Craniocerebral Trauma

▶ Extradural haematoma
- Aetiology: Trauma
- Between internal table of skull and dura
- Rapid intracranial pressure increase
- Mostly arterial haemorrhage (middle meningeal artery), more rarely venous haemorrhage (diploic veins, dural sinus)
- Mostly temporoparietal

- **CT**
  - Hyperdense semiconvex haemorrhage
  - Does not cross cranial sutures
  - Pronounced mass effect
  - Adjacent focal cerebral oedema
  - Often associated fracture
▶ Subdural haematoma
  - Aetiology: Trauma
  - Between dura and arachnoid
  - Slower intracranial pressure increase
  - Mostly venous bleeding (bridging veins)
  - Mostly frontoparietal, more rarely bilateral
  - **CT**
    - Acute subdural haematoma: Hyperdense concave haemorrhage, crosses cranial sutures, mass effect
    - Chronic subdural haematoma: Iso- to hypodense concave haemorrhage, displacement of the cortical veins away from the skull
    - Bilateral chronic subdural haematoma: Contrast agent application for detection if necessary
  - **MR:** Determination of the haematoma age via the signal intensity of the blood degradation products

Cerebral Contusion

▶ Aetiology: Trauma
▶ Predilection sites
  - Anterior inferior frontal lobe
  - Temporal pole
▶ Stages
  - I: Focal traumatic oedema
  - II: Focal contusion haemorrhage
  - III: Multifocal contusion haemorrhages
  - IV: Diffuse traumatic oedema
▶ Headache, nausea, vomiting, dizziness, reduction in consciousness

▶ **CT**
- First hypodense, then hyperdense with hypodense rim (perifocal oedema)
- A few millimetres to several centimetres
- Coup and contrecoup
- Signs of mass effect
  - Cerebral swelling with effacement of sulci
  - Midline shift
  - Compression of the ventricular system, can lead to hydrocephalus

▶ **MR:** T2* Signal drop-out due to bleeding

Shearing Injuries

▶ Aetiology: Trauma, drug abuse
▶ Diffuse axonal damage with rupture of nerve fibres and death of nerve cells
▶ With involvement of the perineural vessels—can also develop petechial haemorrhages
▶ In the late stage, atrophy due to the loss of neurons
▶ Disturbance of consciousness, seizures
▶ Predilection sites
- Subcortical grey-white matter junction
- Splenium of the corpus callosum
- Upper brainstem

▶ Discrepancy between critical clinical findings and mild radiological findings
▶ **CT:** Often normal, may show small foci of haemorrhage, associated traumatic injury
▶ **MR**
- T2* Signal drop-out to bleeding
- Punctate and linear haemorrhage
- Non-haemorrhagic lesions as hyperintense foci on T2/FLAIR
- Areas of restricted diffusion/ ADC reduction

▶ **Differential Diagnosis:** Contusion haemorrhage, subarachnoid haemorrhage

Trauma Consequences

▶ Vascular injury
▶ Infarct
▶ Pneumocephalus
▶ Hydrocephalus
▶ CSF fistula
▶ Infection
  • Meningitis, encephalitis, abscess, empyema, pyocephalus
▶ Hygroma
▶ Atrophy

Paediatric Radiology: Brain

Brain Malformations

▶ Cephalocele
  • Meningocele
  • Encephalocele
  • Meningoencephalocele
▶ Holoprosencephaly
  • Alobar
  • Semilobar
  • Lobar
  • MR: Missing or incomplete division of the brain into two cerebral hemispheres
▶ Chiari malformation
  • Types
    – I: Herniation of the cerebellar tonsils into the foramen magnum by more than 5 mm
    – II: Herniation of the caudal cerebellum, 4th ventricle and medulla oblongata into the cranial cervical canal, spinal myelomeningoceles, syringohydromyelia, hydrocephalus, osseous malformations
    – III: Type II in combination with an occipital cephalocele

- Associations
  - Hydrocephalus
  - Platybasia
  - Basilar invagination
  - Klippel-Feil syndrome
  - Atlanto-occipital assimilation
  - Myelomeningocele
  - Scoliosis
► Dandy-Walker malformation
  - Hypoplastic cerebellar vermis, ballooned 4th ventricle, upward displacement of the tentorium and torcular hydrocephalus
  - Differential Diagnosis: Arachnoid cyst, mega cisterna magna
► Arachnoid cyst
  - Arachnoid fluid accumulation often in the middle cranial fossa
  - Deformation of the cranial vault, pneumatosinus dilatans, rostral displacement of the sphenoid wings
  - No symptoms or recurrent headaches
  - MR: Matches CSF signal on all sequences, no enhancement, CSF flow measurement to check communication between cyst and subarachnoid space
  - Differential Diagnosis: Epidermoid (signal intense in T2 and in DWI), mega cisterna magna
► Empty sella
  - Herniation of the suprasellar subarachnoid space through the diaphragm sellae into pituitary fossa
  - Visual loss and visual field impairment possible due to displacement of the optic nerve junction
  - Can be seen in idiopathic intracranial hypertension
  - Differential Diagnosis: Suprasellar arachnoid cyst
► Cerebellar malformations
  - Lhermitte-Duclos syndrome
  - Dysplastic cerebellar gangliocytoma
  - Associated with Cowden syndrome

- **MR**: T2 alternating hyper- and isointense areas with striped and zebra-like pattern in cerebellum
▶ Rhombencephalosynapsis
  - **MR**: Absence of the vermis, juxtaposition of the cerebellar hemispheres
▶ Joubert syndrome
  - **MR**: Bat-wing configuration of the caudal portion of the 4th ventricle (agenesis of the vermis). Molar tooth appearance of brainstem and superior cerebellar peduncles

Cortex Malformations

▶ Disorders of neuronal proliferation
  - Hemimegalencephaly
    - **MR**: Enlargement of a hemisphere or a partial hemisphere
  - Microlissencephaly
    - **MR**: Decrease in head circumference, decrease in gyration
  - Transmantle cortical dysplasias
    - **MR**: Dysplasia tract from the ventricular surface to the brain surface
  - Dysembryoplastic neuroepithelial tumours (neoplastic)
    - **MR**: Cortical multicystic space lesion with typically wedge-shaped configuration
  - Ganglioglioma (neoplastic)
    - **MR**: Cortical cystic space with peripheral nodular enhancement, often calcifications
  - Gangliocytoma (neoplastic)
    - **MR**: Cortical cystic space with peripheral nodular enhancement, often calcifications
▶ Disorders of neuronal migration
  - Heterotopia
    - Subependymal heterotopia
    - Focal subcortical heterotopia
    - Band heterotopia
    - **MR**: grey matter at atypical locations

- Lissencephaly
  - Agyria: Absence of gyration
  - Pachygyria: Reduction of gyration
▶ Disorders of cortical organisation
  - Polymicrogyria
    - MR: Too many and too small gyri, wavy transition from grey to white matter
  - Schizencephaly
    - Open lip schizencephaly: Cleft completely filled with fluid
    - Closed lip schizencephaly: Cleft lips directly against each other
    - MR: Cleft formation in the brain from the ventricular surface to the brain surface, lining of the entire length of the cleft with grey matter

Corpus Callosum Malformations

▶ Corpus callosum agenesis
  - Association with cortex malformations, lipomas and cysts
    - MR: Colpocephaly, dilated and elevated 3rd ventricle, bull horn configuration of frontal horns, Probst's bundle
▶ Corpus callosum lipoma
▶ Interhemispheric cyst

Leucodystrophies

▶ Adrenoleukodystrophy
  - Adrenal dysfunction
    - MR: Involvement of the occipital and parietal lobes, marginal enhancement of the involved white matter areas
  - Metachromatic leukodystrophy
    - MR: Tigroid pattern, symmetrical periventricular white matter T2 hyperintensity
▶ Alexander's disease
  - Macrocephaly
    - MR: Involvement of the frontal lobe, occasionally enhancement

▶ Canavan disease
- Macrocephaly
  - MR: Diffuse involvement of the entire white matter, pathognomonic MRS (increased N-acetyl aspartate)
▶ Pelizaeus-Merzbacher disease
- Nystagmus
  - MR: Diffuse involvement of the entire white matter
▶ Phenylketonuria
- Newborn screening
  - MR: Non-specific changes in the white matter

Premature Craniosynostoses

▶ Sagittal suture
- Scaphocephaly (narrow, long, high)
▶ Both coronal sutures
- Brachycephaly (short, wide, high)
▶ One coronal suture
- Plagiocephaly (asymmetric, Harlequin eye deformity)
▶ Metopic suture
- Trigonocephaly (triangular)

Macrocephaly

▶ Hydrocephalus
▶ Megencephaly
▶ Chronic subdural haematoma
▶ Skull thickening
- Haemolytic anaemias
- Healed rickets
▶ Neoplasm
▶ Phakomatoses
- Neurofibromatosis 1
- Tuberous sclerosis
- Leucodystrophies
  - Alexander disease
  - Canavan disease

Microcephaly

▶ Brain malformation
▶ Chromosomal abnormality
▶ Hypoxic-ischaemic encephalopathy
▶ TORCH infections—cytomegalovirus
▶ Foetal alcohol syndrome
▶ Craniosynostosis

Hydrocephalus

▶ Causes: Post-haemorrhagic aqueduct stenosis, idiopathic aqueduct stenosis, post-infectious hydrocephalus, intracranial tumours, Chiari malformation II, Dandy-Walker malformation, arachnoid cyst
▶ Symptoms depending on the aetiology
▶ **Diagnosis**: MR

Spinal Cord

Spinal Malformations

▶ Cleavage malformations
  • Spondylolysis
    – Pars defect
    – Defect in the pars interarticularis of the vertebral arch, between the superior and inferior facets
    – L5 level most common
    – Congenital or acquired
    – Bilateral or unilateral
  • Spondylolisthesis
    – Displacement of one vertebra with respect to an adjacent vertebra. Anterolisthesis—cranial vertebra moves anteriorly, retrolisthesis—cranial vertebra moves posteriorly
    – Often secondary to spondylolysis, degenerative changes
    – Classification according to Meyerding

- Grade I: Offset <25%
- Grade II: Offset 25–50%
- Grade III: Offset 50–75%
- Grade IV: Offset >75%
- Grade V: Spondyloptosis

▶ Assimilation processes
- Lumbarisation
- Sacralisation
- Atlas assimilation
- Block vertebrae

▶ Basilar invagination
- Cranial displacement of the cervical spine so that the tip of the odontoid process is located at the level of the foramen magnum or cranial to it
- Dizziness, neck headache, restricted movement
- **X-ray**
  - On the AP view—dens 10 mm or more above the line from mastoid tip to mastoid tip
  - On the lateral view—dens 5 mm or more above the line from the posterior edge of the hard palate to the lowest point of the occiput, or dens above the line from the basion (middle anterior foramen magnum) to the opisthion (middle posterior foramen magnum)

▶ Os odontoideum
- Isolated ossicle at the tip of the dens
- **Differential Diagnosis:** Dens fracture, dens pseudarthrosis

▶ Klippel-Feil syndrome
- Cervical block vertebrae formation
- Often associated with atlas assimilation, cervical spina bifida, cleft palate, omovertebral bone, Sprengel deformity
- Short neck, low hairline, shoulder upright, torticollis, spasticity

Spondylosis

▶ **X-ray:** Osteophyte formation, disc degeneration
▶ **MR:** Osteophytes may contain bone marrow

Degenerative Endplate Changes

▶ **X-ray**: Osteophyte formation, sclerosis near the intervertebral disc, disc degeneration
▶ **MR**
  • Classification according to Modic
    – Type I (acute, oedema): T1 bone marrow hypointense, T2 hyperintense, enhancement
    – **Differential Diagnosis**: Bone marrow metastasis (follow-up), spondylodiscitis (T1 disc hypointense, T2 hyperintense, strong enhancement)
    – Type II (chronic, adipose tissue): T1 bone marrow hyperintense, T2 hyperintense, no enhancement
    – **Differential Diagnosis**: Haemangioma (entire vertebral body or only vertebral body centre affected)
    – Type III (chronic, sclerosis): T1 bone marrow hypointense, T2 hypointense, no enhancement
    – These findings represent sclerosis adjacent to disc—definite finding

Disc Herniation

▶ Prolapse of the intervertebral disc beyond the disc space.
  • Subligamentous: Herniated disc covered by the posterior longitudinal ligament
  • Extra-ligamentous: Disc herniation perforated through posterior longitudinal ligament
▶ Types
  • Protrusion: Widest point of the herniation is less than the width of the base of the herniation in that plane
  • Extrusion: Widest point of the herniation is larger than the base of the herniation
  • Sequestered: Herniated disc without contact with the disc
▶ Axial location
  • Central
  • Subarticular (involves lateral recess)
  • Foraminal

- Extraforaminal (far lateral)
- Anterior/ventral
▶ Special types
  - Intradural prolapse
  - Discal cyst
▶ Cervical disc prolapse: Lateral—severe neck/arm pain, distal paraesthesia, radicular distribution; lateral—incomplete paraplegia, complete paraplegia, cervical myelopathy
▶ **Differential Diagnosis**: Spinal tumours, spinal lesion of multiple sclerosis, amyotrophic lateral sclerosis
▶ Lumbar disc prolapse: Sciatica, sensory disturbances, paralysis
▶ **Differential Diagnosis**: Extramedullary tumour, synovial cyst at facet joints (L4/5, L5/S1), arachnoid root cyst
▶ Cauda equina syndrome: Loss of bowel and bladder control, saddle anaesthesia, bilateral absence of the Achilles tendon reflex
▶ In the cervical region, the exiting nerve roots are numbered the same as the vertebral body below the intervertebral disc level; in the thoracic and lumbar region, exiting nerve roots are numbered the same as the vertebral body above
  - Examples: Foraminal disc prolapse at the level of C4/5 compresses the C5 root, foraminal disc prolapse at the level of L4/5 compresses the L4 root
  - Exception: C8 root between C7 and T1
▶ Postoperative spine
  - Differentiation of disc tissue (residual, recurrence) and scar tissue
    – Intervertebral disc tissue: Clear contact with the disc, sharp delineation, clear mass effect on thecal sac; mild, slow and peripheral enhancement
    – Scar tissue: Lack of contact with the disc, blurred border, hardly any mass effect on the dural sac; avid, rapid and homogeneous enhancement
  - Evidence of complications
    – Discitis
    – Spondylodiscitis
    – Abscess
    – Empyema

Spinal Canal Stenosis

▶ Aetiology
  • Congenital
    – Idiopathic spinal stenosis
    – Down's syndrome
    – Klippel-Feil syndrome
    – Basilar invagination
    – Achondroplasia
    – Osteopetrosis
  • Degenerative
    – Osteophytes
    – Disc degeneration
    – Synovial cyst
    – Facet joint arthrosis, ligamentum flavum hypertrophy
    – Epidural lipomatosis
    – Spondylolisthesis
    – Vertebral body fractures
    – Calcification of the posterior longitudinal ligament
▶ Low back pain, spinal claudication, paralysis
▶ MR
  • Grade I: Obliteration of the subarachnoid space >50%, no spinal cord compression
  • Grade II: Spinal cord compression without signal change
  • Grade III: Spinal cord compression with signal change
▶ CT/MR
  • Lumbar spinal canal
    – Sagittal diameter: Relative stenosis 10–12 mm, absolute stenosis <10 mm
    – Interpedicular distance: Pathological <15 mm
    – Lateral recess: Probable stenosis 3 mm, definite stenosis ≤2 mm
    – Ligamentum flavum: Pathological ≥5 mm
▶ Diagnosis: MR

Baastrup's Disease

▶ Aetiology: Hyperlordosis, highly developed spinous processes, osteochondrosis
▶ Pain in the area of the lumbar spine due to touching spinous processes (kissing spine)
▶ X-ray: Sclerosis at the points of contact of the spinous processes
▶ MR
  • STIR increased signal between the spinous processes
  • Remodelling of the contact surfaces
  • Significant enhancement of fibrovascular tissue

Myelopathy

▶ Dysfunction of the spinal cord. Wide range of causes
  • Trauma
  • Demyelination
  • Ischaemia
  • Metabolic/ toxic
  • Paraneoplastic
  • Degenerative
  • Radiation-induced
  • Syringomyelia
▶ Paraplegic symptoms, different involvement of sensory and motor pathways, urinary bladder dysfunction
▶ MR
  • Cord distension/ oedema
  • T2 hyperintensity
  • Variable enhancement

Acute Transverse Myelitis

▶ Aetiology: Viral infection, bacterial infection, multiple sclerosis, acute disseminated encephalomyelitis, numerous systemic diseases, paraneoplastic syndrome
▶ Neurological dysfunction of motor, sensory, and autonomic pathways due to focal spinal cord inflammation

▶ Leg weakness, urinary bladder dysfunction, paraesthesia, back pain
▶ Lesion in MR with simultaneous pleocytosis or increased IgG in the CSF
▶ **MR**
  - Distension of the cord
  - Extension of the lesion over more than two thirds of the cross-sectional area of the spinal cord
  - Often extension over several vertebral segments
  - Normal cord between affected segments
  - Frequently delayed, peripheral, irregular, transient enhancement

Radiation Myelitis

▶ Critical dose from about 40 Gy
▶ Types
  - Transient
  - Chronic
▶ Initial irritation symptoms in segmental distribution, later various spinal cord syndromes
▶ **MR**
  - T2 intramedullary hyperintensity and oedema
  - Later circumferential spinal cord atrophy
  - Associated fatty marrow in adjacent vertebral bodies

Acute Spinal Ischaemia

▶ Aetiology: Atherosclerosis, embolism, hypotension, aortic rupture, angiography, vascular interventions, vasculitis, giant cell arteritis
▶ Anterior spinal artery syndrome
  - Anterior 2/3 of the cord, spares dorsal columns
  - Dissociated sensory disturbance caudal to the lesion (pain and temperature sensation lost)
  - Initially flaccid, then spastic paraparesis
  - Sphincter disorders, sexual dysfunction
  - Flaccid paresis and atrophy at the level of the affected segment

▶ Posterior spinal artery syndrome
  • Posterior cord disorder—loss of proprioception and vibration sensation
  • Preserved strength and reflexes
▶ Radicularis magna artery (Artery of Adamkiewicz) syndrome
  • Thoracic paraplegic syndrome
    – Artery of Adamkiewicz from the aorta at the level of T10-L1
▶ **MR**
  • DWI hyperintense signal from an early stage
  • Mostly bilateral paramedian position, T2 hyperintense, only slight enhancement in subacute phase
  • Exclusion of a tumour or an arteriovenous malformation
  • Circumscribed cord atrophy as a permanent residuum
▶ **Differential Diagnosis:** Acute transverse myelitis

Spinal Vascular Malformations

▶ Types
  • Spinal arteriovenous fistula
    – Inflow from radicular arteries, outflow into spinal cord veins, intradural location
    – Risk of bleeding
    – **MR:** Central cord oedema, dilated perimedullary vessels, mild enhancement; in early stages of disease spinal cord swelling, in late stages of disease spinal cord atrophy
  • Spinal arteriovenous malformation
  • Cavernous malformation
    – Inflow from spinal cord arteries, outflow into spinal cord veins, intramedullary position
▶ **IR:** Embolisation

Syringomyelia

▶ Aetiology: Cavity formation in the spinal cord
▶ Types
  • Congenital (Chiari malformation, Dandy-Walker malformation, arachnoid cyst, tethered cord syndrome)

- Acquired (trauma, tumours)
- Idiopathic

▶ Syringobulbia: Dilation in the medulla oblongata
▶ Pain, dissociated sensory disturbance, flaccid paresis of the upper limb, spastic paresis of the lower limb
▶ **Diagnosis**: MR including visualisation of cerebrospinal fluid pulsation

Arachnoiditis

▶ Aetiology: Postoperative, post-traumatic, infectious
▶ Inflammation of the meninges and subarachnoid space
▶ Mostly lumbosacral
▶ Radicular pain
▶ **MR**
- Type I: Nerve root thickening and clumping due to adhesions
- Type II: Image of the "empty" dural sac on axial images due to adhesion of the cauda fibres to the dural sac
- Type III: Soft tissue mass in the dural sac

▶ **Differential Diagnosis**: Leptomeningeal metastasis, neurosarcoidosis, intradural tumour
▶ **Diagnosis**: MR, MR myelography, myelography, CT myelography
▶ **Complications**: Syringomyelia, arachnoiditis ossificans, arachnoid cysts

Spinal Tumours

▶ Types
- Extradural
  - Bone metastasis, bone tumour, plasmacytoma, haemangioma
- Intradural extramedullary
  - Primary: Meningioma, schwannoma, neurofibroma, lipoma
  - Metastatic: Medulloblastoma, glioblastoma, melanoma, breast cancer, lung cancer

- Intradural intramedullary
  - Ependymoma: Adult, often cervical, central location, sharp boundary, very strong enhancement, cap sign (hypointense) on T2 from haemosiderin
  - Astrocytoma: Children, often thoracic, eccentric location, blurred boundary, patchy inhomogeneous enhancement
  - Haemangioblastoma: Flow voids
  - Metastasis: Oncological history
- Pain, paresis, sensory disturbances

Spinal Metastases

▶ Aetiology: Bronchial carcinoma, breast carcinoma, prostate carcinoma, renal cell carcinoma
▶ Pain, paraparesis, paraplegia, urinary bladder disorders

Benign Vertebral Body Tumours

▶ Haemangioma
▶ Bone island
▶ Osteoid osteoma
▶ Osteoblastoma
▶ Aneurysmal bone cyst
▶ Eosinophilic granuloma

Semimalignant and Malignant Vertebral Body Tumours

▶ Giant cell tumour
▶ Chordoma
▶ Plasmacytoma
▶ Osteosarcoma
▶ Chondrosarcoma

Vertebral Body Metastases

▶ Aetiology: Most common, breast carcinoma, bronchial carcinoma, prostate carcinoma, renal cell carcinoma
▶ Affect vertebral bodies and vertebral arches
▶ Osteolytic, osteoplastic, mixed
▶ **MR:** T1 hypointense, STIR hyperintense, enhancement
▶ **Complications**: Pathological vertebral body fracture, spinal cord compression

Phacomatoses

▶ Neurofibromatosis
  • Neurofibromas, optic pathway gliomas, café au lait spots, axillary hyperpigmentation, seizures
  • Progressive radicular or peripheral nerve lesions
  • Cerebellopontine angle tumours, meningiomas
  • **X-ray**
    – Bowing of long bones
    – Pseudoarthrosis of the tibia
    – Tibial dysplasia
    – Scoliosis
    – Scalloping of the vertebrae
    – Rib notching
    – Non-osseous bone fibromas
▶ Tuberous sclerosis
  • Ash leaf spots, adenoma sebaceum, often connective tissue nevi
  • Seizures, reduced intelligence, renal angiomyolipomas
  • **X-ray:** Spotty sclerosis of the skull, lumbar spine and pelvis
    – Scoliosis
▶ Gorlin-Goltz syndrome
  • Basal cell naevus syndrome
  • **X-ray**
    – Large cysts in mandible and long bones
    – Frontoparietal hyperostosis
    – Pronounced falx calcifications

Spinal Trauma

▶ Acute features
  • Cord contusion
  • Cord compression
  • Cord transection
  • Cord haemorrhage
  • Subdural haematoma
  • Epidural haematoma
▶ Late effects
  • Spinal cord atrophy
  • Syringohydromyelia
  • Gliotic changes
  • Cystic degeneration

Spinal Epidural Haemorrhage

▶ Aetiology: Coagulation disorders, anticoagulants, trauma, epidural catheter, lumbar puncture
▶ Bleeding from epidural venous plexus (different from cranial epidural haematoma)
▶ Acute severe, initially local, then radicular pain
▶ Paraplegic syndrome
▶ MR: Detection of bleeding

Spinal Epidural Abscess

▶ Aetiology: Diabetes, alcohol abuse, drug abuse, spondylitis, spondylodiscitis, psoas abscess
▶ Spinal and radicular symptoms
▶ MR: Peripheral enhancement
▶ IR: Puncture and drainage, also for microorganism identification

Paediatric Radiology: Spinal Cord

Spinal Cord Malformations

► Meningocele
  - Often skin covering
  - No neurological deficits
► Meningomyelocele
  - No skin covering
  - Conus syndrome, paraplegia
► Tethered cord
  - Aetiology: Lumbosacral lipoma, lipoma of the filum terminale, lipomyelomeningocele, dermal sinus, intraspinal tumours, adhesions
  - Attachment of the spinal cord to the dura with impairment of the usual ascension of the cord with growth resulting in increasing traction effect
  - Conus depression, conus fixation, conus shape changes
  - Associated changes
    – Segmentation disorders of the vertebral bodies
    – Syringomyelia
    – Scoliosis
    – Rib deformities
    – Diastomatomyelia
  - Pain, sensory disturbances, spastic gait disorder, muscular atrophy, urinary bladder dysfunction
► Dermal sinus
  - Epithelialised duct, which may extend to the intradural compartment, but may also end extradurally
► Diastematomyelia
  - Split cord malformation
  - Division of the spinal canal in sagittal direction by a connective tissue septum or a bony spur
  - Associated changes
    – Vertebral body malformations
    – Syringohydromyelia
    – Lipomas
    – Meningomyelocele

▶ Syringohydromyelia
  • Aetiology: Chiari malformation, Dandy-Walker malformation, arachnoid cyst, tethered cord syndrome

Scheuermann's Disease

▶ Adolescent kyphosis
▶ Hunchback in the case of thoracic manifestation, flat back in the case of lumbar manifestation
▶ X-ray
  • Segmental thoracic vertebral kyphosis
  • At least three contiguous wedge vertebrae
  • Schmorl's nodules
  • Irregular end plates
  • Reduced disc space, particularly anteriorly
▶ MR
  • Reduced-height, dehydrated intervertebral disc
  • Schmorl's nodule as a central intramedullary indentation of the endplate with comparable signal intensity to the surrounding disc tissue even after administration of contrast medium. May be acute with accompanying oedema
  • At least three levels

Eyes, Ears, Nose, Throat

Anatomy

Eye

▶ Parts
- Anterior
  - Sclera, conjunctiva, cornea, iris, ciliary body, lens, anterior chamber, posterior chamber
- Posterior
  - Vitreous chamber, choroid, retina, optic disc
▶ Innervation
- Motor
  - Oculomotor nerve (CN III): Superior rectus muscle, inferior rectus muscle, medial rectus muscle, inferior oblique muscle, levator palpebrae superioris muscle
  - Trochlear nerve (CN IV): Superior oblique muscle
  - Abducens nerve (CN VI): Lateral rectus muscle
  - Facial nerve (CN VII): Orbicularis oculi muscle
- Sensation
  - Trigeminal nerve (CN V)

© The Author(s), under exclusive license to Springer Nature
Switzerland AG 2026
D. Pickuth, J. T. Murchison, *Pocket Guide to Radiology*,
https://doi.org/10.1007/978-3-031-76520-9_11

Orbit

▶ Walls
- Roof
  - Frontal bone (orbital portion)
  - Sphenoid bone
- Medial wall
  - Lacrimal bone
  - Maxilla
  - Ethmoid bone
  - Sphenoid bone
- Floor
  - Maxilla (mainly)
  - Palatine bone
  - Zygomatic bone
- Lateral wall
  - Zygomatic bone—anterior
  - Sphenoid, greater wing—posterior

▶ Pathways
- Optic canal
  - Optic nerve
  - Ophthalmic artery (branch of internal carotid artery)
- Superior orbital fissure
  - Oculomotor, trochlear, trigeminal and abducens nerves
  - Superior ophthalmic vein
- Inferior orbital fissure
  - Trigeminal nerve (CNV)
  - Inferior ophthalmic vein

▶ Bordering structures
- Anterior cranial fossa
- Middle cranial fossa
- Frontal sinus
- Ethmoid sinuses
- Maxillary sinus
- Infratemporal fossa
- Temporalis muscle

Cavernous Sinus

▶ Oculomotor, trochlear, trigeminal and abducens nerves
▶ Internal carotid artery

Visual Pathway

▶ Optic nerve
▶ Optic chiasm
▶ Optic tract
  • Uncrossed fibres of the ipsilateral temporal half of the retina, crossed fibres of the contralateral nasal half of the retina
  • Right optic tract with fibres representing the left half of the visual field of both eyes
  • Left optic tract with fibres representing the right half of the visual field of both eyes
▶ Lateral geniculate body
▶ Optic radiation
▶ Primary visual cortex in the region of the calcarine sulcus

Neck Muscles

▶ Platysma
▶ Sternocleidomastoid muscle
▶ Digastric muscle
▶ Longus colli muscle
▶ Longus capitis muscle
▶ Anterior scalene muscle
▶ Middle scalene muscle
▶ Posterior scalene muscle
  • Scalene triangle
    – Between anterior and middle scalene muscles
    – Brachial plexus, subclavian artery

Cervical Lymph Nodes

▶ Level I: Floor of the mouth
▶ Level II: Upper jugular group, from the base of the skull to the hyoid bone
▶ Level III: Middle jugular group, from the hyoid bone to the cricoid cartilage
▶ Level IV: Lower jugular group, from the cricoid cartilage to the supraclavicular fossa
▶ Level V: Lateral neck triangle (posterior to the sternocleido-mastoid muscle)
▶ Level VI: Trachea, larynx, thyroid gland
▶ Level VII: Trachea, oesophagus, mediastinum

Salivary Glands

▶ Parotid gland
  • Superficial and deep lobes which are divided by the facial nerve
  • Topography
    – Anterior: Ramus of the mandible, masseter muscle, medial pterygoid muscle
    – Posterior: Auricle, mastoid process, sternocleidomastoid muscle, digastric muscle
    – Medial: Styloglossus muscle, internal jugular vein, internal carotid artery
▶ Submandibular gland
▶ Sublingual gland
▶ Minor salivary glands

Pharynx

▶ Nasopharynx
▶ Oropharynx
▶ Hypopharynx. Subsites:
  • Piriform sinus
  • Postcricoid
  • Posterior wall

Waldeyer Tonsillar Ring

▶ Adenoid tonsils (adenoids/pharyngeal tonsils)
▶ Palatine tonsils
▶ Lingual tonsils
▶ Tubal tonsils
▶ Posterior pharyngeal wall

Larynx

▶ Laryngeal framework
  • Epiglottis
  • Thyroid cartilage
  • Cricoid cartilage
  • Arytenoid cartilage
    – Vocal process
    – Muscular process
    – Superior process
▶ Laryngeal interior
  • Supraglottic space: Laryngeal inlet to superior surface of true vocal cords
  • Glottic space: Between the vocal cords
  • Subglottic space: Vocal cords to lower edge of cricoid cartilage
▶ Laryngeal muscles
  • Vocal cord tensors: Cricothyroid muscle, vocalis muscle
  • Vocal cord abduction: Posterior cricoarytenoid muscle
  • Vocal cord adduction: Lateral cricoarytenoid muscle, transverse arytenoid muscle

Nose and Sinuses

▶ Nasal passages
  • Superior nasal meatus: Sphenoid sinus, posterior ethmoid air cells
  • Middle nasal meatus: Frontal sinus, maxillary sinus, anterior ethmoid air cells
  • Inferior nasal meatus: Nasolacrimal duct

▶ Nasal conchae
  • Concha bullosa: Pneumatisation of the middle concha and protrusion into the middle nasal meatus
▶ Sinus pneumatisation
  • Ethmoid air cells: 6th month of life
  • Maxillary sinus: 1st year of life
  • Sphenoid sinus: 4th year of life
  • Frontal sinus: 6th year of life
  • Sinuses fully formed around time of puberty
▶ Topography
  • Orbits
  • Anterior cranial fossa
  • Middle cranial fossa
  • Pharynx
  • Pterygopalatine fossa
  • Teeth

Ear

▶ Parts
  • Outer ear: Pinna, external auditory canal
  • Middle ear: Tympanic membrane, Eustachian tube, tympanic cavity
    – Epitympanum: From tegmen tympani to lower edge of scutum
    – Mesotympanum: From lower edge of scutum to lower edge of bony external ear canal
    – Hypotympanum: From lower edge of bony external auditory canal to floor of middle ear
  • Inner ear: Labyrinth, cochlea, vestibule, semicircular canals, auditory nerve
▶ Topography
  • External auditory canal
    – Anterior: Temporomandibular joint, infratemporal fossa
    – Posterior: Mastoid process
    – Cranial: Middle cranial fossa
    – Caudal: Parotid gland, facial nerve
    – Medial: Tympanic cavity

- Tympanic cavity
  - Anterior: Carotid canal, Eustachian tube
  - Posterior: Mastoid antrum
  - Cranial: Tegmen tympani
  - Caudal: Jugular bulb
  - Medial: Labyrinth
  - Lateral: Tympanic membrane

Hearing Tests

Hearing test	Conductive hearing loss (middle ear deafness)	Sensorineural hearing loss (sensorineural and neural hearing loss)
Speech audiometry	No loss of discrimination	Often loss of discrimination
Rinne	Negative	Positive
Weber	Heard in the affected ear	Heard in the healthy ear
Sound audiogram	Difference between bone conduction and air conduction	Hearing loss often in the high range
Tympanogram	Change in the shape of the curve	Normal curve

Taste Pathway

▶ Afferent sensory signalling
- From the anterior two-thirds of the tongue (fungiform papillae) via lingual nerve, chorda tympani, nervus intermedius to geniculate ganglion of facial nerve
- From the posterior third of the tongue (foliate papillae and circumvallate papillae) via the glossopharyngeal nerve to the caudal glossopharyngeal nerve ganglion
- From the base of the tongue, pharynx and laryngeal inlet via the vagus nerve

▶ Nucleus of tractus solitarius
▶ Contralateral thalamus
▶ Frontal and parietal operculum and limen insulae

Olfactory Pathway

► Olfactory nerve
► Olfactory bulb
► Olfactory tract
► Olfactory trigone
► The medial olfactory stria crosses the paraterminal gyrus, the olfactory trigone and the anterior perforated substance
► The lateral olfactory stria crosses the gyrus semilunaris, the gyrus ambiens and the amygdala
  • The olfactory pathway extends uncrossed to the ipsilateral cortex
  • However, the olfactory centres on both sides are connected via the anterior commissure
  • The secondary cortical fields of the rhinencephalon are closely connected via tertiary cortical fields, especially with the limbic system

Auditory Pathway

► Cochlear ganglion
► Cochlear nerve
► Dorsal and ventral cochlear nucleus
► Lateral lemniscus
► Inferior colliculus
► Medial geniculate body
► Acoustic radiation
► Transverse temporal gyri
  • Most of the central auditory pathway crosses to the contra-lateral side in the secondary neuron
  • However, since part of it also runs ipsilaterally, each organ of Corti is connected to the auditory cortex on both sides
  • The cortical auditory spheres are interconnected via nerve fibres

Vestibular Pathway

▶ Vestibular ganglion
▶ Vestibular nerve
▶ Vestibular nuclei
  • Superior vestibular nucleus (Bechterew)
  • Inferior vestibular nucleus
  • Medial vestibular nucleus (Schwalbe)
  • Lateral vestibular nucleus (Deiters)
▶ Inferior cerebellar peduncle
▶ Cerebellar nuclei and flocculonodular lobe

Thyroid Gland

▶ Sections
  • Right lobe
  • Left lobe
  • Isthmus
    – Pyramidal lobe
▶ Arteries
  • Superior thyroid artery (from external carotid artery)
  • Inferior thyroid artery (from the thyro-cervical trunk of the subclavian artery)
▶ Topography
  • Trachea
  • Oesophagus
  • Recurrent laryngeal nerve

Eyes

Sonography

▶ **US pachymetry**
  • Assessment of the corneal thickness
▶ **US biomicroscopy**
  • Assessment of the anterior chamber angle, iris and ciliary body

▶ **B-scan US**
- Assessment of muscle thickness in endocrine orbitopathy
- Assessment of the retina in case of vitreous haemorrhage or cataract (ophthalmoscopy not possible)
- Assessment of the optic nerve in papilloedema

▶ **Colour duplex US**
- Assessment of central retinal artery, central retinal vein, posterior ciliary artery and ophthalmic artery

Diseases of the Lacrimal Gland

▶ Inflammation
- Dacryoadenitis—inflammation of the lacrimal gland
- Dacryocystitis—inflammation of the lacrimal sac

▶ Lacrimal duct stenosis
- Aetiology: Primary, secondary (infectious, inflammatory, neoplastic, traumatic, mechanical)
- **Dacryocystography**
  - Differentiation of the level of obstruction—canalicular, lacrimal sac, nasolacrimal duct
  - Indications—inflammation, dacryoliths, dacryoceles, fistulas, foreign bodies, tumours

▶ **Diagnosis**: Fluorescein dye test, probing, irrigation, dacryocystography, CT, MR

▶ **IR**: Dacryocystography-guided balloon dilatation, stent implantation

▶ Tumours
- Benign
  - Pleomorphic adenoma
- Malignant
  - Adenoid cystic carcinoma, mucoepidermoid carcinoma, lymphoma

Intraocular Foreign Body

Foreign body material	X-ray	Ultrasound	CT	MR
Metal	Visible	Highly echogenic structure with dorsal acoustic shadow, exclusion of a foreign body not possible, confusion with air bubbles possible	Particularly useful if the foreign body is located close to the orbit wall	Contraindicated, additional injury possible due to migration of the foreign body. Artefacts
Plastic	Mostly invisible	Useful (research context)	Method of choice, different window settings necessary	Alternative to CT
Wood	Invisible	Useful (research context)	Method of choice, different window settings necessary	Alternative to CT
Glass	Can be seen depending on size and lead content	Not useful	Method of choice	Alternative to CT

Retinal Detachment

Cause of detachment	Ultrasound	MR
Rhegmatogenous retinal detachment	Detached retina visible as membrane structure, aftermovements provide information about mobility	Detached retina visible as a membrane structure, at the interface of the vitreous cavity and the subretinal cavity
Traction-related (with retinal fibrosis)	Tensioned membrane structures visible, interaction of fibrous vitreous strands and detached retina visible	Stretched membrane structures can be displayed
Exudative	Detached retina visible as membrane structure, search for cause (e.g. tumour, metastasis, pseudotumour, angioma)	Detached retina can be seen as a membrane structure, the high protein content in the subretinal cavity can mimic a tumour

Benign Intraocular Tumours (Less Common)

▶ Hamartoma
▶ Choroidal naevus
  • Flat, small base diameter, lack of growth
▶ Haemangioma
  • Idiopathic or in Sturge-Weber syndrome or von Hippel-Lindau syndrome
  • MR: Strong enhancement

Malignant Intraocular Tumours (More Common)

▶ Retinoblastoma
  • Most common primary eye tumour in childhood, usual age of onset 1–2 years
  • Both eyes affected in 25%
    – Bilateral occurrence mostly in hereditary form, unilateral occurrence in sporadic form

- Presentation—leucocoria, strabismus, inflammation
- Whitish, bulbous tumour
- Extrabulbar extension, meningeal metastasis
- US: Inhomogeneous internal structure, calcifications
- CT: Density increased due to exudative vitreous fluid, calcifications
- MR: T1 hyperintense, T2 hypointense, marked enhancement, careful assessment of the distal optic nerve to exclude tumour infiltration

▶ Melanoma
- Most common primary eye tumour in adults
- Pigmented protrusion at the back of the eye with irregular surface, orange pigment deposits, serous retinal detachment
- Subretinal haemorrhage, scleral infiltration, extrabulbar extension
- US: Visualisation of the tumour height, and any accompanying retinal detachment located above the tumour and the vessels
- CT: Hyperdense
- MR: T1 hyperintense, variable signal characteristics of any associated haemorrhage, contrast enhancement
    - Metastasis to liver, lung

▶ Metastases to the eye
- Origin: Carcinoma of lung, breast and GI tract
    - Primary intraocular lymphoma
        - Often bilateral, may be accompanied by primary lymphoma of the central nervous system

Causes of Orbital Diseases by Location

▶ Optic nerve/optic sheath
- Optic glioma
- Optic sheath meningioma

▶ Intraconal
- Cavernous haemangioma
- Lymphoma
- Metastasis

- Lymphangioma
- Idiopathic orbital inflammation (orbital pseudotumour)
- Endocrine orbitopathy
- Orbital venous varix
▶ Extraconal
  - Capillary haemangioma
  - Lymphoma
  - Metastasis
  - Lymphangioma
  - Idiopathic orbital inflammation (orbital pseudotumour)
  - Meningioma
  - Phlegmon
▶ Subperiosteal
  - Dermoid
  - Epidermoid
  - Metastasis
▶ Lacrimal gland
  - Inflammation
  - Adenoma
  - Carcinoma
  - Lymphoma
  - Idiopathic orbital inflammation (orbital pseudotumour)

Optic Nerve Enlargement

▶ More common causes
  - Optic nerve glioma
  - Optic sheath meningioma
  - Idiopathic orbital inflammation (orbital pseudotumour)
  - Papilloedema
▶ Rarer causes
  - Sarcoidosis
  - Erdheim-Chester disease
  - Metastases
  - Haemangioblastoma

Orbital Calcifications

▶ Neoplastic
  • Retinoblastoma
  • Hamartoma
  • Haemangioma
  • Osteoma
▶ Non-neoplastic
  • Foreign body
  • Hypercalcaemia
  • Post-traumatic
  • Orbital venous varix

Endocrine Exophthalmos

▶ Aetiology: Autoimmune
▶ Bilateral in 90% of those affected
▶ Most frequent extrathyroidal manifestation of Graves' disease
▶ In rare cases it is also seen in autoimmune thyroiditis
▶ Women affected 6 times more often than men
▶ Eyelid retraction, exophthalmos, motility disorder, chemosis, eyelid oedema
▶ Dry eye symptoms (burning of the eye, redness of the eye surface, sensitivity to light)
▶ MR
  • Thickening of the eye muscles, eyelids and lacrimal glands
    – Muscle width on coronal sequences >4 mm
  • Infiltration of the retrobulbar space
  • Proliferation of fatty tissue
  • Medial and inferior rectus muscles initially affected
  • In contrast to idiopathic orbital inflammation (orbital pseudotumour), the tendinous attachment is not affected
▶ Complication: Optic nerve damage with visual loss

Idiopathic Orbital Inflammation

▶ Orbital pseudotumour
▶ Aetiology: Diffuse or focal, idiopathic, lymphocytic inflammation of the orbit
▶ Types
  • Anterior (retrobulbar fat)
  • Diffuse
  • Orbital apex
  • Myositic
  • Dacryoadenitic—lacrimal glands
▶ Pain, proptosis, ocular motility disorder, chemosis, eyelid swelling
▶ MR
  • Diffuse or patchy infiltrates in the retrobulbar space
  • Thickening of the sclera and optic sheath
  • Medial and superior rectus and superior oblique muscles initially affected
  • In contrast to endocrine orbitopathy, the tendinous insertion is also affected
▶ Differential Diagnosis: Endocrine orbitopathy, orbital phlegmon
▶ Complications: Venous sinus thrombosis, meningoencephalitis, brain abscesses

Tolosa Hunt Syndrome

▶ Idiopathic inflammation of the superior orbital fissure, the orbital apex and the cavernous sinus
▶ Visual loss, pain, ophthalmoplegia, cranial nerve palsies
▶ MR
  • Unilateral soft tissue proliferation around the cavernous sinus
  • Increasing narrowing of the adjacent carotid artery
  • Involvement of the orbital apex
  • Involvement of the optic nerve
  • Focal dural thickening
  • Strongly enhancing

Benign Orbital Tumours

▶ Dermoid
   • MR: T1 hyperintense due to fat content, fat-fluid level
▶ Epidermoid
   • MR: T1 slightly hyperintense due to protein content
▶ Orbital Varix
   • Intermittent exophthalmos, increased under Valsalva manoeuvre and in head-down position
   • US: Venous channels dilate along with increased blood flow with the Valsalva manoeuvre
   • CT: Isoattenuating to blood, polycyclic structure, phlebo-liths
▶ Lymphangioma
   • Tendency to haemorrhage
   • US: Cystic cavities
   • MR
     – Signal dependent on past episodes of haemorrhage
     – Typically T1 hyperintense, T2 hyperintense
     – No flow, no enhancement
▶ Cavernous haemangioma
   • Women, middle age
   • Orbital symptoms, pulsatile exophthalmos
   • CT: Sharply demarcated, intraconal, homogeneously hyperdense, phleboliths (uncommon)
   • MR: T1 hypointense, T2 hyperintense, reduced flow, late enhancement
▶ Neurofibroma
   • Associated with neurofibromatosis
▶ Optic glioma
   • Common
   • Children, mean age 5 years
   • More common in females
   • Higher incidence in neurofibromatosis
   • Visual loss, visual field defects, exophthalmos, optic atrophy
   • Later diencephalic symptoms such as polyuria, obesity

- **US:** Spindle-shaped distension of the distal optic nerve
- **CT/MR**
  - Variably enhancing, rarely contains calcifications
  - Dilatation of the optic canal
  - Intracranial extension to the optic chiasm
- ▶ Optic sheath meningioma
  - Rare
  - Mean age 40 years
  - More common in females
  - Visual loss, exophthalmos
  - Obstruction of the central vein with papilloedema
  - **US:** Concentric widening of the distal optic nerve
  - **CT/MR**
    - Linear or punctate calcifications
    - Marked enhancement around the nerve, but not of the nerve itself (tram-track sign)
    - Hyperostosis of the adjacent bones
    - Intracranial expansion at the meninges
  - **Differential Diagnosis:** The optic nerve can still be identified within the tumour in optic meningioma which is not the case with optic glioma

Malignant Orbital Tumours

- ▶ Rhabdomyosarcoma
  - Children
  - Exophthalmos, globe displacement from the sagittal axis, ocular motility disorder
- ▶ Neuroblastoma
  - Children
  - Proptosis, periorbital or eyelid ecchymosis (raccoon eyes)
  - **CT:** Characteristically spreads along the periosteum of the orbit
- ▶ Metastases
  - Origin: Carcinoma of breast, lung and gastrointestinal tract, melanoma, neuroblastoma

▶ Lymphoma
  • Can be isolated or part of more systemic lymphoma
  • Usually low grade malignancy

Other Tumours/Lesions with Possible Orbital Involvement

▶ Paranasal sinus carcinoma
▶ Mucocele
▶ Osteoma
▶ Sphenoid wing meningioma
▶ Basal cell carcinoma

Optic Neuritis

▶ Aetiology: Idiopathic, children with infection, adults with multiple sclerosis
▶ Types
  • Papillitis: Anterior part of the optic nerve affected (ophthalmoscopically positive)
  • Retrobulbar neuritis: Posterior part of the optic nerve affected (ophthalmoscopically negative). Acute retrobulbar neuritis: "the patient sees nothing, and the doctor sees nothing"
▶ Mostly unilateral
▶ Central visual disturbances, rarely visual field disturbances, feeling of pressure, pain on movement
▶ Progressive visual acuity loss, afferent pupil dysfunction, central scotoma, impulse conduction delay
▶ MR
  • Thickened optic nerve
  • Oedematous changes
  • Significant enhancement
▶ Differential Diagnosis: Chiasmatic tumours, diabetes mellitus with retrobulbar circulatory disturbance (posterior ischaemic optic neuropathy)

Diseases of the Visual Pathway

▶ Lesions of the optic nerve
- Blindness
- Abnormal pupillary light reflex
- Optic atrophy

▶ Lesions of the optic chiasm
- Aetiology: Optic glioma, pituitary adenoma, craniopharyngioma, meningioma, aneurysm
- Chiasmal syndrome
  - Bitemporal visual field defects
  - Decrease in visual acuity
  - Desaturation of colour perception
  - Moderate optic atrophy

▶ Lesions above the optic chiasm
- Homonymous visual field defect
- Optic atrophy

▶ Lesions above the lateral geniculate nucleus
- Aetiology: Infarction of the visual cortex
- Homonymous visual field defect
- No optic atrophy

Ears

Ear Malformations

▶ Congenital malformations of the external, middle or inner ear
▶ Types
- Auditory canal atresia: Soft tissue or bony obstruction of the external auditory canal in the presence of a normal inner ear.
- Goldenhar syndrome: Range of abnormalities including hemifacial microsomia often affecting the ear
- Inner ear malformations
  - Cochlear aplasia
  - Mondini malformation: Abnormal cochlea missing turns, enlarged vestibule, enlarged vestibular aqueduct

– Michel aplasia: Complete lack of development of the inner ear-labyrinthine aplasia

Necrotising Otitis Externa

▶ Cause: Infection with Pseudomonas aeruginosa
▶ Necrotising auditory canal inflammation with spread to the bone, spread along the skull base and involvement of cranial nerves
▶ Especially in diabetes, old age and after radiotherapy
▶ Pain, purulent otorrhoea, granulation tissue in external auditory canal, often facial paresis
▶ CT: Bony erosion of the external auditory canal
▶ **Complications**: Meningitis, venous sinus thrombosis, vein thrombosis, intracranial abscess

Otitis Media

▶ Types
  • Acute—with good Eustachian tube function (childhood), good mastoid pneumatisation (later in life). Middle ear effusion, mastoiditis
  • Chronic—with poor Eustachian tube function or poor mastoid pneumatisation. CT can show air-fluid level, bony erosion, mastoid air cell sclerosis. Can lead to acquired cholesteatoma
▶ Acute otitis media does not turn into chronic otitis media with good Eustachian tube function and pneumatised mastoid

Mastoiditis

▶ Cause: Often as a complication of acute otitis media
▶ Purulent erosion of the bony cells of the mastoid process
▶ Pain, tinnitus, conductive hearing loss, ringing in the ears, mastoid pressure pain
▶ Lowering of the posterior superior auditory canal wall

▶ **CT**
- Mastoid effusion (non-specific)
- Eroded bony septa
- Erosion of the mastoid bone cortex

▶ **Differential Diagnosis**: Ear canal furuncle (boil), lymphadenitis, parotitis

▶ **Complications**: Subperiosteal abscess with pus perforation through the lateral cortex of the mastoid, Bezold's abscess with pus perforation at the tip of the mastoid process into and around the sternocleidomastoid muscle, petrous apicitis, labyrinthitis, dural venous sinus thrombosis, meningitis, brain abscess, facial nerve palsy

Cholesteatoma

▶ Types
- Acquired. Pars flaccida of the tympanic membrane is the most common location
- Congenital

▶ Non-neoplastic mass consisting of multi-layered squamous epithelium, keratin-containing cellular detritus and inflammatory cells

▶ Course (pars flaccida cholesteatoma)
- Erosion of the scutum
- Erosion of long process of incus, then head of malleus and body of incus

▶ Tympanic membrane findings alone, insufficient to determine cholesteatoma extension

▶ **CT**
- Well-defined soft tissue hyperdensity
- Opacification of Prussak's space
- Erosion of scutum, ossicles
- Often very extensive bone destruction

▶ **MR**
- Primary diagnosis: Diffusion restriction
- Diagnosis of recurrence: Diffusion restriction. No central contrast enhancement (in contrast to granulation tissue)

▶ **Differential Diagnosis**: Chronic otitis media with ossicular destruction, cholesterol granuloma
▶ Complications due to cholesteatoma pressure and inflammation
▶ **Complications**:
- Preoperative
  - Erosion of the scutum: HR-CT
  - Erosion of the ossicles: HR-CT
  - Erosion of the facial nerve canal: HR-CT
  - Facial nerve neuritis: MR
  - Tegmen tympani defect: HR-CT
  - Cerebral complications: MR
  - Venous sinus thrombosis: MR
  - Cochlear erosion: HR-CT
  - Bony labyrinth erosion: HR-CT
  - Membranous rupture of the labyrinth: MR
  - Acute labyrinthitis: MR
  - Chronic fibrosing labyrinthitis: MR
  - Chronic ossifying labyrinthitis: HR-CT/MR
- Postoperative
  - Recurrent cholesteatoma: HR-CT/MR
  - Erosion of the facial nerve canal: HR-CT
  - Facial nerve neuritis: MR
  - Bony labyrinth fistula: HR-CT
  - Membranous labyrinth fistula: MR
  - Acute labyrinthitis: MR
  - Chronic fibrosing labyrinthitis: MR
  - Chronic ossifying labyrinthitis: HR-CT/MR
  - Meningoencephalocele: MR

Benign Middle Ear Tumours

▶ Glomus tumours
- Cause: Paragangliomas of the parasympathetic nervous system
- Highly vascular, locally destructive tumours

- Glomus jugulare tumour
  - Arise from the glossopharyngeal and vagus nerves in the jugular foramen
  - Jugular foramen, carotid canal, hypotympanum, middle ear
- Glomus tympanicum tumour
  - Arise from Jacobson's nerve in the tympanic cavity
  - Tympanic cavity, cochlear promontory, can cause encasement or destruction of the ossicles
- Pulsatile tinnitus, conductive hearing loss, cranial nerve palsies, reddish eardrum
- Bleeding from the tumour
- **CT**: Soft tissue mass, bone destruction
- **MR**
  - Soft tissue intensity mass, avid enhancement
  - T2 salt and pepper pattern due to flow voids of numerous tumour vessels
- **Angio**: Hypervascularisation
- **IR**: Embolisation

▶ Facial nerve schwannoma
▶ Haemangioma
▶ Dehiscent jugular bulb (tumour mimic)
- Elevation of the jugular bulb with absence of the sigmoid plate
- Bluish tympanic membrane

Malignant Middle Ear Tumours

▶ Types
- Squamous cell carcinoma
- Adenocarcinoma
- Metastases
- Sarcomas
▶ Conductive hearing loss, bleeding granulations, bloody secretions, bone sequestrum, facial nerve palsy
▶ Pain due to dural infiltration

- ▶ Spread to the parotid gland
- ▶ **Diagnosis**: CT (bone erosion), MR (soft tissue infiltration, dural infiltration)

Otosclerosis

- ▶ Cause: Disease of the bony labyrinth capsule of unknown cause due to bone remodelling
- ▶ Types
  - • Fenestral otosclerosis
  - • Retro-fenestral (cochlear) otosclerosis. This occurs both with and as progression of the fenestral form
- ▶ Particularly affects women
- ▶ Mostly bilateral
- ▶ Increasing conductive hearing loss in the fenestral type or sensorineural hearing loss in the cochlear type, often ringing in the ears, no ear pain
- ▶ Carhart notch in the sound audiogram
- ▶ CT
  - • Focus of radiolucency at the oval window, in the fissula ante fenestram
  - • Radiolucency around the cochlea
  - • Later progressive ossification of the oval window
- ▶ Differential Diagnosis
  - • Middle ear malformations, tympanosclerosis
  - • Fibrous dysplasia, Paget's disease

Menière's Disease

- ▶ Cause: Hydrops (fluid accumulation) of the membranous labyrinth
- ▶ Vertigo, tinnitus, hearing loss, fullness in the ears
- ▶ Initially nystagmus, positive Romberg's test
- ▶ MR
  - • Visualisation of the endolymph hydrops with high-resolution examination protocols
  - • Exclusion of a retrocochlear cause (e.g. cerebellopontine angle tumour)

Hearing Loss

▶ Sudden hearing loss, pressure in the ear, often ringing in the ears
▶ MR: Exclusion of a retrocochlear cause (e.g. cerebellopontine angle tumour)

Vestibular Neuritis

▶ Cause: Acute dysfunction of the peripheral vestibular apparatus
▶ Significant vertigo, violent spontaneous nystagmus, no hearing impairment
▶ MR: Exclusion of a retrocochlear cause (e.g. cerebellopontine angle tumour)

Tumours of the Internal Auditory Canal

▶ Vestibular schwannoma
  • Acoustic neuroma
  • Cause: Mostly originating from the inferior vestibular nerve, rarely from the superior vestibular nerve
  • Bilateral vestibular schwannomas typical of neurofibromatosis II
  • Classification according to Koos
    – Grade I: Intracanalicular
    – Grade II: Protrusion into cerebellopontine angle, with a maximum longitudinal diameter of 20 mm. No brainstem contact
    – Grade III: Occupying cerebellopontine cistern with a maximum longitudinal diameter of 30 mm, reaches the brainstem which is not displaced
    – Grade IV: More than 30 mm longitudinal diameter, displaces the brainstem and cranial nerves
  • Many vestibular schwannomas demonstrate slow or static growth (watch and wait)
  • High-frequency hearing loss, tinnitus, dizziness

- **MR**
  - Pencil-shaped configuration (when confined to IAM) or ice cream cone-like morphology (with cerebellopontine angle component)
  - Very avid enhancement
  - Larger tumours may be inhomogeneous
  - Expanded internal auditory canal
- **Differential Diagnosis:** Neurovascular compression syndrome (vascular-nerve contact between mostly AICA or more rarely PICA and the vestibulocochlear nerve at the root entry zone)

▶ Facial schwannoma
▶ Meningioma
▶ Epidermoid
▶ Paraganglioma
▶ Arachnoid cyst
▶ Metastasis

Nose

Epistaxis

▶ Causes: Fracture, foreign bodies, nasal manipulation, septal polyp, nasopharyngeal fibroma, tumours, hypertension, infections
▶ **CT** or **MR** in case of suspected tumour
▶ **IR:** Embolisation

Septum Deviation

▶ Deviation of the septum from the midline position
▶ Impaired nasal breathing, impaired ability to smell, snoring, headaches
▶ Vasomotor conchal swelling, thickening of the posterior ends of the inferior conchae, pathological rhinomanometry
▶ Frequent concomitant finding in CT or MR

Choanal Atresia

- ▶ Cause: Congenital occlusion of the posterior nasal passage (membranous, bony or mixed)
- ▶ Mostly unilateral, rarely bilateral
- ▶ Secretions, rhinitis, feeding problems
- ▶ **Diagnosis**: Endoscopic, CT
- ▶ Associations: CHARGE syndrome, DiGeorge syndrome, Treacher-Collins syndrome, Crouzon syndrome, foetal alcohol syndrome
- ▶ **Complication**: Respiratory distress

Paranasal Sinus Variants

- ▶ Aplasia
  - • Sphenoid sinus or frontal sinus aplasia in about 5%
  - • Maxillary sinus or ethmoidal cell aplasia very rare
- ▶ Nasal septum
  - • Pneumatisation: Narrowing of the nasal cavity, the hiatus semilunaris or the infundibulum of the osteomeatal complex
  - • Deviation: Narrowing of the hiatus semilunaris or the infundibulum
- ▶ Middle turbinate
  - • Paradoxical lateral convexity: Narrowing of the hiatus semilunaris or the infundibulum
  - • Concha bullosa (pneumatisation): Narrowing of the hiatus semilunaris or the infundibulum
- ▶ Uncinate process
  - • Pneumatisation: Constriction of the infundibulum
- ▶ Ethmoid cells
  - • Onodi cells: Anatomical variant with extension of the posterior ethmoidal cells superolateral to the sphenoid sinus; close proximity to the optic nerve and internal carotid artery has relevance for sphenoid surgery
  - • Haller cells: Ethmoidal cell under the orbital floor, can cause constriction of the infundibulum

- Agger nasi cells: Anterolateral and inferior to the frontal recess, can cause constriction of the frontal sinus excretory duct
- Variation in depth of the olfactory fossa/cribriform plate
  - Keros grade I: 1–3 mm
  - Keros Grade II: 4–7 mm
  - Keros grade III: >7 mm (increased risk of damage with sinus surgery)

▶ Sphenoid sinus
- Highly varying degree of pneumatisation

Sinusitis

▶ Acute sinusitis
- Causes: Rhinogenic (rhinitis), odontogenic (dental infection)
- Unilateral maxillary sinusitis typical of odontogenic sinusitis
- Pain, headache, pressure pain, hyposmia, anosmia
- Swelling of the mucous membrane and mucus and pus in the middle nasal passage
- **CT**
  - Mucosal thickening
  - Gas-fluid level
  - Bubbly secretions
  - CT- low dose technique
- **Complications**: Bone erosion with subperiosteal abscess formation, osteomyelitis, orbital involvement (stage I: Orbital oedema, stage II: Orbital periostitis, stage III: Subperiosteal abscess, stage IV: Intraorbital abscess, stage V: Orbital phlegmon), dural venous sinus thrombosis, meningoencephalitis, brain abscess

▶ Chronic sinusitis
- Causes: Multifactorial
- Inflammation of the nose and sinuses lasting more than 12 weeks

- Obstruction of the osteomeatal unit due to polypoidal mucosal swelling
- Predisposing factors include deviated septum, septal spur, concha bullosa, Haller's cells, conchal hyperplasia, and antrochoanal polyps
- Mostly maxillary sinus and ethmoidal cells
- Often nasal polyposis
- Dull headache, blocked nose, rhinophonia (nasal speech), hyposmia, pharyngitis
- **CT**
  - Mucosal thickening
  - Thickened secretions
  - Polyps
  - Sclerosed sinus walls
- **Differential Diagnosis:** In the case of a polyp on the nasal roof, meningoencephalocele; in the case of a antrochoanal polyp, juvenile nasopharyngeal fibroma
▶ Kartagener syndrome
- Chronic sinusitis or polyposis
  - Underdevelopment or non-formation of the paranasal sinuses and mastoid cells
- Bronchiectasis
- Situs inversus

Paranasal Sinus Surgery

▶ Bony variants as a potential hazard in endoscopic sinus surgery
- Paranasal sinus variants
▶ Expected postoperative findings
- Extended osteomeatal unit
- Loss of the individual bony lamellae of the ethmoidal cell system
- Shortened rounded turbinates
▶ Important postoperative complications
- Bleeding
- Infection
- CSF leak

Antrochoanal Polyp

▶ Mucosal polyp of the maxillary sinus with growth towards the nasal cavity and choanae
▶ Extension into the nasopharynx possible
▶ Adolescent patients, unilateral nasal airway obstruction, rarely pain
▶ CT: Soft tissue mass, arising from maxillary sinus and widening ostium
▶ MR: T2 hyperintense mass, no enhancement
▶ Differential Diagnosis: Inverted papilloma, juvenile nasopharyngeal fibroma, encephalocele, nasopharyngeal carcinoma

Mucocele and Pyocele

▶ Causes: Obstruction of the ostium of a paranasal sinus
▶ Sinus cavity filled with mucus (mucocele) or pus (pyocele) and dilated by secretion
▶ CT: Expansile, thinned bone, bony remodelling
▶ MR: T1 initially hypointense, then hyperintense; T2 initially hyperintense, then hypointense (signal reversal due to secretion thickening); no enhancement
▶ Differential Diagnosis: Paranasal sinus papilloma, odontogenic cyst, antrochoanal polyp

Fungal Sinusitis

▶ Types
  • Type I: Acute invasive
  • Type II: Chronic invasive
  • Type III: Fungus mycetoma
  • Type IV: Allergic fungal sinusitis
▶ Invasive forms of progression in immunocompromised, non-invasive forms of progression in immunocompetent patients
▶ Invasive forms often clinically severe
▶ CT
  • Complete obstruction of the paranasal sinuses without fluid level

- Increased density due to metabolic products, mycetoma and calcifications
- Osteodestructive changes in invasive forms
- In allergic fungal sinusitis appearances as in chronic sinusitis

▶ **Differential Diagnosis:** Sinus carcinoma, chronic sinusitis
▶ **Complication:** Fungal sepsis

Granulomatosis with Polyangiitis

▶ Formerly Wegener's disease
▶ Cause: Vasculitis with ulcerating granulomas in the respiratory tract (nose, sinuses, middle ear, oropharynx, lungs) and renal involvement (glomerulonephritis, microaneurysms)
▶ Rhinitis, sinusitis, otitis, oropharyngeal ulcerations, pulmonary nodules
▶ Initially bloody rhinitis, mucosal thickening, septal perforation, septal necrosis, saddle nose, pulmonary infiltrates
▶ May be kidney, liver and joint involvement
▶ Detection of cANCA
▶ **CT**
  - Destruction of the nasal septum, turbinates, medial maxillary sinus wall
  - Sclerosis of the remaining maxillary sinus walls
▶ **MR**
  - Nodular soft tissue proliferation
  - T2 pronounced signal reduction
▶ Avid enhancement
▶ **Differential Diagnosis:** Chronic or fungal sinusitis, sarcoid, lymphoma, tuberculosis, syphilis, actinomycosis
▶ **Diagnosis:** Biopsy

Benign Tumours of the Paranasal Sinuses and the Nasal Cavity

▶ Polyps
▶ Papilloma

- Inverted papillomas
  - Starting from the lateral wall of the nose, extending into the maxillary sinus and ethmoid bone
  - Can cause obstruction of the osteomeatal complex with sinusitis
  - CT/MR: Soft tissue density mass, lobulated surface— cerebriform pattern, serpiginous enhancement
- Exophytic papillomas
  - Starting from the nasal septum
- Oncocytic papillomas
- Differential Diagnosis: Retention cyst, antrochoanal polyp, nasopharyngeal fibroma, carcinoma
- Complications: Malignant transformation, bone destruction, orbital collapse, intracranial involvement, recurrence

▶ Osteoma
- Frontal sinus

Malignant Tumours of the Paranasal Sinuses and Nasal Cavity

▶ Types
- Squamous cell carcinoma
- Adenocarcinoma
  - Squamous cell carcinomas and adenocarcinomas preferentially involve the maxillary sinus antrum, the anterior ethmoid cells and the nasal cavity
- Esthesioneuroblastoma
- Sarcoma
- Lymphoma
- Plasmacytoma

▶ Unilateral nasal obstruction, bloody secretions, double vision, lockjaw
▶ US: Detection of lymph node metastases
▶ CT/MR: Soft tissue dense mass, infiltrative growth, inhomogeneous enhancement
▶ Differential Diagnosis: Fungal sinusitis, granulomatosis with polyangiitis, chronic sinusitis

Salivary Glands

Acute Sialadenitis

▶ Often bacterial infection. Causes: Salivary stones, dehydration, malnourished patients, immunosuppression
▶ Swelling, pain, pus discharge from the papilla when pressure is applied to the gland, erythema of the skin, fever
▶ US
  • Enlarged gland
  • Hypoechoic internal structure
  • Intraglandular lymph nodes
▶ Colour Doppler US: Increased perfusion

Chronic Sialadenitis

▶ Reduction in saliva formation, damage to the glandular parenchyma
▶ Sjögren's syndrome
  • Lymphoepithelial sialadenitis
  • Arthritis, xerostomia, keratoconjunctivitis sicca, parotid enlargement
  • Calcifications on CT
  • US
    – Diffuse small anechoic cysts which increase in size over time
    – Hypoechoic solid masses (aggregates of lymphocytes)
    – Gland enlargement followed by atrophy
  • MRI
    – Salt and pepper micronodular appearance in chronic disease
  • MR sialography
    – Initially punctate, later globular, finally cavitary fluid accumulation
    – Destruction of the glandular parenchyma as the final stage
  • Nuclear Medicine: Salivary gland scintigraphy with 99mTc pertechnetate

- **Complication**: Lymphoma of the parotid gland
▶ Heerfordt syndrome (Heerfordt-Walderström)—rare
  - Form of sarcoidosis
  - Anterior uveitis, parotid gland swelling, fever, facial palsy
▶ Mikulicz syndrome—rare, IgG4 disease associated
  - Painless swelling of the lacrimal glands and salivary glands
  - **US**
    - Multiple hypoechoic areas, high vascularity
    - Dendritically distended vessels
  - **MR sialography:** Diffuse enlargement of lacrimal and parotid glands with reduced apparent diffusion coefficients.

Sialolithiasis

▶ Causes: Stone formation in the excretory duct exacerbated by reduced salivary flow and increased viscosity
▶ Calcium phosphate or carbonate stones
▶ Particularly submandibular glands
▶ Swelling of the gland when eating
▶ **US**
  - Echogenic complexes with dorsal acoustic shadow
  - Obstruction of the excretory duct
▶ **MR sialography:** Low signal stone, pre-stenotic duct dilatation

Sialadenosis

▶ Causes: Endocrine, metabolic, neurogenic, medicinal
▶ Recurrent, non-inflammatory, painless swellings of the salivary glands
▶ Particularly the parotid gland
▶ Hamster-like appearance
▶ **US:** Homogeneous, hypoechoic, diffuse enlargement of the gland
▶ **Differential Diagnosis:** Salivary gland lipomatosis

Ranula

▶ Causes: Mostly acquired, rarely congenital retention cyst of the sublingual gland or the minor salivary glands
▶ Bluish translucent, painless swelling in the floor of the mouth
▶ US: Thin-walled cyst
▶ MR
  • Simple ranula: Sublingual thin-walled cyst, wall may enhance
  • Diving ranula: Into submandibular space, often through a mylohyoid muscle defect. Comet-shaped with a head in the submandibular space and a tail in the collapsed sublingual space
▶ Differential Diagnosis: Retention cyst of the submandibular gland, epidermoid cyst

Benign Tumours of the Salivary Glands

▶ Pleomorphic adenoma
  • Most common benign tumour of the salivary glands
  • Solitary, well demarcated, roundish, rarely bilateral
  • Rough consistency, bumpy surface
  • High tendency to recur, possible malignant degeneration
  • US
    – Well-circumscribed mass
    – Hypoechoic, homogeneous internal structure
    – Dorsal acoustic enhancement
    – Poor vascularity
  • MR
    – T1 iso- to hypointense, T2 hyperintense, low enhancement
    – Possible inhomogeneities due to necrosis, haemorrhages, calcifications in larger tumours
▶ Warthin's tumour
  • Cystadenolymphoma
  • Second most common benign tumour of the salivary glands
  • Epithelial tumour accompanied by lymphoid tissue

- Painless swelling
- Low tendency to recurrence, no malignant degeneration
- **US:** Smooth and sharply circumscribed tumour with solid and cystic components
- **MR:** Like pleomorphic adenoma, but cystic components

▶ Venous malformation (non-neoplastic)
- Children, young people
- Heterogeneous, cystic structure that can be compressed by finger pressure and then fills up again. Flow may not be detectable on Doppler ultrasound. Phleboliths

▶ Lymphatic malformation (non-neoplastic)
- Soft cystic swelling that fills or deflates depending on the inclination of the head
- Growth not only in the gland but also in the surrounding tissues

Malignant Tumours of the Salivary Glands

▶ Mucoepidermoid carcinoma
- Mostly parotid gland

▶ Adenoid cystic carcinoma
- Mostly minor salivary glands
- Perivascular and perineural infiltration
- Facial paresis as an important clinical indication of malignancy
- Lymphogenic and haematogenic metastasis

▶ Acinar cell carcinoma
- Mostly parotid gland

▶ Adenocarcinoma
- Mostly parotid gland

▶ Squamous cell carcinoma
- Mostly parotid gland

▶ Metastases
- Mostly parotid gland
- Head and neck tumours, melanoma

Mandible

Mandible Resorption

▶ Degrees of resorption of the edentulous jaw on radiograph
  • Grade A: Almost intact alveolar process
  • Grade B: Minor resorption of the alveolar process
  • Grade C: Advanced resorption of the alveolar process up to the basal bone
  • Grade D: Incipient resorption of the basal bone
  • Grade E: Extreme resorption of the basal bone

Mandibular Cysts

▶ Developmental odontogenic cysts
  • Dentigerous (follicular) cyst
  • Odontogenic keratocyst
  • Eruption cyst
  • Primordial cyst
  • Lateral periodontal cyst
▶ Developmental non-odontogenic cysts
  • Invasive canal cyst (nasopalatine duct cyst)
  • Nasolabial cyst
▶ Inflammatory cysts
  • Periapical (radicular) cyst
  • Lateral radicular cyst
  • Residual cyst
  • Paradental cyst

Mandibular Inflammation

▶ Acute dental (periapical) abscess
  • Tooth very painful and sensitive to touch
  • X-ray: Blurring of the lamina dura around the root apex, lucency around the tooth apex

► Chronic periapical abscess
  • Often draining fistula to the oral cavity, maxillary sinus or skin surface
  • X-ray: Poorly demarcated defect with irregular rim
► Periapical granuloma
  • Reparative process after the decline of the acute event or after periodontitis
  • Conversion to a periodontal cyst possible
  • X-ray: Round or oval, relatively well demarcated, not distinguishable from a periapical cyst
► Osteomyelitis
  • Causes: Odontogenic, post-traumatic
  • Osteolysis in the alveolar process due to inflammation
  • X-ray: Osteolysis, sequestrum

Mandibular Tumours

► Numerous benign and malignant histological types (odontogenic, osteogenic-medullary, chondrogenic)
► Ameloblastoma
  • X-ray: Multicystic lucency, well-defined scalloped margins, bone expansion and distortion in the lateral part of the mandible
  • Differential Diagnosis: Central giant cell lesions (giant cell reparative cysts)
► Central giant cell lesions (giant cell reparative cysts)
  • X-ray: Similar morphology to ameloblastoma, medial position
► Keratocystic odontogenic tumour
  • Odontogenic myxoma
  • Differential Diagnosis: Odontogenic (radicular and follicular) cysts, non-odontogenic cysts

Neck

Diseases of Compartments of the Neck

Compartment	Content	Diseases
Superficial mucosal compartment	Squamous epithelium, submucosal salivary glands, lymphatic tissue	Squamous cell carcinoma, Tornwaldt's disease, tumours of the minor salivary glands, lymphoma, angiofibroma
Parapharyngeal compartment	Fat, Cranial nerve V, Ascending pharyngeal artery	Hygroma, lipoma, salivary gland tumours, abscess, schwannoma
Carotid compartment	Cranial Nerves IX-XII, sympathetic trunk, lymph nodes, carotid artery, jugular vein	Schwannoma, neurofibroma, paraganglioma, lymph node metastases, lymphoma, abscess, meningioma
Parotid compartment	Parotid gland, lymph nodes, Cranial nerve VII, auriculotemporal nerve, external carotid artery, retromandibular vein	Parotid gland tumours, parotid gland cysts, lymph node metastases, lymphoma
Masticator compartment	Masticatory muscles, mandible, inferior alveolar nerve, maxillary artery, pterygoid plexus, lingual nerve	Dental abscess, lymphoma, neurogenic tumours, sarcoma, invasive squamous cell carcinoma
Retropharyngeal compartment	Lymph nodes, fat	Lymph node metastases, lymphoma, abscess
Prevertebral compartment	Musculature, phrenic nerve	Bone metastases, osteomyelitis, chordoma, abscess

Neck Cysts

▶ Midline neck cyst
- Thyroglossal duct cyst
  - Thyroglossal duct remnant
  - Midline of the neck

- Most commonly at the level of the hyoid bone but can also be suprahyoid or infrahyoid. Can occur anywhere along path of descent of the thyroid from the foramen caecum of the tongue to the thyroid bed
- Fluctuates on palpation
- Cyst displaced by the hyoid bone when swallowing
- Rarely a thyroid tumour can form within them
- **MR**: T1 variable (depending on protein content and inflammatory reactions), T2 hyperintense, possible thin enhancement of the cyst wall (with infection)
- **Differential Diagnosis**: Dermoid cyst

▶ Lateral neck cyst
- Remnants of the second, more rarely the third brachial cleft duct
- Second branchial tract cysts have variable locations, most common location between submandibular gland and sternocleidomastoid muscle lateral to carotid sheath
- May extend between internal and external carotid arteries
- Can form a sinus or fistula, commonly opening at the anterior border of the sternocleidomastoid muscle at the level of the larynx
- **MR**: Finding similar to midline neck cyst

Neck Tumours

▶ Lipoma
▶ Lipomatosis (multiple lipomas)
▶ Carotid body tumour
- Vascular tumour at the carotid bifurcation, with splaying of the ICA and ECA
- Painless swelling, pulsatile
- Later vagus and hypoglossal palsy
- **MRI**: Flow voids, strong early enhancement
- **IR**: Pre-operative embolisation for larger lesions
▶ Venous malformation
▶ Lymphatic malformation
- Ectatic, non-vascularised lymphatic vessels

Cervical Lymphadenitis

▶ Nonspecific
  • Bacterial infection (unilateral), viral infection (bilateral), peritonsillar abscess
▶ Specific
  • Tuberculosis, sarcoidosis, cat-scratch disease, toxoplasmosis, mononucleosis, HIV

Cervical Lymph Node Metastasis

▶ Metastasis frequency is particularly high in carcinomas of the oropharynx, hypopharynx, nasopharynx, salivary glands and oral cavity
▶ US
  • Round shape
    – Solbiati index (long axis/short axis) ≤ 2
    – Short axis ≥ 10 mm
  • Irregular border
  • Indistinct margin
  • Inhomogeneous structure
  • Absent fatty hilum sign
  • Central necrosis
  • Infiltrative growth
  • Immobile
▶ Colour Doppler US
  • Increased vascularity
  • Aberrant vessels
  • Subcapsular vessels
▶ CT
  • Round configuration
  • Loss of fatty hilum
  • Central necrosis
▶ MR
  • Necrosis
  • Extranodal extension

- Lymph node metastases of melanotic melanomas T1 hyperintense
- With ultrasmall superparamagnetic iron oxide (USPIO) contrast injection—Normal high T2 signal in lymph nodes is absent with metastatic infiltration
▶ **FDG-PET**
  - Avid uptake
▶ **Differential Diagnosis**: Lymphoma
▶ **Diagnosis**: Lymph node biopsy and histology

Neck Dissection

▶ Radical neck dissection
  - Removed: All ipsilateral cervical lymph nodes levels I-V, internal jugular vein, sternocleidomastoid muscle, spinal accessory nerve, submandibular gland, fat tissue
  - Remain intact: Carotid artery, vagus nerve, scalene muscles
  - Indication: Lymph node metastases
▶ Selective neck dissection
  - Removed: Known or potentially affected lymph node stations
  - Preserved: Non lymph-node structures

Cervical Tumour Recurrence

▶ Confident radiological diagnosis in the early postoperative phase can be difficult
  - Often hard to distinguish residual tumour, tumour recurrence, inflammatory tissue, granulation tissue and fibrosis in all imaging methods
▶ **MR**: T1 isointense, T2 hyperintense, infiltrative growth, marked enhancement, restricted diffusion
▶ **Diagnosis**: Biopsy

Lymphomas

Criteria	Hodgkin lymphoma	Non-Hodgkin lymphoma
Limited disease (stage I or II)	Frequent	Rare
Nodal involvement	Continuous	Discontinuous
Extranodal involvement	Rare	Common
Mediastinal lymph node involvement	Anterior mediastinum	All compartments
Abdominal lymph node involvement	Rare	Common
Bone marrow involvement	Rare	Common

Pharynx

Tornwaldt Cyst

▶ Disorder in which the invagination of the pharyngeal mucosa into the midline of the nasopharynx leads to accumulation of secretions and cyst formation
▶ Can become inflamed—Tornwaldt Disease
▶ Usually no symptoms, can have foul-smelling breath
▶ **MR**: T1 isointense to hyperintense, T2 hyperintense, no enhancement unless inflamed
▶ **Differential Diagnosis**: Adenoids

Base of Tongue and Floor of Mouth Abscess

▶ Swelling of the tongue, pain when speaking, tenderness, lockjaw
▶ Diagnosis with cross-sectional imaging techniques
▶ Ludwig's Angina
  • Rapidly spreading cellulitis of the floor of mouth, originating from the teeth, tonsils or from the sublingual or submandibular gland
▶ **Complications**: In the case of phlegmon, spread to the mediastinum

Peritonsillar Abscess

▶ Causes: Streptococci, multiple other microorganisms
▶ Spread of inflammation in the connective tissue between the tonsil and the pharyngeal constrictor muscles
▶ A few days after tonsillitis, swallowing difficulties
▶ Fever, trismus
▶ US/CT/MR
  • Diagnosis of the peritonsillar abscess
  • Exclusion of jugular vein thrombosis (Lemierre syndrome)
  • Lymphadenitis
▶ Differential Diagnosis: Lymphoid hyperplasia, tonsillar retention cyst, tonsillar lymphoma
▶ Complications: Retropharyngeal abscess, mediastinitis, sepsis

Parapharyngeal Abscess

▶ Causes: Streptococci, Staphylococci
▶ Spread from the pharyngeal space to the carotid space
▶ Sore throat, neck pain
▶ US/CT/MR
  • Stranding of the parapharyngeal fat
  • Inhomogeneous fluid collections peripheral enhancement, possibly containing gas
▶ Differential Diagnosis: Parapharyngeal phlegmon, carcinoma, metastatic lymph node
▶ Complications: Laryngeal oedema, retropharyngeal abscess, mediastinitis, jugular vein thrombosis, internal carotid artery mycotic aneurysm

Nasopharyngeal Tumours

▶ Squamous cell carcinoma
  • Epistaxis, nasal obstruction, conductive hearing loss, lymphadenopathy

- **CT/MR**
  - Location of tumour and pattern of local growth
  - Obliteration of fat spaces
  - Infiltration of the musculature
  - Bone destruction
  - Enhancement
  - Lymph node metastases
- **Nuclear Medicine**: 18F-FDG-PET—search for metastases for staging purposes
▶ Juvenile nasopharyngeal angiofibroma
  - Histologically benign, clinically malignant tumour
  - Young males
  - Originate from the region of the sphenopalatine foramen, near the roof of the nasopharynx adjacent to the choanae
  - Spread to nasal cavity, paranasal sinuses, pterygopalatine fossa, skull base, sphenoid wing
  - Supply from the ascending pharyngeal and internal maxillary arteries
  - Obstructed nasal breathing with purulent rhinitis
  - Nosebleeds, headaches, middle ear symptoms due to Eustachian tube blockage
  - Biopsy contraindicated due to risk of bleeding
  - **CT**: Soft tissue mass, widening of sphenopalatine foramen, bone remodelling
  - **MR**
    - T1 isointense, T2 hyperintense, strong enhancement
    - Flow voids due to flow artefacts in highly vascularised tumour tissue
  - **Differential Diagnosis**: Adenoid hyperplasia, nasopharyngeal cyst, choanal polyp, lymphoma, rhabdomyosarcoma
  - **IR**: Embolisation
▶ Nasopharyngeal carcinoma
  - Lateral pharyngeal recess (fossa of Rosenmüller)
  - Infiltrating and destructive growth
  - Lymph node metastasis common
▶ Lymphoma
▶ Sarcomas

▶ Adenoid hyperplasia (non-neoplastic)
  • Childhood and adolescence
  • Lymphatic hyperplasia in the nasopharynx with obstruction of the choanae
  • Nasal obstruction, mouth breathing, snoring, middle ear effusions

Oropharyngeal Tumours

▶ Squamous cell carcinoma
  • Tongue base
  • Tonsil
  • Soft palate
  • Posterior pharyngeal wall
▶ Lymphoma
▶ Lipoma
  • Dermoid
  • Epidermoid

Hypopharyngeal Tumours

▶ Squamous cell carcinoma. Subsites of the hypopharynx that can be affected:
  • Posterior pharyngeal wall
  • Piriform sinus
  • Postcricoid region

TNM Classification Oropharyngeal Cancer

▶ Oropharynx
  • T1: ≤2 cm
  • T2: >2 cm to ≤4 cm
  • T3: >4 cm or spread to the lingual surface of the epiglottis
  • p16-negative carcinomas
    – T4a: Larynx, external muscles of the tongue, medial pterygoid muscle, hard palate, mandible
    – T4b: Lateral pterygoid muscle, pterygoid plates, skull base, encases internal carotid artery

- p16-positive carcinomas
  - T4: Larynx, external musculature of the tongue, pterygoid muscles, hard palate, mandible, skull base,
- p16-negative carcinomas
  - N1: Ipsilateral solitary ≤3 cm without extra-nodal spread
  - N2a: Ipsilateral solitary >3 cm to ≤6 cm without extra-nodal spread
  - N2b: Ipsilateral multiple ≤6 cm without extra-nodal spread
  - N2c: Bilateral, contralateral ≤6 cm without extra-nodal spread
  - N3a: >6 cm without extranodal spreading
  - N3b: Extra-nodal spread (skin, soft tissues, nerves)
- p16-positive carcinomas
  - N1: Ipsilateral ≤6 cm
  - N2: Bilateral or contralateral ≤6 cm
  - N3: >6 cm
- M1: Distant metastases

Larynx

Laryngocele

▶ Causes: Congenital, acquired (obstructing tumour, coughing, glass blowers, wind musicians)
▶ Dilation of the saccule of the laryngeal ventricle
▶ Types
  - Internal laryngocele: Inside larynx, contained by the thyrohyoid membrane. In supraglottis, paraglottic region. Hoarseness, shortness of breath
  - External laryngocele: Outside larynx, extension through the thyrohyoid membrane. Protrusion of the neck, swelling of the neck
  - Mixed: Contains both internal and external components
▶ US/CT/MR
  - Internal laryngocele: Air- or fluid-filled lesion in the paraglottic space, communicating with the laryngeal ventricle
  - External laryngocele: Air- or fluid-filled lesion in the lower submandibular space with herniation through the thyrohyoid membrane

- Exclude obstructing tumour as a cause of the laryngocele
▶ **Differential Diagnosis**: Thyroglossal cyst, hypopharyngeal diverticulum, branchial cleft cyst
▶ **Complication**: Pyolaryngocele (infected, pus-filled)

Glottic Oedema

▶ Causes: Infection, Ludwig's angina, allergy, insect bite
▶ Oedema or abscess of the epiglottis
▶ Inspiratory stridor, hoarse voice, severe pain on swallowing, salivation, fever, shortness of breath
▶ **US**: Epiglottis thickening, abscess formation

Laryngeal Perichondritis

▶ Causes: Tumours, tracheotomy, intubation, nasogastric tube, relapsing polychondritis
▶ Inflammation of the cartilaginous membrane of the thyroid and cricoid cartilage with fusion of the cartilage
▶ Hoarseness, severe pain, shortness of breath
▶ **CT**: Laryngeal oedema, cartilage erosion, abscess
▶ **Complications**: Cartilage destruction, scar, stenosis

Benign Laryngeal Tumours/Lesions

▶ Vocal fold polyp
▶ Vocal fold nodule
▶ Laryngeal papillomatosis
▶ Chondroma

Malignant Laryngeal Tumours

▶ Squamous cell carcinoma
  - Causes: Smoking, alcohol, asbestos, leucoplakia, papilloma
  - Types
    – supraglottic
    – glottic
    – subglottic
  - Particularly older men

- Clinically persistent hoarseness as the most important presenting symptom
- Laryngoscopy—abolition of the normal vocal fold configuration, adhesion to surrounding structures, tumour crossing the anterior commissure
- When breaking into the cartilage, tumour perichondritis due to infection
- Lymphatic metastasis to the cervical lymph nodes (supraglottic tumours)
- CT/MR
  - Asymmetric soft tissues
  - Inhomogeneous internal structure
  - Significant enhancement
  - Look for involvement of the paraglottic and pre-epiglottic fat, cartilage erosion, extra-laryngeal extension (staging)
- Diagnosis: Laryngoscopy, excision biopsy
▶ Chondrosarcoma
- CT: Mass arising from cartilage (usually cricoid), typical calcifications (arc and ring or popcorn)

Thyroid Gland

Sonography

▶ Enlarged thyroid
- Goitre
  - Thyroid volume >18 ml in women or >25 ml in men
▶ Diffuse hypoechogenicity
- Graves' disease
  - Autoimmune hyperthyroidism
  - Enlarged thyroid, heterogeneous, increased vascularity
  - Other findings: Hyperthyroidism, TSH receptor antibodies
- Subacute thyroiditis- de Quervain
  - Ill-defined hypoechoic hypovascular areas, unilateral or bilateral
  - Other findings: Thyroid pain, elevated ESR

- Hashimoto's thyroiditis
  - Autoimmune thyroiditis
  - Small hypoechoic nodules and echogenic septations (giraffe patterns)
  - Initially enlarged thyroid, later atrophic
  - Variable vascularity
  - Other findings: Usually hypothyroid, elevated anti-TPO antibody, antithyroglobulin antibodies
- ▶ Diffusely hyperechoic
  - Goitre
- ▶ Focal hypoechogenicity
  - Adenoma
  - Carcinoma
- ▶ Focal inflammation
  - Haemorrhagic cyst
- ▶ Focal hyperechogenicity
  - Scar
- ▶ Focal anechoic lesion
  - Cyst
- ▶ Doppler ultrasound hyperperfusion
  - Graves' disease
  - Acute thyroiditis
- ▶ Thyroid adenoma
  - Usually a solitary nodule in otherwise normal thyroid
  - Often isoechoic, can be hypo- or hyperechoic
  - Well-defined
  - Hypoechoic or anechoic halo (capsule)
- ▶ Adenomatous nodule
  - Often multiple nodules present
  - Thin hypoechoic halo
  - Less well-defined than thyroid adenoma
  - Degenerative changes
    - Cysts
    - Coarse calcifications
- ▶ Features suspicious for malignancy
  - Solid nodule
  - Hypoechoic internal structure
  - Irregular outline

- Ill-defined
- No hypoechoic halo (can be seen with benign nodules)
- Microcalcifications
- Hypervascularity
- Rapid growth
- Regional lymph node enlargement
  - Risk stratification and management of nodules according to TIRADS

Nuclear Medicine

▶ Diagnosis made in conjunction with knowledge of laboratory parameters (T3, T4, TSH, thyroid antibodies, calcitonin) and ultrasound findings

▶ 99mTc pertechnetate
- Indications: Finding the cause of hyperthyroidism, evaluating function of thyroid nodules, thyroiditis
- Provides information about iodide clearance
- Increased technetium uptake in functional autonomy with TSH suppression
- Lowered technetium uptake in cold nodules

▶ 123I sodium iodide, 131I sodium iodide
- Indications: Differentiated (papillary or follicular) thyroid carcinoma
  - Staging
  - Diagnosis of recurrence
  - Radioiodine therapy
- Additionally 124I-sodium iodide PET can be used during restaging

▶ 18F-DOPA-PET
- Indications: Medullary thyroid carcinoma

▶ 18F-FDG-PET
- Indications: Anaplastic thyroid carcinoma

Multiple Endocrine Neoplasia

▶ MEN type 1
- Primary hyperparathyroidism; neuroendocrine tumours of the duodenum and pancreas; hormonally active pituitary adenoma

▶ MEN type 2
- Medullary thyroid carcinoma; phaeochromocytoma
- MEN 2A: Primary hyperparathyroidism
- MEN 2B: Intestinal ganglioneuromatosis

Parathyroid Gland

Parathyroid Gland

▶ Parathyroid adenoma
▶ Imaging in first instance using ultrasound (orthotopic adenomas) or CT (ectopic adenomas)
- Typical location posterior or inferior to the thyroid gland, round or oval shape. Hypoechoic, hypervascular

▶ Localisation with Tc-99m sestamibi
- Persistent storage of the tracer in the parathyroid (seen on early and delayed images) compared to normal thyroid tissue (just seen on early images)

▶ Selective venous blood sampling to detect a local parathyroid hormone gradient